Jean-Noël Bruneton

Imaging of Gastrointestinal Tract Tumors

In Collaboration with
C. Balu-Maestro   J. Drouillard
A. Geoffray   M.-Y. Mourou   A. Rogopoulos
G. Schmutz   P.-J. Valette

Translated by N. Reed Rameau
Foreword by J. Delmont

With 267 Figures and 25 Tables

Springer-Verlag Berlin Heidelberg GmbH

Author

Dr. Jean-Noël Bruneton
Service de Radiologie, Centre Antoine-Lacassagne
36, Voie Romaine, 06054 Nice Cedex, France

Translator

Nancy Reed Rameau
Centre Antoine-Lacassagne
36, Voie Romaine, 06054 Nice Cedex, France

ISBN 978-3-642-83827-9   ISBN 978-3-642-83825-5 (eBook)
DOI 10.1007/978-3-642-83825-5

Library of Congress Cataloging-in-Publication Data
Bruneton, J. N.
Imaging of gastrointestinal tract tumors/Jean-Noël Bruneton, in collaboration with
C. Balu-Maestro ... [et al.]; translated by N. Reed Rameau: foreword by J. Delmont.
p. cm. Includes bibliographical references.
ISBN 978-3-642-83827-9 (U.S.)
1. Gastrointestinal system-Tumors-Imaging. I. Title.
[DNLM: 1. Diagnostic Imaging. 2. Gastrointestinal Neoplasms-radiography. 3. Gastro-
intestinal Neoplasms-radionuclide imaging. WI   149   B895i]   RC280.D5B78
1990   616.99'4330754-dc20   DNLM/DLC   89-26287

© Springer-Verlag Berlin Heidelberg 1990
Softcover reprint of the hardcover 1st edition 1990

The use of registered names, trademarks, etc. in this publication does not imply, even in the
absence of a specific statement, that such names are exempt from the relevant protective
laws and regulations and therefore free for general use.

Product Liability: The publisher can give no guarantee for information about drug dosage
and application thereof contained in the book. In every individual case the respective user
must check its accuracy by consulting other pharmaceutical literature.

2121/3140-543210 – Printed on acid-free paper.

The authors wish to thank
Christine Rostagni and Françoise Fein
for their assistance in the preparation of this book.

Foreword

This new book by Jean-Noël Bruneton demonstrates once more his numerous talents and expertise in both the practice and the teaching of radiology. Numerous readers will undoubtedly have the same pleasure I did from reading it straight through, from cover to cover, especially those chapters on topics not covered elsewhere, such as that on metastases of the gastrointestinal tract. *Imaging of Gastrointestinal Tumors* will be most highly valued as an atlas and a reference book; in this respect, it will prove of special interest to all radiologists and medical and surgical specialists in gastroenterology and occupy a privileged place in their library.

As an atlas, the high quality illustrations are of outstanding exemplary value. The many young gastroenterologists who have entered the field since the rapid development of digestive endoscopy, and are less familiar with the interpretation of barium contrast films, will profit from the expertise of Jean-Noël Bruneton, who himself was privileged to work with the illustrious radiologist Paul Lecomte. A superb iconography has also been compiled covering the numerous state-of-the-art imaging techniques that have enriched modern radiology.

As a practical reference book, the logical histopathologic approach and detailed index facilitate the location of information on topics of current interest, such as Kaposi's sarcomas in AIDS, and on such infrequent pathologies as aberrant pancreas and gastrointestinal endometriosis.

When dealing with any gastrointestinal tract tumor, today's physician has two equally important and inseparable obligations: histologic diagnosis and tumor staging (local, regional, distant); such information is essential for evaluating tumor resectability, a major concern in the case of these lesions.

Since a positive diagnosis of gastrointestinal tract tumors requires histopathologic confirmation, gastrointestinal endoscopy is of prime importance. The three-dimensional endoscopic view of the tumor in actual size and natural color can be likened to a gross histopathologic examination. By contrast, to use the terms of the renowned Parisian radiologist X. Porcher, barium contrast radiology is never more than the study of silhouettes (two-dimensional black and white images).

Endoscopy also widens the possibilities for microscopic analysis of biopsy material. Although the use of biopsy forceps is often sufficient other stratagems are sometimes useful, especially for submucosal tumors, including serial biopsies at a given site, needle aspiration biopsy, macrobiopsies with an electrosurgical snare, and cytology brushes. The classic means of histology have been enriched by the advent of techniques such as immunofluorescence, and thanks to electron microscopy, the muscular origin of the "bizzare tumors" of Stout has been recognized since 1969 (P. Laffargue, H. Monges, J. Delmont (1969) Etude ultrastructurale d'une tumeur myoïde de l'estomac. *Annales d'Anatomie Pathologique* 14:295). Similarly, modern monoclonal antibody techniques (anticytokeratin antibodies for epithelial cancer, panleukocytic antibodies for malignant lymphomas, etc.) now facilitate classification of difficult cases. Until fairly recently, tumor staging was hampered by the fact that gastrointestinal endoscopy merely provided a "bird eye" view and was of no assistance in evaluating the depth of lesion penetration. Miniaturization of ultrasonic probes that can be inserted through fiberscope biopsy channels has partly overcome this problem and represents a link between modern radiology and gastroenterology. Other more specifically radiologic techniques continue to provide irreplaceable information, however, and ultrasonography, computed tomography, and MRI are all extensively reviewed in this excellent book by Jean-Noël Bruneton, which will soon undoubtedly become a classic.

Jean P. Delmont
Hepato-gastroenterologist, Nice Regional Hospitals
Vice-Dean, University of Nice Medical School

Contents

Collaborators

Catherine Balu-Maestro
Service de Radiologie, Centre Antoine-Lacassagne
36, Voie Romaine, 06054 Nice Cedex, France

Jacques Drouillard
Service de Radiologie, Hôpital du Haut Lévèque
Avenue Magellan, 33600 Pessac, France

Anne Geoffray
Service de Radiologie, Centre Antoine-Lacassagne
36, Voie Romaine, 06054 Nice Cedex, France

Michel-Yves Mourou
Service de Tomodensitométrie, Hôpital Princesse Grace
Avenue Pasteur, 98000 Principauté de Monaco

André Rogopoulos
Service de Radiologie, Centre Antoine-Lacassagne
36, Voie Romaine, 06054 Nice Cedex, France

Gérard Schmutz
Service de Radiologie Médico-Chirurgicale B, Hôpital Central
1, Place de l'Hôpital, 67091 Strasbourg Cedex, France

Pierre-Jean Valette
Service de Radiologie, Hôpital Edouard Herriot
Place d'Arsonval, 69374 Lyon Cedex 03, France

Collaborators

Benign Tumors

1 Benign Epithelial Tumors*

The term "polyp" is merely the gross description of a tumor that projects above the surface of the mucous membrane. In the gastrointestinal tract, and especially in the colon and rectum, numerous lesions of different origins and pathologic significance share this morphologic appearance. Histologic examination is mandatory for identification of the type of polyp, which cannot be determined from the radiologic or gross appearance. While certain types of polyps have no malignant potential, adenomas, which are benign epithelial tumors found from the stomach to the rectum, can undergo malignant degeneration.

Benign gastrointestinal epithelial tumors are represented by papillomas in the esophagus, and by adenomas in the stomach, the small intestine, and the colon and rectum. Radiologic examination usually cannot differentiate these lesions from other non-neoplastic polyps (discussed at each level of the gastrointestinal tract as differential diagnoses): hamartomas (Peutz-Jeghers, juvenile polyp), hyperplastic (metaplastic) polyp, inflammatory polyp. Polyposis is discussed separately (see Chap. 2).

1.1 Esophagus

1.1.1 General Features

Papillomas and adenomas, the two forms of benign epithelial tumors in the esophagus, account for 4.4% of all benign tumors of this organ (Plachta 1962; Schmidt et al. 1961). There are approximately three papillomas for every adenoma. These lesions are usually smaller than 1 cm (Montesi et al. 1983). Papillomas may occur at any point in the esophagus whereas adenomas tend to occur in the lower third (Ming 1973); this site predilection appears related to the possible presence of gastric mucosa in the lower esophagus.

Histologically, squamous cell papilloma is a benign neoplastic tumor. Adenomas are often hard to diagnose because inflammatory lesions in a zone of glandular epithelium may have the same appearance (Ming 1973).

The evolutionary potential of benign epithelial tumors of the esophagus is poorly understood because of the rarity of these lesions. For this same reason, a papilloma-cancer sequence is improbable. Moreover, the gross appearance of papillomas is completely different from that of early esophageal cancer (Itai et al. 1978).

Average patient age at diagnosis is 50 years; there is no sex predominance. Owing to the small size of lesions, a period of clinical latency is common. On rare occasions, the patient complains of dysphagia, retrosternal pain, or nausea. Endoscopic localization and biopsy of these small lesions are generally compatible with curative resection, especially for papillomas, which have a sessile, polypoid appearance (Montesi et al. 1983).

1.1.2 Imaging

The radiologic features of these small lesions correspond to sessile polyps; polyps smaller than 1 cm may exhibit a ring shadow. Endoscopy and biopsy are not always diagnostic because the biopsy material must include a fragment of the fibrovascular core of the papilloma for positive diagnosis (Montesi et al. 1983). Intraluminal filling defects are rare (Parnell et al. 1978). The radiologic differential diagnosis for small lesions includes leiomyoma, a vascular tumor, or a fibrovascular polyp. In practice, the differential diagnosis is not of

---

* Written in collaboration with G. Schmutz.

capital importance because these lesions have no malignant potential.

1.2 Stomach

1.2.1 General Features

Hyperplastic polyps are by far the most common polyp in the stomach, followed by adenomas. Literature reports thus frequently associate hyperplastic and adenomatous etiologies. These two pathologies are therefore discussed together, without considering hyperplastic polyps as a differential diagnosis.

These two types of polyp account for 12%–41% of all benign gastric tumors (Bognel et al. 1986; Ming 1973) and 3.1% of all gastric tumors (Ming 1973). The radiologic incidence is 1.7%. They are the most frequent benign tumors of the stomach. The incidence rises with age, and the increased number of cases in literature reports is due to the improvement of diagnostic techniques. The relative frequency with respect to cancer of the stomach has changed because of the decline in the frequency of gastric adenocarcinoma.

At diagnosis, 85%–93.8% of these lesions are under 2 cm (Ming and Goldman 1965; Feczko et al. 1985). Lesions smaller than 1 cm almost always have a hyperplastic etiology; similarly, hyperplastic polyps are rarely larger than 2 cm. Size is of no real value for determining the etiology of "intermediate-size" lesions (Joffe and Antonioli 1978; Smith and Lee 1983). Regardless of the type of polyp, the antrum is the site of predilection (Rosato and Noto 1966). Hyperplastic and adenomatous polyps rarely coexist (Tomasulo 1971), whereas multiple lesions are common, especially with hyperplastic polyps. For McNeer and Pack (1967), the presence of six or more polyps suggests the diagnosis of polyposis.

For Feczko et al. (1985), hyperplastic polyps account for 97.3% of all gastric polyps. These lesions are multiple in 63.5% of cases. Malignant degeneration of hyperplastic polyps is rare (Papp and Joseph 1976). Focal foveolar hyperplasia is a specific form that may occur after partial gastrectomy (Domellof et al. 1977) or be associated with an ulcer or cancer (Elster 1976).

The relative frequency of adenomatous polyps is thus much lower than that of hyperplastic polyps (2.7% for Feczko et al. 1985). These solitary lesions (Sleyster et al. 1986) can be divided into three histologic forms: tubular, villous, and tubulovillous. Whether villous or non-villous, 8.4%–9.6% of all gastric adenomas degenerate (Bognel et al. 1986; Ghazi et al. 1984) once they exceed 2 cm (Marshak and Feldman 1965; Monaco et al. 1962). Non-villous gastric adenomas may change size (enlarge or occasionally disappear) without undergoing histologic modification (Seifert et al. 1983; Tsukamoto et al. 1977). Clinical follow-up of gastric adenomas reveals malignant change in 1%–2% of cases (Seifert et al. 1983).

Villous gastric adenomas are rare, representing only 1.2%–2% of all gastric polyps (MacDonald et al. 1985; Snorer 1985). These lesions are generally much larger than hyperplastic polyps (2–6 cm long) at diagnosis (Gaitini et al. 1988). Villous adenomas have a high propensity for malignant degeneration: the incidence in literature reports ranges from 40% to 100% of all cases (Meltzer et al. 1966; Miller et al. 1980; Robbins and Cotran 1979). Of all gastric adenocarcinomas, 7.5% are reportedly associated with an adenomatous polyp (Morson and Dawson 1972).

Hyperplastic and adenomatous polyps tend to occur in patients over 60 years of age; there is no sex predominance. Clinical latency is the rule for lesions under 2 cm. Dyspepsia, pain, or hemorrhage can be major complications. Villous adenomas may be revealed by hypoalbuminemia, which has been attributed to exudative protein loss (Gaitini et al. 1988).

Endoscopy can identify small lesions and be combined with ultrasound examination (Caletti et al. 1986; Strohm and Classen 1986). Small polyps (less than 2 cm in largest dimension) are amenable to curative endoscopic polypectomy (Feczko et al. 1985; Hughes 1984; Papp and Joseph 1976). Surgical resection is reserved for atypical or malignant forms.

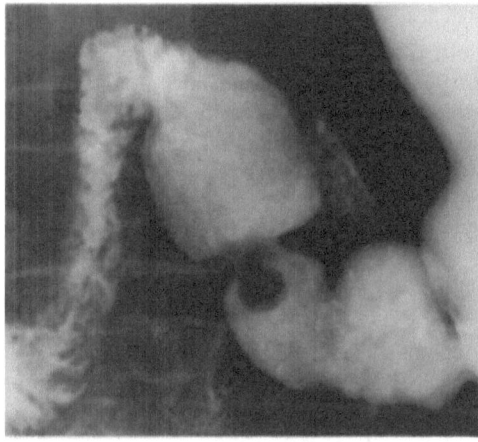

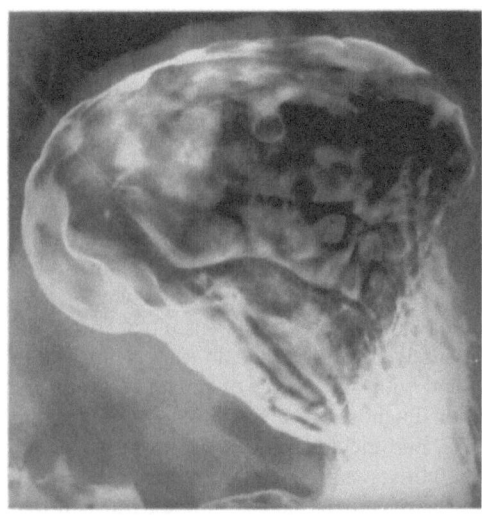

Fig. 1.1. Non-villous adenoma of the gastric antrum

Fig. 1.2. Small hyperplastic gastric polyp

1.2.2 Imaging

Radiologic studies, and preferentially double-contrast examinations, provide interesting but not determinant information. Such studies have a sensitivity of 85.5% and a specificity of 99.6% for diagnosis of polyps (Feczko et al. 1985); however, there is no radiologic difference between hyperplastic and adenomatous polyps. Only the presence of multiple small lesions suggests the diagnosis of hyperplastic polyps. Small lesions appear sessile; larger ones may have a stalk (Figs 1.1 and 1.2). Villous adenomas are generally imaged as a cauliflower-like polypoid mass with a superimposed reticular pattern due to coating of the intervillous interstices of the frond-like tumor (Fig. 1.3). Large polycyclic masses with a fine reticular pattern are infrequent. Regardless of the type of polyp, none of the following features has any value for distinguishing between benign and malignant lesions: lesion margins, size, shape, or pattern of the adjacent mucosa.

1.2.3 Differential Diagnosis

Aside from a gastric fold, the differential diagnoses for small polyps include an inflammatory polyp, a hamartomous polyp, a non-epithelial polyp, and polypoid adenocarcinoma.

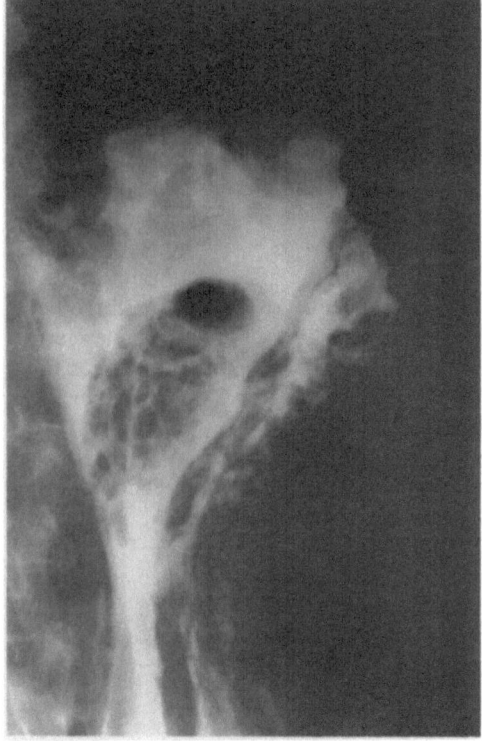

Fig. 1.3. Degenerated villous adenoma of the stomach

Inflammatory gastric polyps account for 4.7% of all benign gastric tumors (Ming 1973). Lesions of the gastroesophageal junction are a rare complication of esophagitis (Rabin et al. 1980). An inflamed gastric fold may progressively evolve into a polyp as the result of continuous irritation (Bleshman et al. 1978). Polyps on the Z line (gastroesophageal junction) are a specific, localized form of gastritis (Styles et al. 1985). Clinical features in favor of this etiology may exist before histologic proof is obtained: gastroesophageal reflux is not usually seen with other types of polyps. The differential diagnoses for inflammatory polyps on the Z line include varices, leiomyoma, a foreign body, and epithelial tumors. The radiologic appearance suggests the diagnosis if the patient has a history of reflux, and a prominent, straight gastric fold terminating in a smooth polypoid expansion is imaged near the squamocolumnar junction. Lesions in the body and antrum of the stomach also probably have a chronic inflammatory etiology (Johnston and Morson 1978; Justrabo et al. 1985; Shimer and Helwig 1984). There are no clinical signs suggestive of the diagnosis. These lesions usually occur in patients older than 60 years, without any sex predominance. A polypoid radiologic appearance is more common than a regular filling defect or a malignant-appearing mass. The antrum is by far the most common site (95% for Justrabo et al. 1985) and over 50% of inflammatory gastric polyps are larger than 2 cm. These lesions follow a benign course and do not recur after treatment.

Gastric hamartomatous polyps, which have an incidence of less than 0.1% in endoscopic series (Iida et al. 1984), represent 11% of all gastric polyps for Sato et al. (1988). They always measure under 1 cm in diameter and are almost constantly smaller than 5 mm. The site of predilection, the fundus, differentiates hamartomatous lesions from other gastric polyps and is of considerable diagnostic value. Hamartomatous polyps may be associated with polyposis.

Histologic confirmation may not be possible for other small *polypoid masses.* Aberrant pancreas, leiomyoma, and endometriosis can all be imaged as small intraluminal filling defects (Feczko et al. 1985).

Polypoid adenocarcinoma, a very rare entity (Gold et al. 1984), corresponds to a lobulated, early gastric cancer. There are no radiologic patterns that suggest or confirm this diagnosis, and endoscopic examination is indispensable.

1.3 Small Intestine

1.3.1 General Features

Adenomas account for 20.4%–34.4% of all benign intestinal tumors; their incidence is thus comparable to that of leiomyomas (Carlson and Good 1973; Wood 1967).

Size can be used to differentiate two forms: non-villous adenomas often measure less than 2 cm (50% in the duodenum) whereas villous adenomas of the duodenum are larger than 2 cm in 86.5% of cases (Delpy et al. 1983). Duodenal sites predominate, and 20%–50% of benign duodenal tumors are of epithelial origin (Hoffman and Grayzel 1945; Raiford 1932; River et al. 1956). Villous adenomas, in particular, are found essentially between the first and third duodenal segments (D1 and D3); non-villous adenomas usually occur between the bulb and the second duodenal segment (Delpy et al. 1983). Adenomatous involvement of the jejunum and ileum is less common and always corresponds to Lieberkühnian adenomas (Osborne et al. 1973).

Multiple lesions are rare. In the duodenum, 3.8% of all villous adenomas and 6.5% of all non-villous adenomas (Brunnerian or non-villous Lieberkühnian) are multiple (Delpy et al. 1983).

Brunner's gland adenomas are thought to exist in 1% of the population (Karkas et al. 1980). These duodenal lesions are always benign (Wood 1967).

Lieberkühnian adenomas are rare; only 100 cases had been reported in the literature up until 1973 (Osborne et al. 1973). These tubular, villous, or tubulovillous lesions may occur at any point in the small intestine. Non-villous Lieberkühnian adenomas have a very low risk of malignant degeneration (2.2% for Delpy et al. 1983) whereas 60% of all villous adenomas (also referred to as papillary adenomas, adenomatous papillomas, or papillary tumors) degenerate (Delpy et al. 1983). The propensity

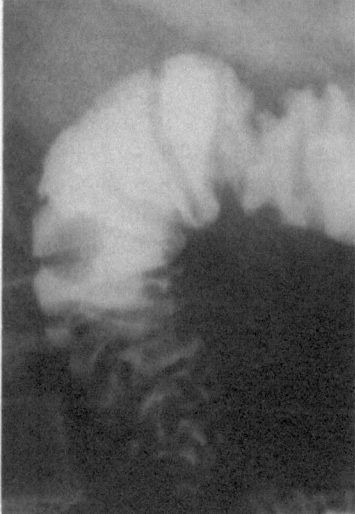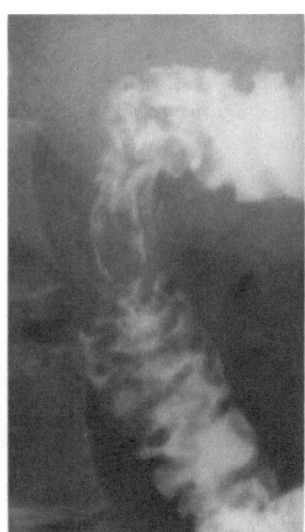

Fig. 1.4. Brunnerian adenoma
of the duodenum

for malignant change does not appear correlated with any particular site in the small intestine, although ampullary villous adenomas
have a higher frequency of degeneration than
non-ampullary villous adenomas (Ryan et al.
1986). Of all lesions greater than 4 cm in diameter, 87.5% are malignant (Delpy et al.
1983).

Regardless of the type of adenoma, duodenal
lesions cause bleeding in over half of all cases.
Other clinical symptoms include pain, vomiting, and weight loss; 4.7%-25% of all patients
are asymptomatic (Delpy et al. 1983; Mouli-
nieer et al. 1975). Pedunculated adenomas in
the jejunum or ileum may undergo intussusception that prompts diagnosis.

Endoscopic examination of duodenal lesions
allows etiologic diagnosis and treatment by
polypectomy. Endoscopic removal is not always possible for lesions over 2 cm, which
may require surgical resection (Delpy et al.
1983; Eklof et al. 1960; Moulinier et al. 1975).

1.3.2 Imaging

Barium studies were negative in 7.7% of the
cases reviewed by Delpy et al. (1983). Duodenal adenomas may be sessile or pedunculated;
there are no specific radiologic features. Barium examinations correctly identify adenoma

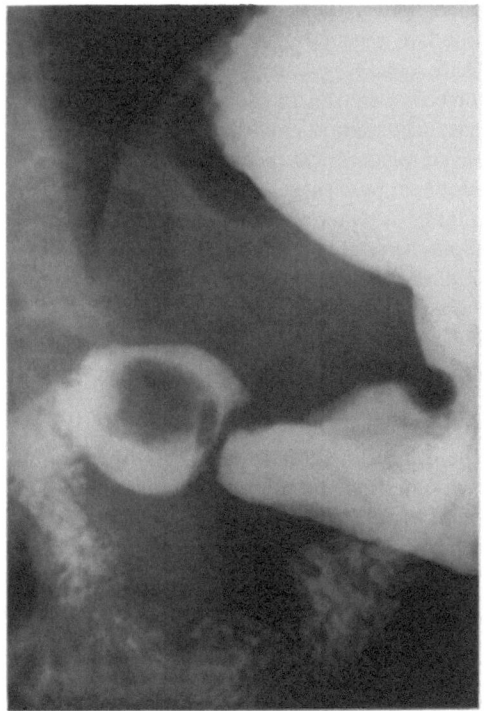

Fig. 1.5. Brunnerian adenoma of the duodenal bulb

in only one-third of cases (Delpy et al. 1983). Multiple coalescing polyps may, on rare occasions, cause intussusception or stenosis following dilatation of the suprajacent tract: such lesions can be visualized sonographically (Brambs et al. 1986). There are no radiologic patterns indicative of partial degeneration of a polyp (Figs. 1.4 and 1.5).

1.3.3 Differential Diagnosis

The *hamartomatous polyps* encountered in Peutz-Jeghers syndrome are more frequent than adenomas in the jejunum and the ileum, and represent 76.6% of all intestinal polyps for Gannon et al. (1962). Multiple hamartomatous polyps are more common than multiple adenomas.

Inflammatory fibroid polyps of the small intestine are much less frequent than in the stomach. Fewer than 100 cases have been published in the literature (Olmsted et al. 1987). These usually solitary lesions, sometimes incorrectly referred to as eosinophilic granulomas, occur almost exclusively in the ileum.

Heterotopic gastric mucosa may occur in the duodenal bulb as well as in the Meckel diverticulum, in enteric duplication cysts, or just about anywhere in the gastrointestinal tract (Agha et al. 1988; Wolf 1971). In the duodenal bulb, this abnormality manifests as clusters of 1–3-mm plaques on the base or posterior wall; less often, a coarse nodular mucosa with superficial erosions or an ulcer crater is seen (Agha et al. 1988).

The other differential diagnoses for intestinal adenomas include submucosal tumors that develop within the lumen (leiomyoma, neurogenic tumors, lipoma) and aberrant pancreas.

1.4 Colon and Rectum

1.4.1 General Features

Adenomas are premalignant lesions whereas the other polyps entertained as differential diagnoses (hyperplastic polyps, juvenile polyps, and inflammatory polyps) all remain benign. Adenoma is a neoplastic tumor consisting of a benign epithelial proliferation presenting differing grades of dysplasia, making it more or less similar to cancer. Colorectal adenomas play a major role in carcinogenesis and are thus at the center of colorectal cancer prevention programs.

The frequency of colorectal polyps varies, depending on the examination technique and study population. The incidence of adenomatous polyps in the autopsy and histologic series of Potet et al. (1978) was 14.5% The reported incidence in northern Europe is twice as high (over 30% of subjects) (Hoff et al. 1985; Vatn et al. 1985; Williams et al. 1982). The frequency rises with age up until 70 years, when a plateau is reached. Radiologic estimates of adenomas based on double-contrast examinations range from 5.1% to 17% (Bernstein et al. 1985; Fork et al. 1983). The wide variations in the frequency of polyps as a function of the population and geographic region appear related to environmental rather than genetic factors. Like colorectal cancers, polyps are fairly infrequent in developing countries but very prevalent in northern Europe (Hoff et al. 1985). Increased intake of fats and reduced consumption of fibers have been implicated in the development of colorectal adenomas (Hoff et al. 1986a). Whereas nearly all gastric polyps are of hyperplastic origin, adenomas predominate in the colon and rectum, where they represent 88% of all polyps for Wegener et al. (1986).

For Morson and Konishi (1982), 39.3% of all polyps are smaller than 5 mm; they tend to occur essentially in the rectum. The 29.1% of polyps larger than 10 mm tend to occur in the sigmoid. Even small adenomas predominate over hyperplastic polyps, because 62% of all diminutive polyps (less than 5 mm) are adenomatous (Ott et al. 1986). By contrast, 82% of all lesions over 5 mm have an adenomatous etiology (Hoff et al. 1984). Polyps larger than 2 cm are often encountered in the right colon, in particular in the cecum (22.5% for Bernstein et al. 1985).

The topographic frequencies cited by Morson and Konishi (1982) are as follows: right colon (8.2%), transverse colon (13.6%), descending colon (18.7%), sigmoid colon (47%), and rectum (12.5%).

At least 50% of all patients with an adenoma have at least one other lesion. The frequency of multiple lesions increases with age, rising from 43.6% before 50 years to 56.2% after 70 years (Morson and Konishi 1982).

Colorectal adenomas can be divided into three histologic forms: tubular adenomas (adenomatous polyps), tubulovillous adenomas (villoglandular adenomas), and villous adenomas (villous papillomas). Tubular adenomas are by far the most prevalent (80.7%); tubulovillous (16.4%) and especially villous adenomas (2.9%) are much rarer (Morson and Konishi 1982). The frequency of villous adenomas is higher in the rectum (5.4%).

Analysis of the histologic types and risks of degeneration reveals existence of an adenoma-carcinoma sequence based on the following observations:

- Coexistence of invasive carcinoma and adenomas, and remnants of adenomas in 23% of adenocarcinomas (Eide 1983).
- Virtual absence of cancers smaller than 5 mm in diameter in otherwise normal colons.
- Certainty of malignant degeneration in familial polyposis.
- An 85% reduction in the incidence of rectosigmoid cancer in individuals who undergo yearly proctosigmoidoscopy (Ott et al. 1986b).

Analysis of histologic sections reveals that the presence of severe dysplasia is correlated with certain parameters:

- The location of the polyp: sigmoid lesions have an increased risk of malignant degeneration; for Morson and Konishi (1982), 9.5% of sigmoid lesions exhibit severe dysplasia versus only 1% of right colon lesions.
- Histologic type: severe dysplasia occurs in 20.6% of all villous adenomas versus only 4.1% of tubular adenomas (Morson and Konishi 1982).
- Size: severe dysplasia is absent in all lesions under 5 mm but present in 17% of lesions over 2 cm (Wegener et al. 1986).

This adenoma-adenocarcinoma sequence is also associated with other particularities. For example, 36% of patients with colorectal cancer have synchronous polyps (Chu et al. 1986). Follow-up of patients who have undergone

surgery for colorectal cancer should include not only local recurrent disease workups at the anastomosis, but also searches for polyps, whose degree of dysplasia is correlated with size and a risk of developing a second cancer (Girodet et al. 1985; Morson and Konishi 1982).

Most adenomas are asymptomatic. Even very large, distal lesions do not cause obstruction, pain, or problems with defecation. Likewise, adenomas within reach of digital examination may not be recognized. The only clinical manifestation specific to polyps is rectal bleeding. Often minimal, or even occult, bleeding is the predominant symptom in over one-half of all symptomatic cases. Rectosigmoid polyps which are voluminous typically cause intermittent rectal bleeding. Occult blood can be detected by fecal occult blood tests. Pedunculation, villous growth, size, and location in the left colon are all factors correlated with hemorrhagic phenomena (Sobin 1985).

Endoscopy is, of course, associated with polypectomy (Wilcox et al. 1986). Colonoscopy is superior to double-contrast enema examination for the left colon. By contrast, the overall accuracy of endoscopy is comparable to that of the double-contrast enema examination for the right colon (80% versus 82%). Combined use of both modalities increases accuracy to 97% (Thoeni and Petras 1982). Endoscopy does not detect all polyps, because 25% of lesions smaller than 5 mm and 5% of polyps greater than 5 mm are missed (Hoff and Vatn 1985). Polypectomy is a simple procedure that provides material for histopathologic examination. Discovery of cancer near the margin of excision, malignant cells in the lymphatic channels or veins, a poorly differentiated tumor, a sessile polyp, or incomplete resection all warrant further surgical resection. Postpolypectomy hemorrhagic complications are rare (only 0.2% for Lambot et al. 1982). Massive hemorrhage can be effectively controlled by infusion of vasopressin into the inferior mesenteric artery (Sanchez et al. 1986). The risk of recurrence rises with the diameter of the resected adenoma, in particular for rectal lesions. Likewise, villous adenomas have a higher recurrence rate (10%–30%) than tubular adenomas (Galandiuk et al. 1987). Matek et al. (1985) recommend the following surveillance policy: (a) simple adenomas should be followed up by fiberoptic endoscopy every 4 years because of the 6% risk of occurrence of another polyp within this period; (b) multiple adenomas, which are associated with a 5.7% risk of a new polyp within 2 years, should be followed up endoscopically every 2 years.

1.4.2 Imaging

1.4.2.1 Value of Barium Studies

Radiologic studies may be performed with either single-contrast or, better yet, a double-contrast method. The overall value of a double-contrast barium enema examination is 97% for Fork et al. (1983); for Teefey and Carlson (1983), the sensitivity is 94% and the specificity is 86%. Comparison of single-contrast and double-contrast studies for the colon reveal a sensitivity of 54%–80% for the first technique versus 89%–91% for the second technique (Ott et al. 1986a; De Roos et al. 1985). For lesions smaller than 1 cm, the sensitivity of single-contrast studies drops to 60% and that of the double-contrast method drops to 74%.

1.4.2.2 Radiologic Patterns and Diagnostic Problems (Figs. 1.6–1.9)

On double-contrast films, sessile polyps are seen as rounded radiodense images on anteroposterior projections; on lateral films, the image is hemispheric, with parietal indentation or amputation. On three-quarter views, the superposition of crescent-shaped loops produces the so-called bowler hat sign. Pedunculated polyps are generally seen as round images with a stalk. When the pedicle is superposed, a target image is seen.

Several diagnostic problems warrant mention. The bowler hat sign, for example, is not always reliable, because it is also seen in diverticular disease (Simms 1985; Tobin and Young 1987). Actually, thorough and careful interpretation of films often corrects the diagnosis (Keller et al. 1984). The diverticulum images as an opacification owing to the thin coating

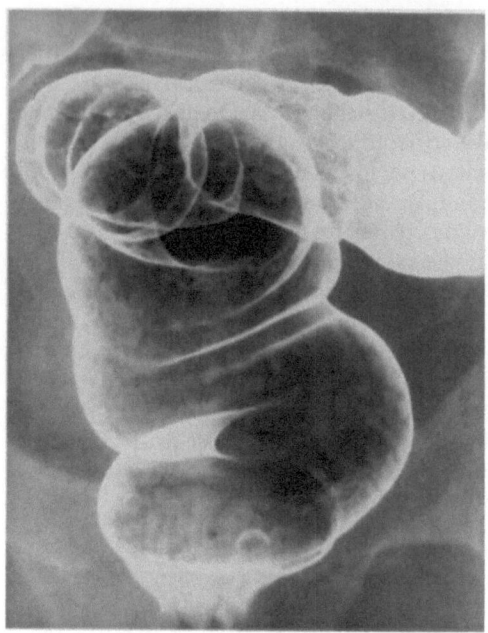

Fig. 1.6. Sessile rectal polyp

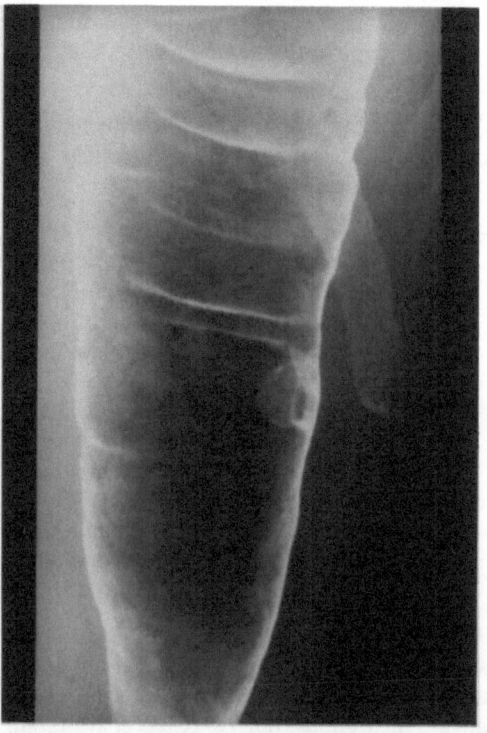

Fig. 1.7. Left colon polyp (lateral view)

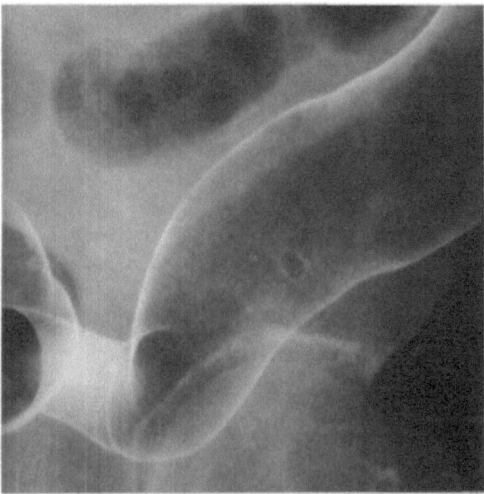

Fig. 1.8. Left colon polyp (anteroposterior view)

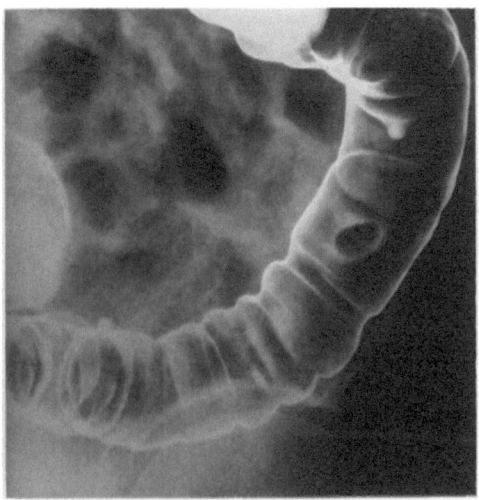

Fig. 1.9. Left colon polyp (anteroposterior view): presence of diverticula

of barium within the diverticular cavity; an extraluminal projection can be seen on tangential double-contrast films. On anteroposterior projections, a ring shadow or double ring shadow pattern is seen, with the base of the diverticulum projecting in the center. The partially filled diverticulum may contain an air-fluid level. The meniscus sign may occur after partial opacification of the diverticulum. Complete filling of the diverticulum is also possible, especially on single-contrast studies.

Sessile polyps may be demonstrated as a bowler hat, where a ring of barium (angle between the bowel wall and the base of the polyp) and a curvilinear density (dome of the polyp) are seen tangentially. The meniscus sign may be visualized, with a ring of barium around the polyp. Single-contrast films may show a filling defect. The stalk sign may be identified. The pedicle can result in the Mexican hat sign (a meniscus of barium around the stalk is surrounded by a second ring of barium around the dome of the polyp).

However, a diverticulum may present the appearance of a polyp in the following cases:

- Stool impaction.
- Edema of the bowel mucosa at the mouth of the diverticulum.
- Thrombus secondary to hemorrhage, filling the diverticulum.

- Inversion of a diverticulum into the intestinal wall, creating a true filling defect (Freeny and Walker 1979; Hugues 1975).

Other possible causes of diagnostic errors with barium enemas, occurring either alone or in combination, include, in order of decreasing frequency: small diameter polyps, air bubbles, overlapping intestinal loops, feces, spasm, excessive barium, poor coating of the barium (Rex et al. 1986).

Villous adenomas have a high propensity for malignant degeneration, which may be identified on double-contrast films when over 75% of the adenoma is affected (Iida et al. 1988). In these cases, the following signs exist:

- Reticular and granular patterns: the frequency of these patterns increases as the percentage of villous tissue rises.
- A nodular pattern: the frequency of this pattern decreases as the percentage of villous tissue rises (Figs. 1.10, 1.11).
- Feathery margins whose presence is directly correlated with the amount of villous tissue. On CT scans, villous adenomas show up as homogeneous, water-density masses lying in an eccentric position with respect to the rectal lumen (Coscina et al. 1986).

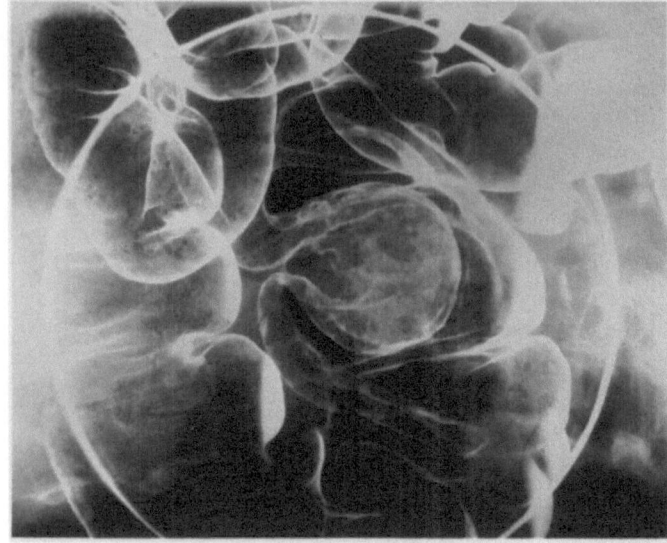

Fig. 1.10. Bulky non-villous colon adenoma

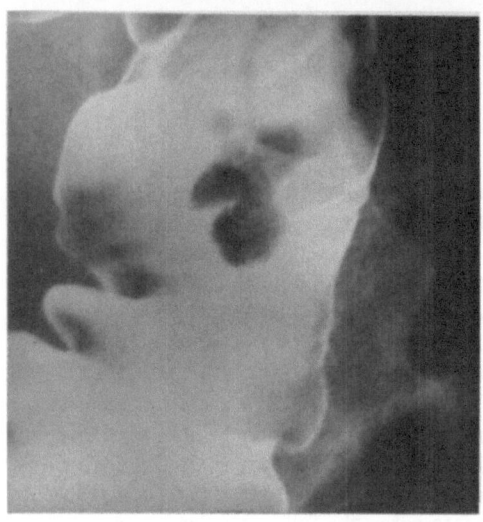

family history of disease, multiple lesions (22% malignancy for multiple lesions versus only 13% for solitary adenomas for Galandiuk et al. 1987), and greatest diameter over 4 cm. Signs of malignancy are difficult to detect on lateral projections because submucosal invasion does not cause peritumoral deformation; such deformation exists only when the tunica muscularis is invaded (Iida et al. 1988). This is particularly true for villous adenomas, which are often malignant.

1.4.2.4 Follow-up After Polypectomy (Fig. 1.12)

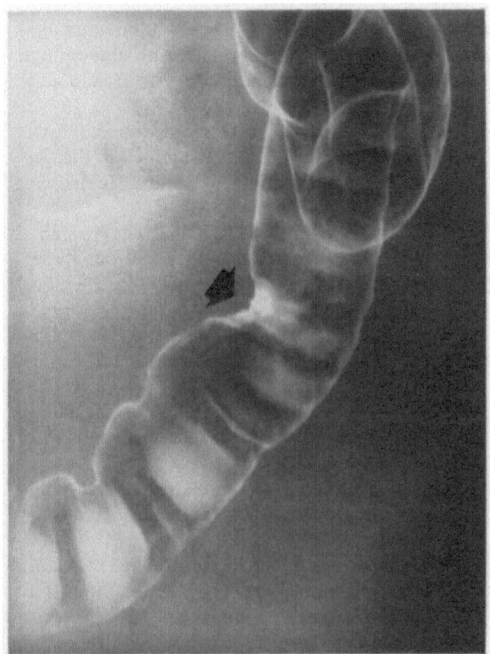

Fig. 1.12. Postpolypectomy examination: focal wall irregularity due to postoperative edema *(arrow)*. No malignant elements were found in the polypectomy specimen.

which have a very low risk of malignant degeneration. A good quality double-contrast barium examination will constantly detect lesions over 8 mm.

1.4.3 Differential Diagnosis

Hyperplastic polyps are frequently encountered in the rectum and throughout the colon. The incidence of these almost always multiple lesions increases with age. Hyperplastic polyps, which very rarely measure more than 10 mm, have no specific symptoms or risk of malignancy (Fenoglio and Pascal 1982), although this affirmation has been questioned by Morson and Konishi (1982).

Hamartomas occur in connection with Peutz-Jeghers syndrome and the juvenile polyp. Most hamartomas in patients with Peutz-Jeghers syndrome occur in the small intestine, although colonic sites are possible. Juvenile polyps are most common in children, with a peak frequency between the ages of 2 and 8 years.

Rare reports have been made in adults. The rectosigmoid is the preferential site (85% of cases) and 75% of these lesions are solitary. The gross appearance suggests the diagnosis: a short pedicle, smooth spherical mass, cystic formation filled with mucus and pus on cut histologic sections. Hemorrhage is common. Lesions low in the rectum may prolapse into the anus. Hamartomatous polyps rarely recur and have no malignant potential.

Inflammatory polyps are often multiple; solitary lesions of this type are rare. These focal, intraluminal masses of tissue are the result of mucosal inflammation during inflammatory bowel disease. The most frequent etiology is ulcerative colitis; granulomatous colitis is a less frequent cause. Inflammatory polyps are not a premalignant condition, and the frequency of carcinoma in patients with ulcerative colitis appears unrelated to the presence or absence of inflammatory polyps (Olmsted et al. 1986).

Postinflammatory polyps correspond to re-epithelialization and healing of the mucosa. They occur after both ulcerative colitis and granulomatous colitis; distribution may be diffuse, segmental, or focal. No association has been found with cancer.

Connective tissue polyps are rare submucosal lesions that develop intraluminally in connection with a lipoma, lymphangioma, hemangioma, or benign neurogenic or muscular tumor.

1.4.4 Conclusion

Owing to the frequency of adenomas in the colon and rectum and their well-recognized relation with colorectal cancer, screening programs and systematic eradication have been advocated. However, application of this policy to all persons at risk, in other words all individuals over 40 years of age, makes such screening impractical. High-risk patients must thus be identified using such generally recognized criteria as family history and especially personal history of colorectal cancer, chronic inflammatory bowel disease, epidemiologically related cancer, history of polyps, and especially the presence of multiple polyps.

Systematic mass screening programs must currently rely on the only selection method available at this time, the guaiac test: this test can detect colorectal lesions but its efficacy is low for small polyps. Regardless of the method of patient selection, screening procedures for colorectal polyps usually include proctosigmoidoscopy and double-contrast barium enema examination.

1.5 References

Agha FP, Ghahremani GG, Tsang TK, Victor TA (1988) Heterotopic gastric mucosa in the duodenum: radiographic findings. AJR 150: 291–294

Bernstein MA, Feczko PJ, Halpert RD, Simms SM, Ackerman LV (1985) Distribution of colonic polyps: increased incidence of proximal lesions in older patients. Radiology 155: 35–38

Bleshman MH, Banner MP, Johnson RC, De Ford JW (1978) The inflammatory esophagogastric polyp and fold. Radiology 128: 589–593

Bognel JC, Hadchouel P, Potet F (1986) Tumeurs bénignes de l'estomac. In: Bernier JJ (ed) Gastroentérologie, 2nd edn, vol 1. Flammarion Médecine Sciences, Paris, pp 387–392

Brambs HJ, Spamer C, Volk B, Holstege A (1986) Diagnostic value of ultrasound in duodenal stenosis. Gastrointest Radiol 11: 135–138

Caletti GC, Bolondi L, Zani L, Labo G (1986) Technique of endoscopic ultrasonography investigation: esophagus, stomach and duodenum. Scand J Gastroenterol 21 (Suppl 123): 1–5

Carlson HC, Good CA (1973) Neoplasms of the small bowel. In Margulis AR, Burhenne HJ (eds) Alimentary Tract Roentgenology, 2nd edn, vol 2. Mosby, Saint Louis, p 865–902

Chu CZJ, Giacco G, Martin RG, Guinee VF (1986) The significance of synchronous carcinoma and polyps in the colon and rectum. Cancer 57: 445–450

Coscina WF, Arger PH, Herlinger H, Levine MS, Coleman BG, Mintz MC (1986) CT diagnosis of villous adenoma. J Comput Assist Tomogr 10: 764–766

Delpy JC, Bruneton JN, Drouillard J, Lecomte P (1983) Non-Vaterian duodenal adenomas: report of 24 cases and review of the literature. Gastrointest Radiol 8: 135–141

De Roos A, Hermans J, Shaw PC, Kroon H (1985) Colonic polyps and carcinomas: prospective comparison of the single- and double-contrast examination in the same patients. Radiology 154: 11–13

Domellof L, Ericsson S, Janunger KG (1977) Carcinoma and possible precancerous changes of the gastric stump after Billroth II resection. Gastroenterology 73: 462–468

Eide TJ (1983) Remnants of adenomas in colorectal carcinomas. Cancer 51: 1866–1872

Eklof O, Eriksson E, Sahlin O (1960) Benign epithelial tumours of the stomach and duodenum. Diagnosis and treatment. Acta Chir Scand 255: 1–32

Elster K (1976) Histologic classification of gastric polyps. In: Morson BC (ed) Pathology of the gastro-intestinal tract. Springer, Berlin, Heidelberg, New York, pp 77–93

Farkas I, Patko A, Kovacs L, Koller O, Preisich P (1980) The brunneroma, the adenomatous hyperplasia of the Brunner's glands. Acta Gastroenterol Belg 63: 179–186

Feczko PJ, Halpert RD, Ackerman LV (1985) Gastric polyps: radiological evaluation and clinical significance. Radiology 155: 581–584

Fenoglio CM, Pascal RR (1982) Colorectal adenomas and cancer. Pathologic relationship. Cancer 50: 2601–2608

Ferin P, Skucas J (1983) Inflammatory fibroid polyp of the colon simulating malignancy. Radiology 149: 55–56

Fork FT, Lindstrom C, Ekelund GR (1983) Reliability of routine double-contrast examination (DCE) of the large bowel in polyp detection: a prospective clinical study. Gastrointest Radiol 8: 163–172

Freeny PC, Walker JH (1979) Inverted diverticula of the gastrointestinal tract. Gastrointest Radiol 4: 57–59

Gaitini D, Kleinhaus U, Munichor M, Duek D (1988) Villous tumors of the stomach. Gastrointest Radiol 13: 105–108

Galandiuk S, Fazio VW, Jagelman DG, Lavery IC, Weakley FA, Petras RE, Badhwar K, Mc Gonagle B, Eastin K, Sutton T (1987) Villous and tubulovillous adenomas of the colon and rectum. A retrospective review, 1964–1985. Am J Surg 153: 41–47

Gannon PG, Dahlin DC, Bartholomew LG, Beahrs OH (1962) Polypoid glandular tumors of the small intestine. Surg Gynecol Obstet 114: 666–672

Gelfand DW, Chen YM, Ott DJ (1987) Detection of colonic polyps on single-contrast barium enema study: emphasis on the elderly. Radiology 164: 333–337

Ghazi A, Ferstenberg H, Shinya H (1984) Endoscopic gastroduodenal polypectomy. Ann Surg 200: 175–180

Girodet J, Salmon RJ, Asselain B (1985) Dépistage coloscopique des polypes chez les sujets opérés d'un cancer colorectal. Etude prospective. Presse Med 14: 1819–1821

Gold RP, Green PHR, O'Toole KM, Seaman WB (1984) Early gastric cancer: radiographic experience. Radiology 152: 283–290

Harned RK, Consigny PM, Cooper NB, Williams SM, Woltjen AJ (1982) Barium enema examination following biopsy of the rectum and colon. Radiology 145: 11–16

Hoff G, Vatn M (1985) Epidemiology of polyps in the rectum and sigmoid colon. Endoscopic evaluation of size and localization of polyps. Scand J Gastroenterol 20: 356-360

Hoff G, Foerster A, Vatn MH, Gjone E (1984) Epidemiology of polyps in the rectum and sigmoid colon. Histological examination of resected polyps. Scand J Gastroenterol 20: 677-683

Hoff G, Vatn M, Gjone E, Larsen S, Sallar J (1985) Epidemiology of polyps in the rectum and sigmoid colon. Scand J Gastroenterol 20: 351-355

Hoff G, Moen IE, Trygg K, Frolich W, Sallar J, Vatn M, Gjone E, Larsen S (1986) Epidemiology of polyps in the rectum and sigmoid colon. Evaluation of nutritional factors. Scand J Gastroenterol 21: 199-204

Hoffman BP, Grayzel DM (1945) Benign tumors of the duodenum. Am J Surg 3: 394-400

Hughes LE (1975) Complications of diverticular disease: inflammation, obstruction and bleeding. Clin Gastroenterol 4: 147-170

Hughes RW Jr (1984) Gastric polyps and polypectomy: rationale, technique, and complications. Gastrointest Endosc 30: 101-102

Iida M, Yao T, Watanabe H, Itoh H, Iwashita A (1984) Fundic gland polyposis in patients without familial adenomatosis coli: its incidence and clinical features. Gastroenterology 86: 1437-1442

Iida M, Iwashita A, Yao T, Kitagawa S, Sakamoto K, Tanaka K, Fujishima M (1988) Villous tumor of the colon: correlation of histologic, macroscopic and radiographic features. Radiology 167: 673-677

Itai Y, Kogure T, Okuyama Y, Akiyama H (1978) Superficial esophageal carcinoma. Radiology 126: 597-601

Joffe N, Antonioli DA (1978) Atypical appearance of benign hyperplastic gastric polyps. AJR 131: 147-152

Johnstone JM, Morson BC (1978) Inflammatory fibroid polyp of the gastrointestinal tract. Histopathology 2: 349-361

Justrabo E, Dusserre L, Dusserre P, Bordes M (1985) Polypes fibro-inflammatoires de l'estomac. Revue de la littérature à propos de 2 cas. Ann Gastroenterol Hepatol (Paris) 21: 291-294

Keller CE, Halpert RD, Feczko PJ, Simms SM (1984) Radiologic recognition of colonic diverticula simulating polyps. AJR 143: 93-97

Kelvin FM, Gardiner R (1987) Clinical imaging of the colon and rectum. Raven, New York

Kjaergard H, Nordkild P, Hennild V, Moller-Pedersen V, Geerdsen J (1986) Follow-up study after colorectal polypectomy. The predictive value of a negative double-contrast barium enema. Scand J Gastroenterol 21: 353-356

Lambot G, Pelletier M, Deck M, Camatte R (1982) Intérêt de la polypectomie endoscopique. A propos d'une série personnelle de 409 polypectomies. Ann Gastroenterol Hepatol (Paris) 18: 195-198

Lev-Toaff AS, Levine MS, Herlinger H (1987) Ring-like rectal ulcers after biopsy or polypectomy. AJR 148: 285-286

Mac Donald JS, Cohn I Jr, Gunderson LL (1985) Cancer of the stomach. In: De Vita VT Jr, Hellman S, Rosenberg SA (eds): Cancer, principles and practice of oncology, 2nd edn. Lippincott, Philadelphia, pp 659-690

Marshak RH, Feldman F (1965) Gastric polyps. Am J Dig Dis 10: 909-935

Matek W, Guggenmoos-Holzmann I, Demling L (1985) Follow-up of patients with colorectal adenomas. Endoscopy 17: 175-181

McNeer G, Pack GT (1967) Neoplasms of the stomach. Lippincott, Philadelphia

Meltzer AD, Ostrum BJ, Isard HJ (1966) Villous tumors of the stomach and duodenum. Report of three cases. Radiology 87: 511-513

Miller JH, Gisoold JJ, Weiland LH, Melbrath DC (1980) Upper gastrointestinal tract: villous tumors. AJR 134: 933-936

Ming SC (1973) Tumors of the esophagus and stomach, 2nd series, fasc 7. Atlas of tumor pathology, AFIP, Washington

Ming SC, Goldman H (1965) Gastric polyps. A histogenetic classification and its relation to carcinoma. Cancer 18: 721-726

Monaco AP, Roth SI, Castleman B, Welch CE (1962) Adenomatous polyps of the stomach. A clinical and pathological study of 153 cases. Cancer 15: 456-467

Montesi A, Pasaresi A, Graziani L, Salmistraro D, Dini L, Bearzi I (1983) Small benign tumors of the esophagus: radiological diagnosis with double-contrast examination. Gastrointest Radiol 8: 207-212

Morson BC (1974) The polyp-cancer sequence in the large bowel. Proc R Soc Med 67: 451-457

Morson BC, Dawson IMP (1972) Gastrointestinal pathology. Blackwell Scientific, Oxford

Morson BC, Konischi F (1982) Contribution of the pathologist to the radiology and management of colorectal polyps. Gastrointest Radiol 7: 275-281

Moulinier B, Faivre J, Marchat F, Lesbros F, Lambert R (1975) Endoscopic removal of benign gastroduodenal tumours. Endoscopy 7: 121-125

Olmsted WW, Ros PR, Sobin LH, Dachman AH (1986) The solitary colonic polyp: radiologic – histologic differentiation and significance. Radiology 160: 9-16

Olmsted WW, Ros PR, Hjermstad BM, Mc Carthy MJ, Dachman AH (1987) Tumors of the small intestine with little or no malignant predisposition: a review of the literature and report of 56 cases. Gastrointest Radiol 12: 231-239

Osborne R, Toffler R, Lowman RM (1973) Brunner's gland adenoma of the duodenum. Am J Dig Dis 18: 689-694

Ott DJ, Gelfand DW, Wu WC, Ablin DS (1983) Colon polyp morphology on double-contrast barium enema: its pathologic predictive value. AJR 141: 965–970

Ott DJ, Chen YM, Gelfand DW, Wu WC, Munitz HA (1986a) Single-contrast vs double-contrast barium enema in the detection of colonic polyps. AJR 146: 993–996

Ott DJ, Gelfand DW, Wu WC, Munitz HA, Chen YM (1986b) How important is radiographic detection of diminutive polyps of the colon? AJR 146: 875–878

Papp JP, Joseph JL (1976) Adenocarcinoma occurring in a hyperplastic gastric polyp. Removal by electrosurgical polypectomy. Gastrointest Endosc 23: 38–39

Parnell SAC, Peppercorn MA, Antonioli DA, Cohen MA, Joffe M (1978) Squamous cell papilloma of the esophagus. Report of a case after peptic esophagitis and repeated bougienage with review of the literature. Gastroenterology 74: 910–913

Plachta A (1962) Benign tumors of the esophagus. Review of literature and report of 99 cases. Am J Gastroenterol 38: 639–652

Potet F, Brousse N, Soullard J (1978) Precancerous lesions of colonic mucosa. Epidemiological study and histological analysis of polyps. Eur J Cancer 1 (Suppl): 59–63

Rabin MS, Bremner CG, Botha JR (1980) The reflux gastroesophageal polyp. Am J Gastroenterol 73: 451–453

Raiford TS (1932) Tumours of the small intestine. Arch Surg 25: 122–177

Rex DK, Lehman GA, Lappas JC, Miller RE (1986) Sensitivity of double-contrast barium study for left-colon polyps. Radiology 158: 69–72

River L, Silverstein J, Tope JW (1956) Benign neoplasms of the small intestine. A critical comprehensive review with reports of 20 new cases. Int Abstr Surg 102: 1–38

Robbins SL, Cotran RS (1979) Pathologic basis of disease, 2nd edn. Saunders, Philadelphia

Rosato FE, Noto JA (1966) Gastric polyps. Am J Surg 111: 647–650

Ryan DP, Schapiro RH, Warshaw AL (1986) Villous tumors of the duodenum. Ann Surg 203: 301–306

Sanchez FW, Rogers JM, Vujic I, Chuang VP (1986) Transcatheter control of post-polypectomy hemorrhage. Gastrointest Radiol 11: 254–256

Sato T, Sakai Y, Ishiguro S, Fujita M, Kuriyama K, Narumi Y (1988) Gastric hamartomatous polyp without polyposis coli: radiologic diagnosis. Gastrointest Radiol 13: 19–23

Schmidt HW, Clagett OT, Harrison EG (1961) Benign tumors and cysts of the esophagus. J Thorac Cardiovasc Surg 41: 717–732

Seifert E, Gail K, Weismuller J (1983) Gastric polypectomy: long-term results (survey of 23 centers in Germany). Endoscopy 15: 8–11

Shimer GR, Helwig EB (1984) Inflammatory fibroid polyps of the intestine. Am J Clin Pathol 81: 708–713

Simms SM (1985) Differential diagnosis of the bowler hat sign. AJR 144: 585–587

Sleyster TJW, Abegg P, Yap SH, Schillings P, Rosenbusch G (1986) Magenpolypen und ihre Beziehung zum Magenkarzinom. Fortschr Roentgenstr 145: 678–680

Smith HJ, Lee EL (1983) Large hyperplastic polyps of the stomach. Gastrointest Radiol 8: 19–23

Snorer DC (1985) Benign epithelial polyps of the stomach. Pathol Annu 20: 303–329

Sobin LH (1985) The histopathology of bleeding from polyps and carcinomas of the large intestine. Cancer 55: 577–581

Strohm WD, Classen M (1986) Benign lesions of the upper GI tract by means of endoscopic ultrasonography. Scand J Gastroenterol 21 (Suppl 123): 41–46

Styles RA, Gibb SP, Tarshis A, Silverman ML, Scholz FJ (1985) Esophagogastric polyps: radiographic and endoscopic findings. Radiology 154: 307–311

Sundblad AS, Paz RA (1982) Mucinous carcinomas of the colon and rectum and their relation to polyps. Cancer 50: 2504–2509

Teefey SA, Carlson HC (1983) The fibroscopic barium enema in colonic polyp detection. AJR 141: 1279–1281

Thoeni RF, Petras A (1982) Double-contrast barium-enema examination and endoscopy in the detection of polypoid lesions in the cecum and ascending colon. Radiology 144: 257–260

Tobin KD, Young JWR (1987) The bowler hat: a valid sign of colonic polyps? Gastrointest Radiol 12: 250–252

Tomasulo J (1971) Gastric polyps. Histologic types and their relationship to gastric carcinoma. Cancer 27: 1346–1355

Tsukamoto Y, Nishitani H, Oshiumi Y, Okawa T (1977) Spontaneous disappearance of gastric polyps: report of four cases. AJR 129: 893–897

Vatn MH, Myren J, Serck-Hanssen A (1985) The distribution of polyps in the large intestine. Ann Gastroenterol Hepatol (Paris) 21: 239–245

Wegener M, Borsch G, Schmidt G (1986) Colorectal adenomas. Distribution, incidence of malignant transformation, and rate of recurrence. Dis Colon Rectum 29: 383–387

Wilcox GM, Anderson PB, Colacchio TA (1986) Early invasive carcinoma in colonic polyps. A review of the literature with emphasis on the assessment of the risk of metastasis. Cancer 57: 160–171

Williams AR, Balasooriya BAW, Day DW (1982) Polyps and cancer of the large bowel: a necropsy study in Liverpool. Gut 23: 835–842

Wolf BS (1960) Roentgen diagnosis of villous tumors of the colon. AJR 84: 1093–1104

Wolf M (1971) Heterotopic gastric epithelium in the rectum: report of three new cases with a review of 87 cases of gastric heterotopia in the alimentary tract. Am J Clin Pathol 55: 604–616

Wood DA (1967) Tumors of the intestines. Atlas of tumor pathology. Fasc 22. AFIP, Washington

2 Polyposis*

Hereditary syndromes, by far the most prevalent form of gastrointestinal polyposes, correspond to multiplication of the main varieties of common polyps in both the colon and other segments of the gastrointestinal tract.

Polyposis, and especially rectocolic polyposis, is hard to define accurately: the term generally refers to the presence of a large number of polyps (over ten for some authors, but more than 100 for others; Bussey 1975). In any case, the number of polyp elements is generally quite high, and these pathologies are easily classified as polyposes. In addition to hereditary forms (familial multiple polyposis, Peutz-

---

* Written in collaboration with J. Drouillard.

Jeghers syndrome, juvenile polyposis), numerous other pathologies exhibit the macroscopic and radiographic features of polyps. Hyperplastic polyps, connective tissue polyps, and pseudopolyps, for example, involve problems for differential diagnosis, because their prognosis and management are quite different.

2.1 Hereditary Polyposis Syndromes
(Table 2.1)

2.1.1 Familial Multiple Polyposis

This hereditary, autosomal dominant disease with a high degree of penetrance (approximately 80%) accounts for 80% of all hereditary

Table 2.1. General features of hereditary polyposes

	Frequency	Histology	Location (in order of frequency)	Malignant potential	Associated lesions
Familial polyposis	80%	Adenoma	Colon Duodenum Stomach	100%	—
Gardner's syndrome	Rare	Adenoma	Colon Duodenum Stomach	100%	Connective tissue tumors
Turcot syndrome	Rare	Adenoma	Colon	<90%	CNS malignancy
Peutz-Jeghers syndrome	10%	Hamartoma	Small intestine Stomach/colon	10%	Mucocutaneous pigmentation (oral mucosa)
Juvenile polyposis	10%	Juvenile polyposis	Colon Stomach/small intestine	Rare	Congenital malformations
Cowden's disease	Rare	All types	Colon Stomach/small intestine Esophagus	Uncertain	Mucocutaneous lesions; thyroid and breast malignancies

polyposis syndromes (Bussey et al. 1978; McConnell 1980). The incidence of familial multiple polyposis is between 1:3000 and 1:6850 (Bussey 1975). Onset of clinical symptoms usually occurs between the ages of 15 and 30 years. Only 5.8% of cases are diagnosed in children under 15, and only 10.7% are detected in patients aged 45 years or more (Bussey 1975). There is no sex predominance.

Familial multiple polyposis usually affects the entire colon, from the rectum to the cecum. Ileal involvement is rare, and ileal polypoid elements actually consist of small foci of nodular hyperplasia. The number of polyps increases from the proximal to the distal colon. Certain distribution patterns have been referred to as segmental or multiple polyposis, but these descriptions are actually not justified. Most polyps are small sessile lesions under 5 mm. Polyps over 10 mm, which account for 1% of cases, tend to be pedunculated. Larger tumors (up to 5 cm) and one or more carcinomas can also occur. The polyp elements in familial multiple polyposis present the histologic features of solitary adenomatous polyps: tubular, tubulovillous, and sometimes villous (Bognel 1985; Dreyfuss 1980; Jagelman 1983; Loygue and Adloff 1977). Severe dysplasia is common, and patients 30 years or older should be examined for signs of malignant degeneration. Three major forms of hereditary polyposis syndromes have been identified: familial multiple polyposis, Gardner's syndrome, and Turcot syndrome.

While the exact incidence of small bowel adenomatous polyposis remains unclear, gastric involvement occurs in 65% of cases, and 60%-90% of patients have duodenal lesions (Nishiura et al. 1984; Sarre et al. 1987a). Gastric polyps are not always adenomatous, whereas duodenal polyps are adenomatous and have malignant propensity.

Gardner's syndrome is an association of multiple adenomatous polyps, soft tissue tumors (fibromas, desmoid tumors, epidermoid cysts), and osteomas (Naylor and Lebenthal 1980; Richards et al. 1981). Desmoid tumors, which tend to develop on abdominal scars and mesenteric or retroperitoneal fibromatosis, are an adverse factor. The invasive nature of fibromatosis and the tendency for recurrence after resection complicates therapy. Osseous lesions (osteomas) characteristically affect the jaw and skull. Along with colorectal adenomas, nearly 50% of patients have gastric and duodenal lesions as well. Owing to its genetically linked nosology (completely expressed tare or double tare), Gardner's syndrome has been likened to pathologies associating familial multiple polyposis with multiple endocrine neoplasia syndrome (Demos et al. 1983; Schneider et al. 1983).

Turcot syndrome is a rare hereditary disease in which colonic polyposis coexists with primary central nervous system (CNS) tumors. The purely colorectal sites are associated essentially with glioblastoma multiforme and occasionally astrocytoma or medulloblastoma (Radin et al. 1984; Todd et al. 1981; Turcot et al. 1959).

All of these hereditary polyposes manifest in variable ways in the gastrointestinal tract. Family screening programs often elicit a history of clinical latency (26.8% of cases for Loygue and Adloff 1977). Clinical symptoms include rectal bleeding (60%-79% of patients), diarrhea (45.6%-70%), and pain (26.6%-40%) (Bussey 1975; Loygue and Adloff 1977).

Endoscopy, which is useful for biopsy and detection of malignancy, demonstrates the lesions as adenomas measuring an average of 1-3 mm. It is an easy diagnostic technique for family screening programs.

An essential characteristic of hereditary polyposis is the constant predisposition for malignant degeneration. Multiple cancers ultimately develop in 25%-50% of patients and affect individuals while young (35-40 years). In a third of cases, the cancers are discovered on the colectomy specimen; the percentage is markedly higher in symptomatic patients than in individuals with early disease identified by systematic screening programs. Upper gastrointestinal polyposes, and in particular those in the duodenum, can also degenerate. This risk is especially specific for Gardner's syndrome (Bognel 1985).

Management of hereditary polyposes is dominated by prevention of these often multiple, early cancers that have a poor prognosis. Radical surgery (prophylactic colectomy) is the standard procedure; the only questions concern the timing of the operation and whether or not to preserve the rectum (Gingold et al. 1979; Jagelman 1983; Jarvinen 1985). The decision to perform surgery should be made before the age of 30-35 years, and earlier intervention may be advisable for symptomatic patients with numerous large polyps.

Total colectomy, including resection of the rectum, is theoretically always indicated because of the rectal involvement and high risk of degeneration, but it constitutes a major mutilation for young individuals. The rectum can be preserved if all rectal polyps can be destroyed endoscopically or surgically; certain techniques result in true rectal mucosectomy (Bess et al. 1980; Sarre et al. 1987b; Watne et al. 1983). Spontaneous regression of rectal polyposis has been reported after colectomy. Recurrence is common, making careful follow-up and repeat eradication by cautery necessary (Heimann et al. 1986). Ileorectal anastomosis currently provides good oncologic control while preserving sphincter function.

Barium examinations should be performed using a double-contrast technique because topographic workup must be as accurate as possible; single-contrast studies are insufficient. Most polyps are between 2 and 5 mm. Although some polyps are larger, they generally do not exceed 1 cm unless they have become malignant. These essentially sessile lesions are scattered throughout the entire colon.

Barium enema examinations of the colon allow rather effective follow-up. The risk of hereditary polyposis must not be overlooked in young individuals even if they present fewer than ten polyps (Bartram and Thornton 1984; Dodds 1976; Kelvin and Gardiner 1987; Marshak et al. 1963). Accurate quantification of the number of polyps is an important prognostic factor (Maeda et al. 1984). The differential diagnoses for multiple polyps include fecal matter, gas bubbles, undigested food, lymphoid follicular hyperplasia, lymphoma, metastases, pneumatosis intestinalis, and deep cystic colitis (Kelvin and Gardiner 1987). Less often, adenomas may present umbilication (Smith and Lee 1986). Barium enema examinations have two other purposes:

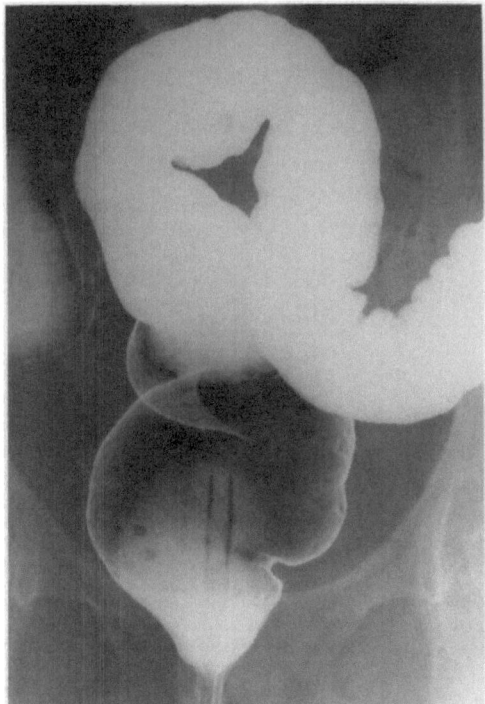

Fig. 2.1. Multiple rectosigmoid polyps

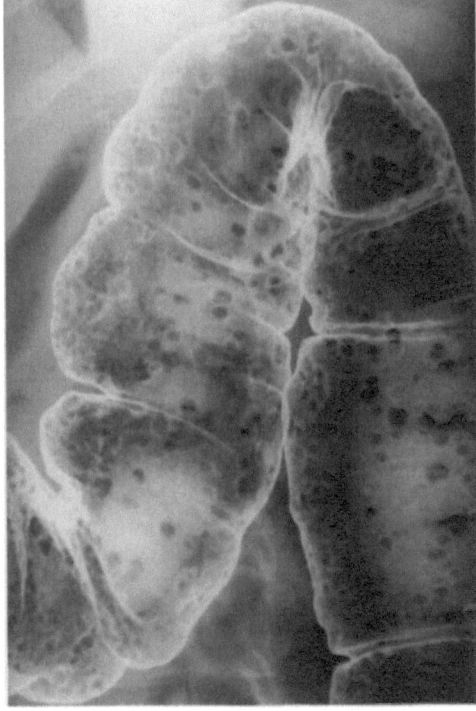

Fig. 2.2. Polyposis coli: spot film of the splenic flexure

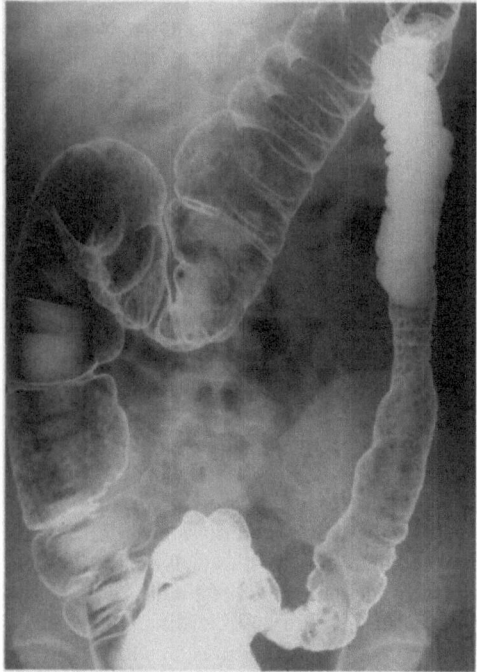

Fig. 2.3. Diffuse involvement of the entire colon and rectum in a patient with familial colorectal polyposis

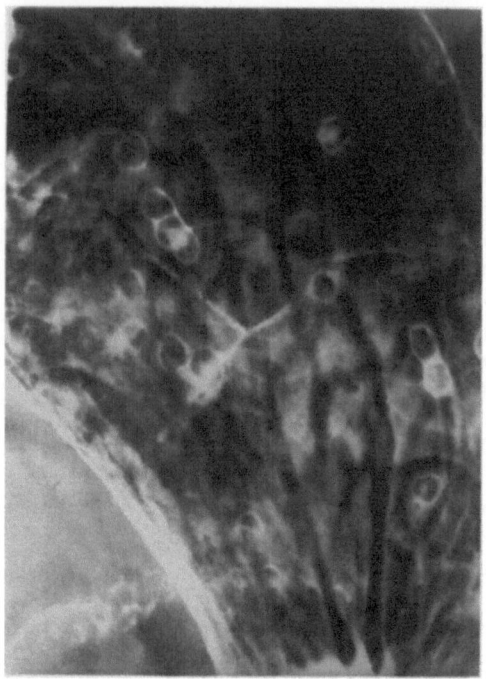

Fig. 2.4. Gastric lesions of familial polyposis

- Document the extent of polyposis in the entire gastrointestinal tract, and in particular the stomach and the duodenum (Figs. 2.1–2.6).
- Search for malignant degeneration or radiologically suspicious features warranting surgery (especially in the colon and the duodenum) (Fig. 2.7).

CT provides valuable data when there are signs of degeneration, and can demonstrate the extent of lesions. In Gardner's syndrome, CT can visualize an apparently primary desmoid tumor in the mesentery or a desmoid tumor occurring on a colectomy scar, for example (Kelvin and Gardiner 1987). These tumors present as a solid, sometimes necrotic mass that enhances moderately after injection of contrast medium.

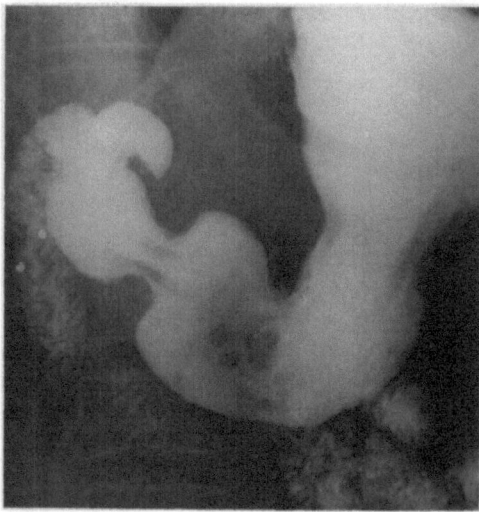

Fig. 2.5. Moderate gastric lesions of colorectal polyposis

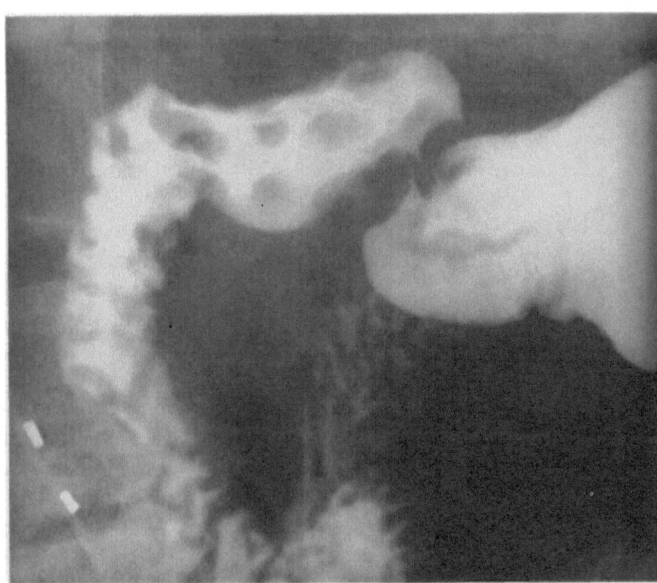

Fig. 2.6. Duodenal bulb lesions of familial polyposis

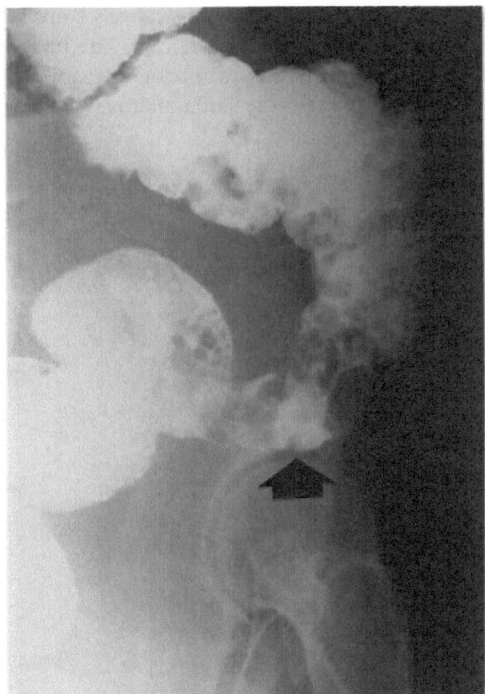

Fig. 2.7. Malignant degeneration in the left colon *(arrow)* in a patient with colorectal polyposis

2.1.2 Other Hereditary Polyposes

Peutz-Jeghers syndrome is a hamartomatous gastrointestinal polyposis associated with mucocutaneous pigmentation predominantly affecting the buccal and anal mucosa. The relatively few polyp elements are large and occur essentially in the upper small intestine; they are less common in the stomach, colon, and rectum. The risk of malignancy has been estimated at 10% (Crochet 1979; Kelvin and Gardiner 1987). Several hundred cases of this infrequent polyposis, which can affect all parts of the gastrointestinal tract, have been published. It usually develops during early childhood and adolescence, and the natural history is marked by obstructive complications and gastrointestinal bleeding. In addition to the risks of malignant degeneration, ovarian and testicular tumors may develop. Because this type of polyposis has a low malignant potential, treatment is essentially aimed at intestinal lesions which may require repeat operations. Colonic polyps can be treated by endoscopic resection (Figs. 2.8, 2.9).

Ruvalcaba-Myhre-Smith syndrome, which is similar to Peutz-Jeghers syndrome (Foster and Kilcoyne 1986; Ruvalcaba et al. 1980), is a hamartomatous polyposis characterized by

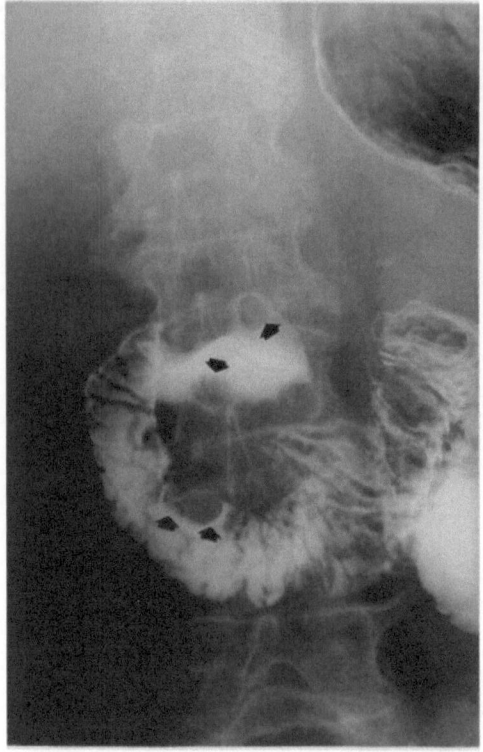

Fig. 2.8. Duodenal polyps *(arrows)* in a patient with Peutz-Jeghers syndrome

macrocephaly and hyperpigmented genital macules.

Juvenile polyposis, which occurs at about the same frequency as Peutz-Jeghers syndrome, includes two subgroups: juvenile polyposis coli and generalized juvenile gastrointestinal polyposis. The latter subgroup, characterized by involvement of the entire gastrointestinal tract and associated adenomatous gastrointestinal lesions, especially in the colon, involves a slight risk of malignant degeneration (Nisard et al. 1981; Rozen and Baratz 1972; Stemper et al. 1975). Various congenital abnormalities may occur in individuals with juvenile polyposis: cardiopathies, intestinal malrotation, hydrocephalus, etc. The affection starts early, between 7 and 15 years. The polyposis essentially affects the colon; other gastrointestinal sites are rare. The histologic features of juvenile polyps associate cysts, abundant and inflammatory connective tissue, and reorganized glands, but there are no neoplastic features (Veale et al. 1966). Clinical symptoms are usually minor; large polyps occasionally cause obstruction after intestinal intussusception. The prognosis is benign, and no major therapy is required. However, the adenomatous polyps

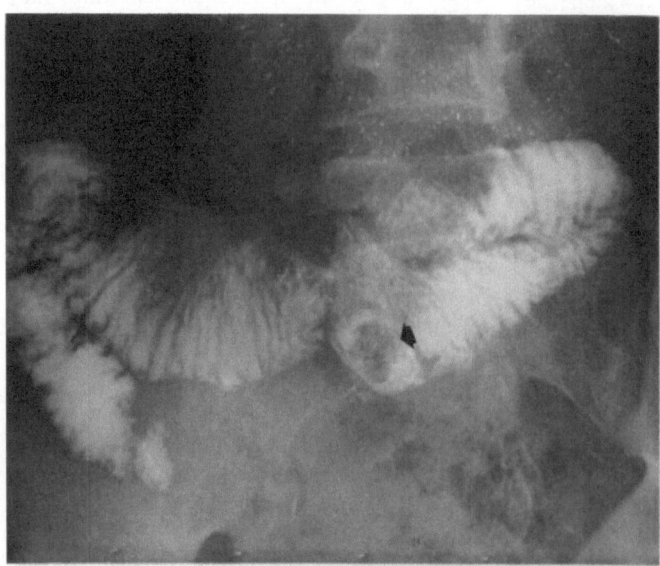

Fig. 2.9. Apparently solitary polyp *(arrow)* discovered during staging of a patient with Peutz-Jeghers syndrome

associated with juvenile polyposis require follow-up because of their risk of malignant degeneration.

Cowden's disease is a very rare pathologic entity affecting the stomach and colon; one-half of patients present with gastrointestinal polyposis. The multiple associated abnormalities occur at variable frequencies: characteristic mucocutaneous manifestations (papular, verrucous, and papillomatous), and abnormalities of the thyroid and mammary glands. The polyps have an inflammatory and adenomatous appearance; malignant degeneration is rare (Chen et al. 1987; Lloyd and Dennis 1963). The prognosis depends on the existence of associated visceral malignancies (thyroid gland, breast, ovary) rather than on degeneration of the gastrointestinal polyps themselves.

The radiologic features of these various polyposes are nonspecific, and barium examinations serve essentially for localization of lesions.

2.2 Non-hereditary Polyposes

Non-hereditary polyposes are rare and involve very different problems from those of familial colonic polyposis. The main concern is ruling out the possibility of adenomatous polyposis, owing to the prognosis and therapeutic implications of this pathology (Erbe 1976).

2.2.1 Proliferation of Hyperplastic Polyps

Hyperplastic polyps are often multiple (Williams et al. 1980); they generally measure 3–5 mm in diameter, but some can reach 15 mm and appear pedunculated. These polyps have no malignant potential, and there is no familial incidence. The radiologic features are identical to those for hereditary polyps (Cohen et al. 1981) (Fig. 2.10).

2.2.2 Cronkhite-Canada Syndrome (Cronkhite and Canada 1955; Canada Diner 1971)

This non-hereditary syndrome is also rare. There is no sex predominance, and the diagnosis is usually made in a 60-year-old individ-

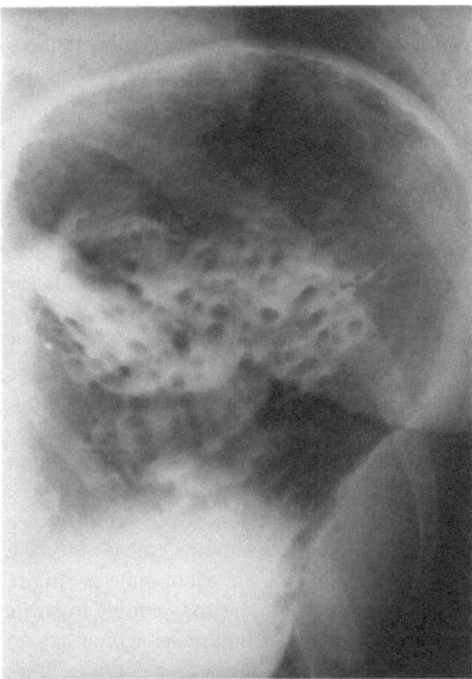

Fig. 2.10. Gastric polyposis (multiple hyperplastic polyps). Owing to the absence of malignant potential, this patient has been merely followed up by radiologic examinations and endoscopy for 10 years

ual with no contributory family history. Multiple polyps occur throughout the stomach, small intestine, and colon. Although described as adenomatous, these polyps have no malignant predisposition. Clinical symptoms include diarrhea and ectodermal abnormalities (hypertrophic nail changes, skin hyperpigmentation, alopecia). Hypoprotidemia leads to cachexia, with a fatal outcome in 6–18 months.

2.2.3 Differential Diagnosis

Various pathologies resemble polyps both endoscopically and radiologically, but actually have other etiologies.

Connective tissue polyposes are polyps of non-epithelial origin (intraluminal lesions of submucosal origin) corresponding to lipoma, leiomyoma, or neurofibroma.

Lymphoid polyposes correspond to lymphomatous polyposis of the benign reactional nodular hyperplasia type (Ranchod et al. 1978). In this pathology, pedunculated or sessile polyps (lymphoid nodules with a clear center) tend to occur in the terminal small intestine or the rectum. These lesions correspond to an inflammatory or immunologic response. Although primarily seen in children, several cases have been reported in adults (Ranchod et al. 1978). Another type of lymphoid polyposis occurs with certain malignant hemopathies, which, in addition to the more common tumoral forms, can mimic polyposis (Williams et al. 1984).

Inflammatory lesions presenting as polyposis are rare and have variable etiologies: inflammatory, parasitic (bilharziosis), secondary to necrotizing colitis (Bernstein et al. 1978; Jalan et al. 1969; Lumb 1961; Munyer et al. 1982). The radiologic and endoscopic features are confusing, and biopsy remains essential to rule out the possibility of an adenomatous origin. Inflammatory pathologies may evolve towards giant intestinal pseudopolyposis, which has an uncertain frequency (Archibald et al. 1988; Margulis 1972). Barium enema examination can demonstrate pseudopolyps measuring over 1.5 cm grouped together in a conglomerate hyperplastic mass. CT allows analysis of the intestinal wall, which is always thickened in this disease (Archibald et al. 1988; Gore et al. 1984). CT may be helpful for management of patients who are poor surgical candidates and cannot always be followed up endoscopically.

2.3 References

Archibald GR, Scholz FJ, Larsen CR (1988) Computed tomographic findings of giant intestinal pseudopolyposis. Gastrointest Radiol 13: 155–159

Bartram CI, Thornton A (1984) Colonic polyp patterns in familial polyposis. AJR 142: 305–308

Bernstein JR, Ghahremani GG, Paige ML, Rosenberg JL (1978) Localized giant pseudopolyposis of the colon in ulcerative and granulomatous colitis. Gastrointest Radiol 3: 431–435

Bess MA, Adson MA, Elveback LR, Moertel CG (1980) Rectal cancer following colectomy for polyposis. Arch Surg 115: 460–466

Bognel JC (1985) Polyposes familiales diffuses. Ann Gastroenterol Hepatol (Paris) 21: 347–350

Bussey HJR (1975) Familial polyposis coli: familial studies, histopathology, differential diagnosis and results of treatment. John Hopkins University Press, Baltimore

Bussey HJR, Veale AMO, Morson BC (1978) Genetics of gastrointestinal polyposis. Gastroenterology 74: 1325–1330

Canada Diner W (1971) The Cronkhite-Canada syndrome. Radiology 105: 715–716

Chen YM, Ott DJ, Wu WC, Gelfand DW (1987) Cowden's disease: a case report and literature review. Gastrointest Radiol 12: 325–329

Cochet B (1979) Peutz-Jeghers syndrome associated with gastrointestinal carcinoma. Gut 20: 169

Cohen SM, Brown L, Janower ML, McCready FJ (1981) Multiple metaplastic (hyperplastic) polyposis of the colon. Gastrointest Radiol 6: 333–335

Cronkhite LW, Canda WJ (1955) Generalized gastrointestinal polyposis: an unusual syndrome of polyposis, pigmentation, alopecia and onychotrophia. N Engl J Med 252: 1011–1015

Demos TC, Blonder J, Schey WL, Braithwaite SS, Goldstein PL (1983) Multiple endocrine neoplasia (MEN) syndrome type IIb: gastrointestinal manifestations. AJR 140: 73–78

Dodds WJ (1976) Clinical and roentgen features of the intestinal polyposis syndromes. Gastrointest Radiol 1: 127–142

Dreyfuss JR (1980) The polyposis disorders. In: Dreyfuss JR, Janower ML (eds) Radiology of the colon. Williams and Wilkins, Baltimore, pp 406–422

Erbe RW (1976) Inherited gastrointestinal polyposis syndromes. N Engl J Med 294: 1101–1104

Foster MA, Kilcoyne RF (1986) Ruvalcaba-Myhre-Smith syndrome: a new consideration in the differential diagnosis of intestinal polyposis. Gastrointest Radiol 11: 349–350

Gingold BS, Jagelman D, Turnbull RB (1979) Surgical management of familial polyposis and Gardner's syndrome. Am J Surg 137: 54–56

Gore RM, Marn CS, Kirby DF, Vogelzang RL, Neiman HL (1984) CT findings in ulcerative, granulomatous, and indeterminate colitis. AJR 143: 279–284

Heimann TM, Bolnick K, Aufses AH (1986) Results of surgical treatment for familial polyposis coli. Am J Surg 152: 276–278

Jagelman DG (1983) Familial polyposis coli. Surg Clin North Am 63: 117–128

Jalan KN, Sircus W, Card WI, McManus JPA, Prescott RJ (1969) Pseudopolyposis in ulcerative colitis. Lancet 1: 555–559

Jarvinen HJ (1985) Time and type of prophylactic surgery for familial adenomatosis coli. Ann Surg 202: 93–97

Kelvin FM, Gardiner R (1987) Clinical imaging of the colon and rectum. Raven, New York

Lloyd KM, Dennis M (1963) Cowden's disease. A possible new symptom complex with multiple system involvement. Ann Intern Med 58: 136–142

Loygue J, Adloff M (1977) Les polyposis recto-coliques. Masson, Paris

Lumb G (1961) Pathology of ulcerative colitis. Gastroenterology 40: 290–298

Maeda M, Iwama T, Ustonomiya J, Aoki N, Suzuki S (1984) Radiological features of familial polyposis coli: grouping by polyp profusion. Br J Radiol 57: 217-221

Margulis AR (1972) Radiology of ulcerative colitis. Annual oration in memory of Robert G Stone, MD, 1891-1966. Radiology 105: 251-263

Marshak RH, Moseley JE, Wolf BS (1963) The roentgen findings in familial polyposis with special emphasis on differential diagnosis. Radiology 80: 374-382

McConnel RB (1980) Genetics of familial polyposis. In: Winawer S, Schottenfeld D, Sherlock P (eds) Colorectal cancer: prevention, epidemiology, and screening. Raven, New York, pp 69-71

Munyer TP, Montgomery CK, Thoeni RF, Goldberg HI, Margulis AR (1982) Postinflammatory polyposis (PIP) of the colon: the radiologic-pathologic spectrum. Radiology 145: 607-614

Naylor BW, Lebenthal E (1980) Gardner's syndrome. Recent developments in research and management. Dig Dis Sci 25: 945-959

Nisard A, Nemeth J, Rambaud JC, Bitoun A, Galian A, Hautefeuille P (1981) Polypose juvénile associant polypes juvéniles et adénomateux et adénocarcinomes développés sur les deux types de polype. A propos d'un cas. Gastroenterol Clin Biol 5: 1160-1165

Nishiura M, Hirota T, Itabashi M, Ushio K, Yamada T, Oguro Y (1984) A clinical and histopathological study of gastric polyps in familial polyposis coli. Am J Gastroenterol 79: 98-103

Radin DD, Fortgang KC, Zee CS, Mikity VG, Halls JM (1984) Turcot syndrome: a case with spinal cord and colonic neoplasms. AJR 142: 475-476

Ranchod M, Lewin KJ, Dorfman RF (1978) Lymphoid hyperplasia of the gastrointestinal tract. A study of 26 cases and review of the literature. Am J Surg Pathol 1: 383-400

Richards RC, Rogers SW, Gardner RJ (1981) Spontaneous mesenteric fibromatosis in Gardner's syndrome. Cancer 47: 597-601

Rozen P, Baratz M (1982) Familial juvenile colonic polyposis with associated colon cancer. Cancer 49: 1500-1503

Ruvalcaba RHA, Myrhe S, Smith DW (1980) Sotos syndrome with intestinal polyposis and pigmentary changes of the genitalia. Clin Genet 18: 413-416

Sarre RG, Frost AG, Jagelman DC, Petras RE, Sivak MV, McGannon E (1987a) Gastric and duodenal polyps in familial adenomatous polyposis: a prospective study of the nature and prevalence of upper gastrointestinal polyps. Gut 28: 306-314

Sarre RG, Jagelman DG, Beck GJ, McGannon E, Fazio VW, Weakley FL, Lavery IC (1987b) Colectomy with ileorectal anastomosis for familial adenomatous polyposis: the risk of rectal cancer. Surgery 101: 20-26

Schneider NR, Cubilla AL, Chaganti RSK (1983) Association of endocrine neoplasia with multiple polyposis of the colon. Cancer 51: 1171-1175

Smith JH, Lee EL (1986) Umbilicated adenomas in familial polyposis coli: radiologic and histologic correlation (case report). AJR 147: 61-62

Stemper TJ, Kent TH, Summers RW (1975) Juvenile polyposis and gastrointestinal carcinoma. Ann Intern Med 83: 639-646

Todd DW, Christoferson LA, Leech RW, Rodolf L (1981) A family affected with intestinal polyposis and gliomas. Ann Neurol 10: 390-392

Turcot J, Despres JP, S Pierre F (1959) Malignant tumors of the central nervous system associated with familial polyposis of the colon: report of two cases. Dis Colon Rectum 2: 465-468

Veale AMO, McColl I, Bussey HR, Morson BC (1966) Juvenile polyposis coli. J Med Genet 3: 5-16

Watne AL, Carrier JM, Durham JP, Hrabovsky EE, Chang W (1983) The occurrence of carcinoma of the rectum following ileoproctostomy for familial polyposis. Ann Surg 197: 550-554

Williams GT, Arthur JF, Bussey HJR, Morson BC (1980) Metaplastic polyps and polyposis of the colorectum. Histopathology 4: 155-170

Williams SM, Berk RN, Harned RK (1984) Radiologic features of multinodular lymphoma of the colon. AJR 143: 87-91

3 Leiomyoma*

Approximately 1% of all gastrointestinal tract tumors are of smooth muscle origin (Buxton 1960; Morton et al. 1956). Leiomyoma, the most prevalent type, has variable clinical manifestations depending on the gastrointestinal segment affected. As for other tumors that develop intramurally, ultrasonography, endosonography, and CT all provide valuable information. Ultrasonography can be hampered by overlying intestinal gas, but can demonstrate the apparently solitary and solid nature of these gastrointestinal wall tumors. CT can assess the size, location, and especially the vascularity of these muscle tumors, but cannot determine their benign or malignant nature. Sonoendoscopy accurately analyzes the lesion location within the wall and has become an excellent means of exploration for this type of tumor. Owing to the different possibilities of imaging techniques depending on the gastrointestinal segment involved, the various localizations are discussed with their general features and imaging patterns.

3.1 Esophagus

3.1.1 General Features

Smooth muscle tumors of the esophagus have been studied extensively (Daniel and Williams 1950; Flavell 1953; Serementis et al. 1976). Leiomyomas are the most frequent benign esophageal tumor; they are six times more common than leiomyosarcomas (Baker and Good 1955) and are discovered in 0.087%–0.14% of autopsies (Griff and Cooper 1967; Harrintong and Moersch 1944; Postlethwait and Musser 1976; Serementis et al. 1976)

and approximately 0.3% of barium studies (Nahum et al. 1972).

Leiomyomas are almost always intramural (Gray et al. 1961) and are very rarely ulcerated (Baker and Good 1955). Multiple lesions are also unusual (Barreiro et al. 1976; Barrett 1964; Bollack et al. 1960; Bradford et al. 1947; Cornell et al. 1950; Godard and MacCrane 1973; Haber and Winfield 1974; Lueders and Tiscenco 1945; Rose 1936; Roussel et al. 1986; Schiebel and Cleaver 1955; Shaffer 1976; Sweet et al. 1956), being found in only 4% of cases (Gray et al. 1961). Calcifications are rare (Worton 1963). Association with a diverticulum is fortuitous (Gray et al. 1971), but leiomyomas in the lower third of the esophagus are often accompanied by a hiatal hernia or gastroesophageal reflux (Domergue et al. 1986; Jost et al. 1986). The locations of 249 cases reviewed (Abrescia et al. 1985; Bruneton et al. 1981; Domergue et al. 1986; Jost et al. 1986; Preda et al. 1986; Solomon et al. 1984) were as follows: upper third 9.6%, middle third 43.6%, lower third 42.7%, diffuse lesions 4%. Average patient age in the literature was 55 years, and males predominated (58.7%).

Clinical symptoms are summarized in Table 3.1. Leiomyomas are asymptomatic in one out of five cases. Respiratory symptoms (5.4%) and hemorrhage (2.9%) are uncommon. Rare clinical manifestations include hypertrophic osteoarthropathy (Kaymakcalan et al. 1980). The duration of leiomyoma-related symptoms is generally under 1 year, but can extend over 17 years (Deverall 1968). The preferred therapy for large leiomyomas is surgery (Cornell et al. 1950; Gray et al. 1961; Haber and Winfield 1974; Serementis et al. 1976); extramucosal enucleation is possible for smaller lesions (Gray et al. 1961; Jost et al. 1986; Naouri et al. 1986; Preda et al. 1986). Certain authors, however, have proposed radiologic

---

* Written in collaboration with J. Drouillard.

surveillance alone for this type of tumor (Brombart 1973; Glanz and Grunebaum 1977; Naouri et al. 1986; Solomon et al. 1984). Recurrence after surgical resection appears exceptional (Standerfer and Paneth 1982).

Table 3.1. Clinical manifestations of gastrointestinal leiomyomas (716 cases reported in the literature)

	Esophagus (237 cases)	Stomach (202 cases)	Small intestine (271 cases)	Colon/ rectum (6 cases)
Pain	35.8%	30.2%	66.8%	33.3%
Hemorrhage or anemia	2.9%	44%	58.7%	50%
Weight loss	–	2%	–	–
Dysphagia	50.2%	–	–	–
Palpable mass	–	8.4%	22.1%	33.3%
Weakness	21.1%	23.7%	7.4%	–
Obstruction	–	1%	32.4%	–
Asymptomatic	21.1%	22.7%	–	–

3.1.2 Imaging (Figs. 3.1 and 3.2)

Chest radiographs reveal a posterior mediastinal opacity in 47.5% of cases and calcification in 3.8% (Barrett 1964; Ghahremani et al. 1978; Graham et al. 1972; Huddy and Griffiths 1972; Merlier et al. 1977). The radiologic appearances of leiomyomas have been well described by Schatzki and Howes (1942). The radiologic patterns and the diameter of lesions observed during barium examination are summarized in Table 3.2. Leiomyomas are usually smaller than 10 cm and tend to be intramural. Ulceration is uncommon (1.4%). Proximal obstruction is also exceptional, being mentioned in connection with only 1.4% of the cases reviewed (Barreiro et al. 1976; Nahum et al. 1972).

Radiologic studies remain interesting for esophageal muscle tumors because biopsies are often negative (Davies 1978; Deverall

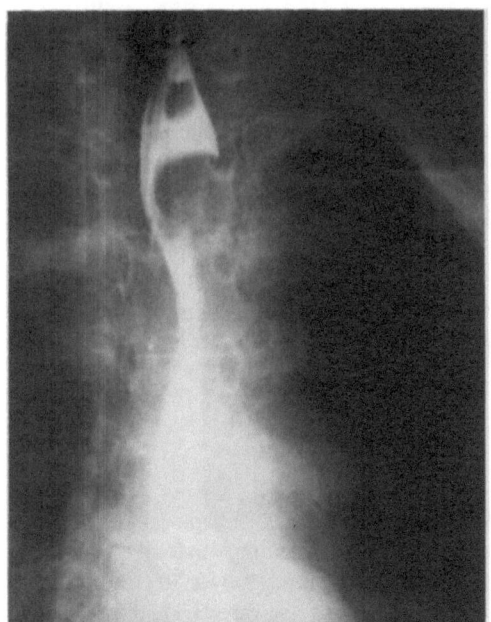

Fig. 3.1. Leiomyoma of the upper third of the esophagus

Fig. 3.2. Leiomyoma of the esophagus: double-contrast study showing the intramural nature of the lesion ▶

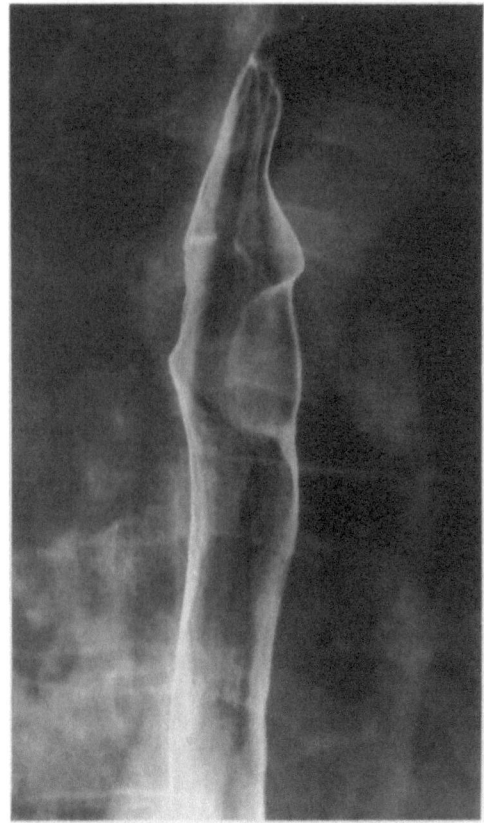

Table 3.2. Diameter (407 cases) and barium findings (557 cases) for gastrointestinal tract leiomyomas

	Esopha-gus	Stomach	Small intestine	Colon/rectum
Diameter				
<5 cm	41.9%	37.6%	71.4%	50%
5–10 cm	40.3%	41.6%	20.9%	16.7%
>10 cm	17.8%	20.8%	7.7%	33.3%
Barium pattern				
Intramural	79%	69.3%	17.8%	50%
Intraluminal	8.4%	5.8%	27.4%	33.3%
Subserosal	9.8%	21.2%	42.6%	16.7%
Dumbbell	2.8%	3.7%	12.2%	–
Ulceration	1.4%	24.7%	5%	16.7%
Negative	0.2%	7%	11.3%	–

1968; Glanz and Grunebaum 1977; Huddy and Griffiths 1972; Moser et al. 1978; Preda et al. 1986). This is especially true for leiomyomas. However, endoscopy nearly always demonstrates the tumor or its endoluminal consequences (Preda et al. 1986; Solomon et al. 1984). Differential diagnosis of leiomyomas can be difficult; it is sometimes impossible to rule out other benign tumors, in particular adenomas and schwannomas (Bernatz et al. 1958). Giant myomatous lesions are rare (Gallinger et al. 1983; Kramer et al. 1986) and may be confused with achalasia (Kramer et al. 1986).

Sonoendoscopy will undoubtedly become a very useful means of diagnosing esophageal leiomyoma in patients who do not require surgery and are followed up instead by imaging studies.

Few *CT* studies have been published on esophageal leiomyomas (Abrescia et al. 1985; Domergue et al. 1986; Nicolas and Schlolaut 1987; Solomon et al. 1984); they can demonstrate tumor size and the integrity of the remainder of the mediastinum, but do not have the sensitivity of sonoendoscopy for precise tumor localization within the esophageal wall.

Six angiographic studies were available for review; examination was completely negative in one case (Ribet et al. 1973), but the other five tumors were all avascular (Ben Benachem et al. 1977; Gothlin et al. 1975; Mouchet et al. 1969; Ribet et al. 1973).

3.2 Stomach

3.2.1 General Features

Whereas leiomyosarcomas represent only 0.51% of all malignant stomach tumors (Skandalakis et al. 1960), leiomyomas are among the most frequent benign gastric tumors (Good 1965; Salmela and Kohler 1969) and account for 2.5% of all gastric tumors (Skandalakis et al. 1960). Leiomyomas are four times as frequent as leiomyosarcomas.

Pathologic features include the possibility of clusters of calcifications (Crummy and Juhl 1962; Ghahremani et al. 1978), the rarity of perforation, and obstructive syndromes caused by intraluminal and antral tumors (Barnett 1925; Grignani et al. 1985; Grundy et al. 1984; Short and Young 1968; Skandalakis et al. 1960). Multiple lesions are exceptional (Braczkowski et al. 1976). Mean patient age was 47 years, and male predominance was noted (67.1%).

The clinical findings for 202 cases reviewed are listed on Table 3.1. One-fifth of all gastric leiomyomas are asymptomatic. For Kavlie and White (1972), gastric leiomyomas do not manifest clinically unless they are at least 3 cm in size or ulcerated. Hemorrhage is the most frequent symptom; pain is less common. As for esophageal leiomyomas, and owing to the submucosal nature of leiomyomas, endoscopic biopsy is often negative (Grimoud et al. 1974). Surgery (resection or partial gastrectomy) is nearly always indicated owing to the risk of hemorrhage with lesions over 5 cm in diameter (Christinaz et al. 1984).

3.2.2 Imaging

On *abdominal plain films*, tumoral opacity was visible for 11% of leiomyomatous lesions and corresponded to tumors over 10 cm in diameter. Calcifications are rare (3%) (Boijsen et al. 1966; Crummy and Juhl 1962; Herlinger 1966; Worton 1963). Intussusception of an intraluminal mass through the duodenal bulb can cause upper gastrointestinal obstruction (Barnett 1925; Short and Young 1968).

Barium studies are rarely negative (7%). Most gastric leiomyomas are intramural, occasional-

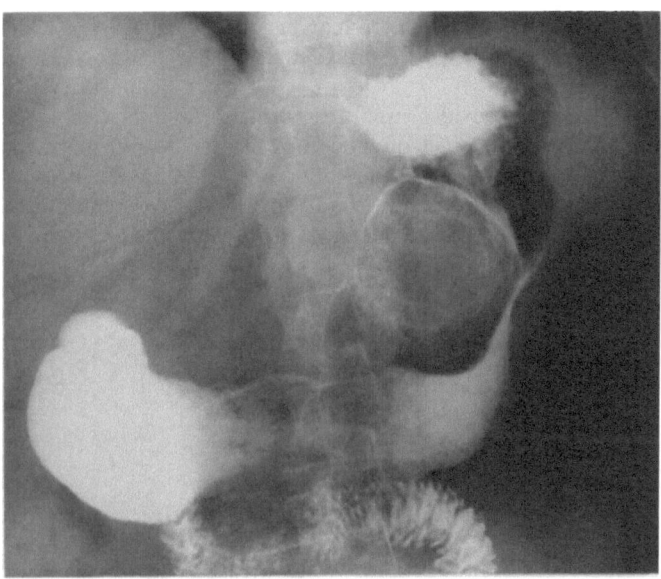

Fig. 3.3. Bulky gastric leiomyoma

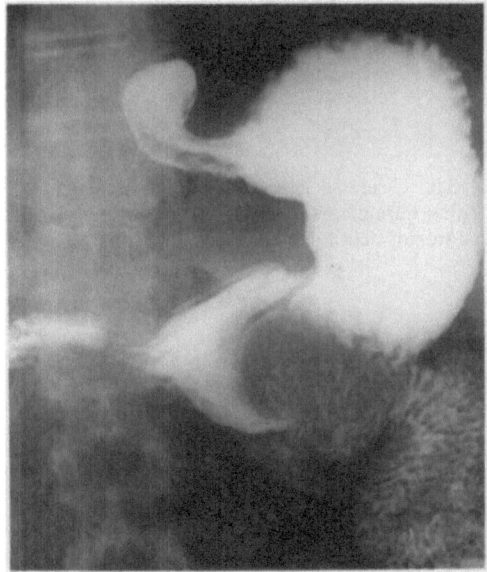

Fig. 3.4. Leiomyoma of the gastric antrum

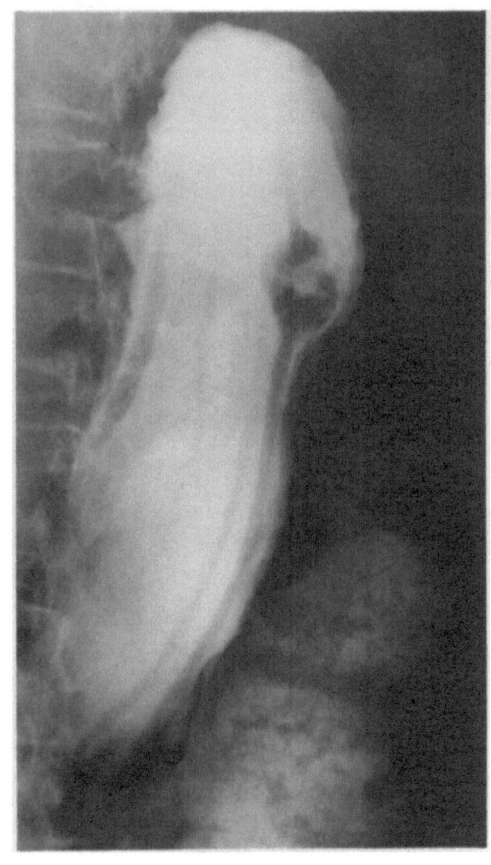

Fig. 3.5. Small ulcerated leiomyoma of the upper ▶
third of the stomach

ly ulcerated lesions. Ulceration may disappear with medical treatment (O'Riordan et al. 1985) (Figs. 3.1–3.6).

Sonoendoscopy provides useful information owing to the low efficacy of endoscopy for diagnosis of leiomyoma. By revealing the lesion's origin within the gastric wall (mucosal muscle, proper muscle), sonoendoscopy can suggest the diagnosis of a muscular tumor (Fig. 3.7). However, differentiation of a small leiomyoma from a small leiomyosarcoma is not possible (Yasuda et al. 1986). Sonoendoscopy will undoubtedly acquire a major role for the diagnosis of intramural gastric tumors. As for other localizations, CT can demonstrate the exact size of the tumor and the gastric ori-

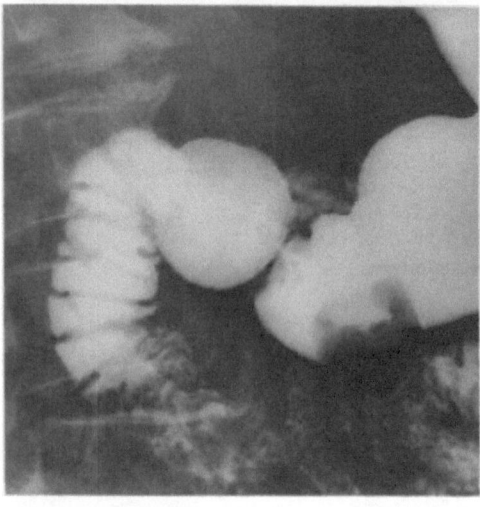

Fig. 3.6. Ulcerated leiomyoma of the gastric antrum

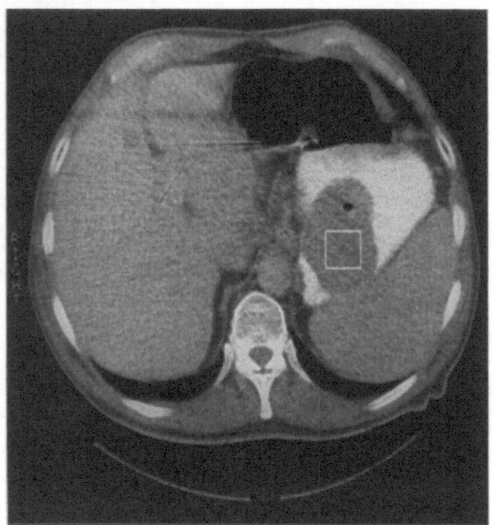

Fig. 3.8. Ulcerated leiomyoma of the stomach exhibiting intraluminal growth, as shown by the CT scan (tumor density 27 HU within the square)

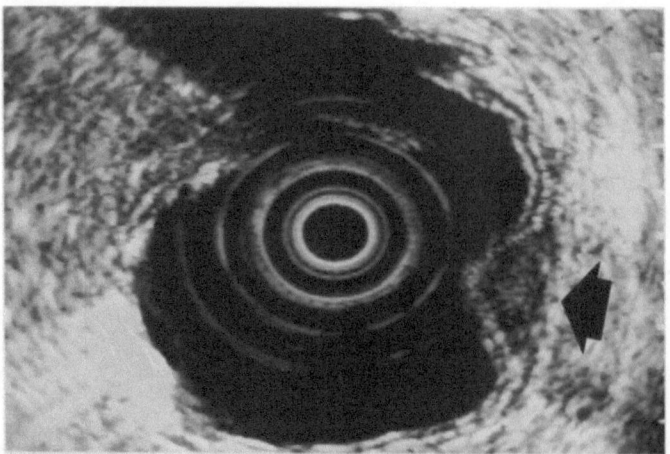

Fig. 3.7. Gastric leiomyoma: the surface of this well-circumscribed lesion *(arrow)* is covered by three layers, including the submucosa, and appears continuous with the muscularis propria

gin of a lesion poorly analyzed by endoscopy and barium examination (Coscina et al. 1986; Solomon et al. 1987) (Fig. 3.8).

Of 21 gastric leiomyomas studied by *angiography* (Boijsen et al 1966; Fujii et al. 1972; Kaude et al. 1972; Kavlie and White 1972; Reuter et al. 1970; Schoembaum et al. 1973; Shibata and Iwasaki 1970), two of the examinations proved normal (Reuter et al. 1970); in one case, the lesion was hypovascular; the other tumors all exhibited hypervascularity with blushing during periods of hemorrhage (Schoembaum et al. 1973). Venous return through a large-diameter drainage vein was noted in eight cases. These images usually only allow presumptive diagnosis of a connective tissue tumor because benign neurogenic tumors and leiomyosarcomas have a comparable appearance.

CT findings in favor of a benign pathology include a solitary lesion without adenopathies or hepatic metastasis (metastatic lymph nodes would indicate lymphoma while liver metastases would indicate leiomyosarcoma).

3.3 Small Intestine

3.3.1 General Features

Leiomyomas and leiomyosarcomas of the small intestine occur with similar frequencies (54% for leiomyomas versus 46% for leiomyosarcomas for Baker and Good 1955). Leiomyomas represent approximately 15.5% of all benign tumors of the small intestine (Botsford et al. 1962; Brief and Botsford 1963; Cohen et al. 1971; Croom and Newsome 1975; Ebert et al. 1953,1965; Hauswald and Griffen 1977; Olsson 1972; Ostermiller et al. 1966; River et al. 1956). The site of predilection is the jejunum (Good 1963). Involvement of the appendix (Cullen and Voss 1972) and Meckel's diverticulum (Blamey and Woods 1986; Swinnen et al. 1986; Weinstein et al. 1963) are exceptional, but leiomyomas are the most common tumors of Meckel's diverticulum. In a review of 373 cases of intestinal leiomyomas, the distribution was as follows: duodenum 20.5%, jejunum 42.2%, ileum 36.3%, appendix 0.2%, Meckel's diverticulum 0.8% (Bruneton et al. 1981).

Multiple leiomyomatous lesions of the small intestine occurred in 1.8% of patients in our literature review (Allen 1971; Han and Aldrete 1977; River et al. 1956; Starr and Dockerty 1955). Subserosal intestinal involvement occasionally occurs in patients with leiomyomatous peritonealis disseminata (Minassian et al. 1986; Renigers et al. 1985). Mean patient age is 52 years, and there is slight male predominance (51.3%). As shown in Table 3.1, intestinal leiomyomas are rarely asymptomatic (Botsford et al. 1962; Myre 1963; Wilson et al. 1975). The most common clinical manifestations are hemorrhage and pain. Exceptionally, a pulsatile mass may occur (Kaude et al. 1972).

3.3.2 Imaging (Figs. 3.9–3.13)

Calcifications are rare (Ghahremani et al. 1978). The radiologic features observed during barium examinations are summarized in Table 3.2; these studies are often negative. Furthermore, the radiologic appearances of leiomyoma and leiomyosarcoma are similar (see Chap. 15). Few studies have been conducted with ultrasonography: the sonographic

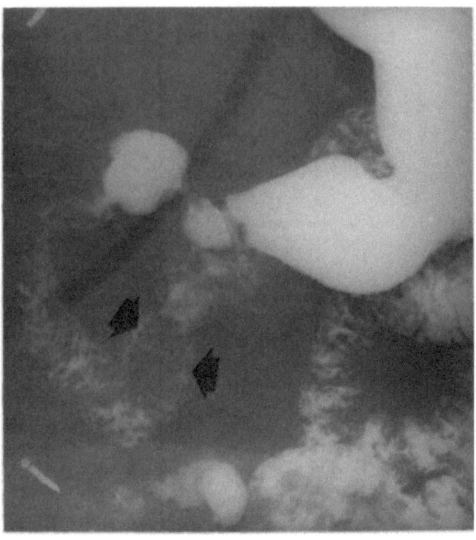

Fig. 3.9. Intraluminal duodenal leiomyoma *(arrows):* this bulky tumor did not cause suprajacent digestive stasis

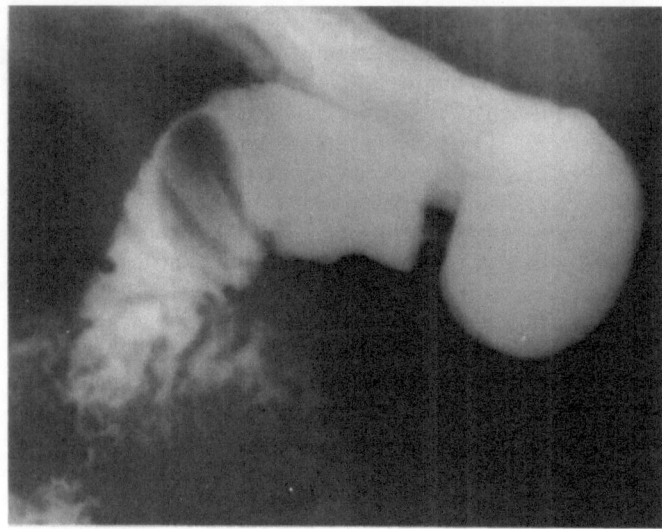

Fig. 3.10. Duodenal leiomyoma: the radiologic image is comparable to that of an adenoma

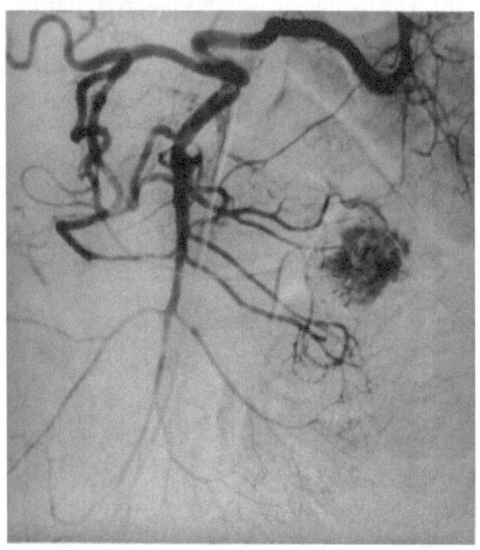

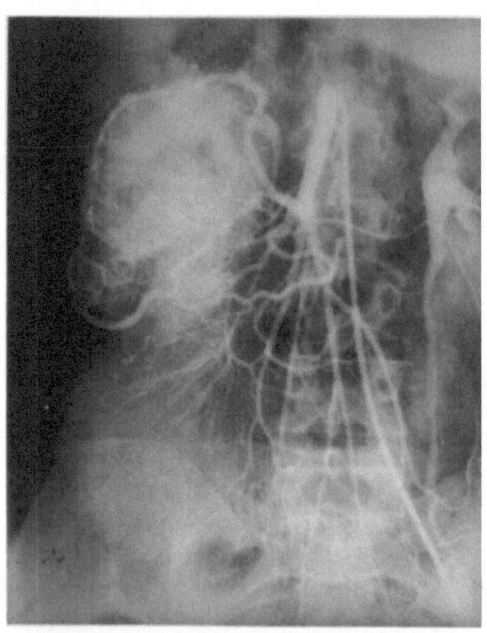

Fig. 3.11. Angiographic study of a jejunal leiomyoma: massive tumoral hypervascularity

Fig. 3.12. Angiographic study of an intestinal leiomyoma with discretely homogeneous tumoral hypervascularity. Angiography suggested a connective tissue tumor, but the absence of signs of invasion made it impossible to determine its benign or malignant nature

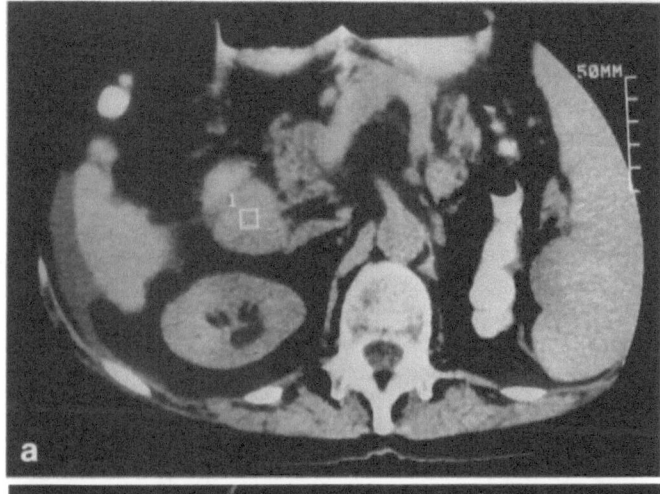

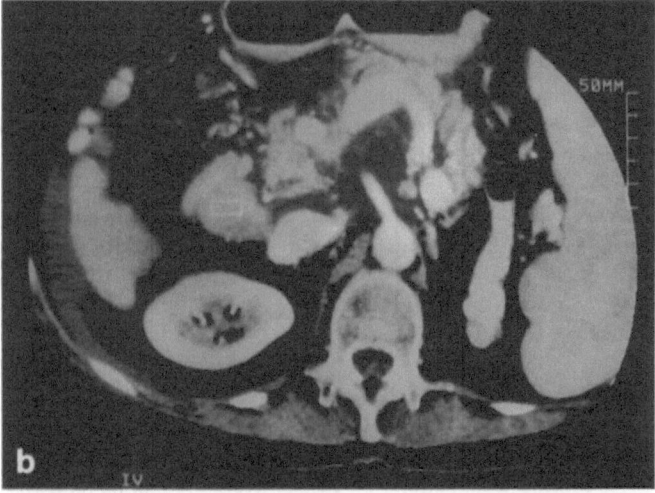

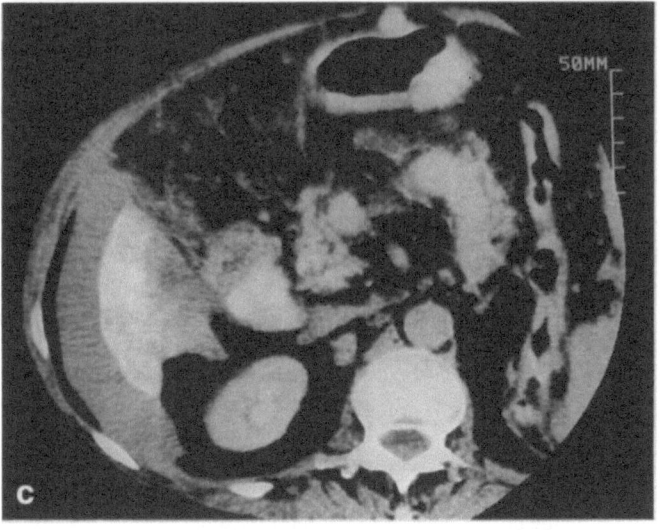

Fig. 3.13a–c. Duodenal leiomyoma: CT study. Before injection **(a)**, solid 40 HU lesion. After iv contrast medium injection **(b)**, the lesion appears hypervascular (93 HU). This cirrhotic patient developed a hepatoma; liver studies were performed by injection of emulsion-form lipiodol into the common hepatic artery. Tumor opacification by the lipiodol on the CT scans reflects tumor hypervascularity **(c)**

pattern corresponds to a well-delimited solid lesion (Kressel et al. 1981; Renigers et al. 1985). CT studies are also rare (Farah et al. 1987; Kressel et al. 1981; Megibow et al. 1985; Scatarige et al. 1987; Swinnen et al. 1986; Zanella et al. 1986). CT scans can show the solitary nature of the lesion; demonstration of hypervascularity by nearly constant enhancement after contrast medium injection suggests a probably benign, connective tissue tumor. In case of bleeding, scans with 99 mTc sulfur colloid may reveal hyperactive areas of purely topographic rather than etiologic interest (Kressel et al. 1981).

Analysis of arteriographic data for 39 leiomyomas revealed that examination was normal in only two cases (Benacerraf 1974; Kressel et al. 1981). Hypervascularity was found in 97.3% of cases, necrosis in 16.1%, and well-demarcated contours in 83.8%. The artery supplying the tumor had increased in size in 97.3% of cases, and a drainage vein was visible in 81%. There are no angiographic differences between leiomyomas and leiomyosarcomas (Bruneton et al. 1981; Zollikofer et al. 1979).

3.4 Colon and Rectum

3.4.1 General Features

As for the rectum (Kusminsky and Bailey 1977), colonic localizations of gastrointestinal muscle tumors are extremely rare, with leiomyosarcomas being slightly more frequent than leiomyomas (55% versus 45%) (Baker and Good 1955). Colorectal leiomyomas represent 1.5%–3% of all leiomyomatous tumors of the gastrointestinal tract (Baker and Good 1955; Good 1963) and colorectal leiomyosarcomas 1.8%–3.4% of all tumors (Baker and Good 1955; Good 1963).

Eight cases of colonic leiomyoma were reviewed (Allen 1971; Delavierre et al. 1975; Freni and Keeman 1977; Kaupp et al. 1964; McKenzie et al. 1954; Spaun and Nielsen 1986; Witt et al. 1983). Mean patient age was 53 years, and males predominated (60%). There are no specific clinical signs with respect to other colon tumors. Sasaki et al. (1985) reviewed 79 cases of rectal leiomyomas: 11.3% were asymptomatic, and 39.2% of patients presented with a history of hemorrhage. In 45.5% of cases, the lesion was smaller than 5 cm diameter.

3.4.2 Imaging

At barium enema examination, leiomyomas are generally intramural whereas leiomyosarcomas tend to be intraluminal or subserosal and frequently present radiologically visible ulcerations.

3.5 Conclusion

Leiomyomas are more common than leiomyosarcomas except in the colon, where the latter predominate, and in the small intestine, where both tumor types occur with similar frequency. From a clinical viewpoint, upper gastrointestinal tract leiomyomas are commonly asymptomatic.

Conventional imaging examinations remain useful for this type of tumor (barium studies, insufficient for the small intestine, or angiography). This strategy allows the diagnosis of small lesions which may explain a hemorrhage. However, no imaging differences have been found between leiomyomas and leiomyosarcomas, and the natural history of these tumors is unpredictable. Supradiaphragmatic lesions tend to be avascular while subdiaphragmatic muscle tumors are usually hypervascular. New imaging techniques, and especially CT, often demonstrate leiomyomas as small, solitary lesions without hepatic metastasis. By contrast, leiomyosarcomas tend to be larger, subserosal lesions with liver involvement. Finally, imaging studies have a role to play for the follow-up of esophageal leiomyomas as various authors (Brombart 1973; Glanz and Grunebaum 1977) advocate radiographic surveillance of these tumors.

3.6 References

Abrescia F, Montresor E, Saggin P, Tenchini P, Sandrini A, Frigo F, Puchetti V (1985) Leiomyomata of the oesophagus: report of four surgically treated cases. Eur J Surg Oncol 11: 333–336

Allen FA (1971) Leiomyomata of gastrointestinal tract. J Kans Med Soc 72: 453–457

Baker HL, Allen Good C (1955) Smooth-muscle tumors of the alimentary tract. Their roentgen manifestations. AJR 74: 246–255

Barnett LE (1925) Myoma of stomach with gastroduodenal intussusception. Br J Surg 12: 615–617

Barreiro F, Seco JL, Molina J, Villamor J (1976) Giant esophageal leiomyoma with secondary megaesophagus. Surgery 79: 436–439

Barrett NR (1964) Benign smooth muscle tumours of the oesophagus. Thorax 19: 185–194

Benacerraf R (1974) Apport de l'artériographie digestive au diagnostic des tumeurs du grêle. Ann Radiol 17: 751–764

Ben Benachem Y, Akhtar M, Duke JH, Harberg BL (1977) Angiographic characteristics of esophageal leiomyoma. AJR 128: 479–482

Bernatz PE, Smith JL, Ellis FH, Andersein HA (1958) Benign pedunculated, intraluminal tumors of the oesophagus. J Thorac Surg 35: 503–512

Blamey SL, Woods SDS (1986) Leiomyoma of Meckel's diverticulum. Med J Aust 145: 232–233

Boijsen E, Wallace S, Kanter IE (1966) Angiography in tumours of stomach. Acta Radiol [Diagn] (Stockh) 4: 306–320

Bollack C, Warter P, Lang G (1960) A propos d'une observation de léiomyomes multiples de l'oesophage thoracique. Arch Fr Mal Appar Dig 49: 1624–1631

Botsford TW, Crowe P, Crocker DW (1962) Tumors of the small intestine. Am J Surg 103: 358–365

Braczkowski Z, Gnarowski H, Solarski J (1976) Case of multiple gastric leiomyomas with prolapse of one myoma into the duodenum and haemorrhage. Pol Przegl Chir 48: 713–714

Bradford ML, Mahon HW, Crow JB (1947) Mediastinal cysts and tumours. Surg Gynecol Obstet 85: 467–491

Brief D, Botsford T (1963) Primary bleeding from small intestine in adults. JAMA 184: 18–22

Brombart M (1973) Radiologie des tumeurs bénignes et malignes de l'oesophage. Ann Gastroenterol Hepatol (Paris) 9: 109–138

Bruneton JN, Drouillard J, Roux P, Lecomte P, Tavernier J (1981) Leiomyoma and leiomyosarcoma of the digestive tract. A report of 45 cases and review of the literature. Eur J Radiol 1: 291–300

Buxton RW (1960) Smooth muscle tumors of the gastrointestinal tract. Am Surg 26: 666–677

Cohen A, Mac Neill D, Terz JJ, Lawrence W (1971) Neoplasms of the small intestine. Am J Dig Dis 16: 815–824

Cornell NW, Shehadi WH, Sharnoff RD (1950) Leiomyomas of esophagus; report of five cases. Surgery 28: 881–886

Christinaz D, Meyer P, Moser G, Rohner A (1984) Etude de 25 cas de tumeurs musculaires lisses gastriques et revue de la littérature. Schweiz Med Wochenschr 114: 708–710

Coscina WF, Arger PH, Levine MS, Herlinger H, Cohen S, Coleman BG, Mintz MC (1986) Gastrointestinal tract focal mass lesions: role of CT and barium evaluations. Radiology 158: 581–587

Croom RD, Newsome JF (1975) Tumors of the small intestine. Am Surg 41: 160–167

Crummy AB, Juhl JH (1962) Calcified gastric leiomyoma. AJR 87: 727–728

Cullen TH, Voss HJ (1972) Leiomyoma of the appendix. Br J Surg 59: 576–580

Daniel RA, Williams RB (1950) Leiomyoma of esophagus. J Thorac Cardiovasc Surg 19: 800–805

Davies PM (1978) Smooth muscle tumours of the upper gastrointestinal tract. Clin Radiol 29: 407–414

Delavierre P, Hureau J, Lasserre D, Bourdais JP (1975) Les léiomyomes bénins ou malins du côlon. Sem Hop 27: 1891–1894

Deverall PB (1968) Smooth muscle tumors of the oesophagus. Br J Surg 55: 457–460

Domergue J, Rouanet P, Joyeux H, Solassol C, Pujol H (1986) Tumeurs musculaires de l'oesophage. A propos de 9 cas et revue de la littérature. J Chir (Paris) 123: 555–558

Ebert PA, Zuidema GD (1965) Primary tumors of the small intestine. Arch Surg 91: 452–455

Ebert RE, Parkhurst GF, Melendy OA, Osborne MP (1953) Primary tumors of the duodenum. Surg Gynecol Obstet 97: 135–139

Farah MC, Jafri SZH, Schwab RE, Mezwa DG, Francis IR, Noujaim S, Kim C (1987) Duodenal neoplasms: role of CT. Radiology 162: 839–843

Flavell G (1953) Leiomyoma of oesophagus. Br J Surg 41: 238–240

Freni SC, Keeman JN (1977) Leiomyomatosis of the colon. Cancer 39: 263–266

Fujii K, Yamagata S, Suzuki J, Sasaki R, Shoji T, Makabe M, Memezawa H, Maesawa S (1972) Angiographic features of submucosal tumours of the stomach. Tohoku J Exp Med 107: 287–299

Gallinger S, Steinhardt MI, Goldberg M (1983) Giant leiomyoma of the esophagus. Am J Gastroenterol 78: 708–711

Ghahremani GG, Meyers MA, Port RB (1978) Calcified primary tumors of the gastrointestinal tract. Gastrointest Radiol 2: 331–339

Glanz I, Grunebaum M (1977) The radiological approach to leiomyoma of the oesophagus with a long term follow-up. Clin Radiol 28: 197–200

Godard JE, MacCrane D (1973) Multiple leiomyomas of the esophagus. AJR 117: 259–262

Good CA (1963) Tumors of the small intestine. AJR 89: 685–704

Good CA (1965) Benign tumors of the stomach and duodenal bulb. J Can Assoc Radiol 16: 92-104

Gothlin J, Bloch R, Sundgren R (1975) Intraphrenic oesophageal leiomyoma associated with diverticula preoperatively diagnosed by angiography. Acta Radiol [Diagn] (Stockh) 16: 673-678

Graham JC, Blanchard IT, Scatliff JH (1972) Calcified gastric leiomyoma presenting as a mediastinal mass. AJR 114: 529-531

Gray SW, Skandalakis JE, Shepard D (1961) Smooth muscle tumours of the esophagus. Collective review. Int Abstr Surg 113: 205-220

Griff LC, Cooper J (1967) Leiomyoma of the oesophagus presenting as a mediastinal mass. AJR 101: 472-481

Grignani G, Pacchiarini L, Gamba G, Rizzo SC (1985) Invaginazione di leiomioma gastrico causante subocclusione duodenale et stasi biliare. Minerva Med 76: 1623-1626

Grimoud M, Toulemonde H, Martinel C (1974) Léiomyomes gastriques et duodénaux. A propos de 13 cas. Chirurgie 100: 125-129

Grundy A, Rayter Z, Shorthouse AJ (1984) Gastrogastric intussuscepting leiomyomas. Gastrointest Radiol 9: 319-321

Haber K, Winfield AC (1974) Multiple leiomyomas of the esophagus. Am J Dig Dis 19: 678-680

Han Sy, Aldrete JS (1977) The radiology corner: angiographic diagnosis of leiomyomas of the small intestine. Am J Gastroenterol 68: 91-94

Harrington SW, Moersch JJ (1944) Surgical treatment and clinical manifestations of benign tumours of oesophagus with report of seven cases. J Thorac Cardiovasc Surg 13: 392-414

Hauswald KR, Griffen WO (1977) Smooth muscle tumors of the duodenum. Rev Surg 34: 64-67

Herlinger H (1966) The recognition of exogastric tumors. Report of 6 cases. Br J Radiol 39: 25-36

Huddy P, Griffiths G (1972) Leiomyoma of the oesophagus with calcification. Br J Surg 59: 239-242

Jost JL, Regnard JF, Merlier M, Vayre P (1986) Léiomyomes de l'oesophage. Presse Med 15: 120

Kaude J, Silseth CH, Tylen U (1972) Angiography in myomas of the gastrointestinal tract. Acta Radiol [Diagn] (Stockh) 12: 691-704

Kaupp HA, Carroll WW, Shields TW (1964) Leiomyomas of the gastrointestinal tract. Trans West Surg Assoc 71: 313-316

Kavlie H, White TT (1972) Leiomyomas of the upper gastrointestinal tract. Surgery 71: 842-848

Kaymakcalan H, Sequeria W, Barretta T, Ghosh BC, Steigmann F (1980) Hypertrophic osteoarthropathy with myogenic tumors of the esophagus. Am J Gastroenterol 74: 17-20

Kramer MD, Gibb SP, Ellis FH (1986) Giant leiomyoma of esophagus. J Surg Oncol 33: 166-169

Kressel HY, Gatenby RA, Troupin RH (1981) Correlative imaging conference: Hospital of the University of Pennsylvania. IV. Abdominal pain and blood loss. AJR 137: 769-775

Kusminsky RE, Bailey W (1977) Leiomyomas of the rectum and anal canal: report of six cases and review of the literature. Dis Colon Rectum 20: 580-599

Lueders HW, Tiscenco E (1945) Benign tumour of oesophagus and its differential diagnosis. Br J Radiol 18: 99-107

McKenzie DA, McDonald JR, Waugh JM (1954) Leiomyoma and leiomyosarcoma of the colon. Ann Surg 137: 67-68

Megibow AJ, Balthazar EJ, Ulnick DH, Naidich DP, Bosniak MA (1985) CT evaluation of gastrointestinal leiomyomas and leiomyosarcomas. AJR 144: 727-731

Merlier M, Le Thoai H, Leguerrier A, Bouquet P, Levasseur P, Vayre P (1977) Les léiomyomes de l'oesophage. A propos de 20 observations. J Chir 113: 249-254

Minassian SS, Frangipane W, Polin JI, Ellis M (1986) Leiomyomatosis peritonealis disseminata. A case report and literature review. J Reprod Med 31: 997-1000

Morton JH, Stabins SJ, Morton JJ (1956) Smooth muscle tumours of the alimentary tract. Ann Surg 144: 487-505

Moser G, Spiliopoulos A, Lecourt AL, Megevand R (1978) Les léiomyomes de l'oesophage. A propos de 16 cas. Helv Chir Acta 45: 657-666

Mouchet A, Chavy A, Daussy M (1969) Léiomyomes de l'oesophage. Arch Fr Mal Appar Dig 58: 541-553

Myre J (1963) Diagnosis of small bowel tumors. Am J Dig Dis 8: 916-922

Nahum H, Reysseguier JC, Prandi D, Conte-Marti J, Benasse S, Lortat-Jacob JL (1972) Les tumeurs bénignes de l'oesophage. Etude radiologique à propos de 11 observations. Ann Radiol 15: 581-590

Naouri A, Naouri C, Tissot E (1986) Léiomyomes et léiomyomatose de l'oesophage. A propos de deux cas. J Chir (Paris) 123: 31-34

Nicolas V, Schlolaut KH (1987) Faszikulares Leiomyom des Osophagus. Fortschr Geb Roentgenstr 146: 101-103

Olsson O (1972) Angiography in the diagnosis of duodenal lesions. II. Benign tumors, ulceration and inflammatory and vascular lesions. Acta Radiol [Diagn] (Stockh) 12: 164-174

O'Riordan D, Levine MS, Yeager BA (1985) Complete healing of ulceration within a gastric leiomyoma. Gastrointest Radiol 10: 47-49

Ostermiller W, Joergenson EJ, Weibel L (1966) A clinical review of tumours of small bowel. Am J Surg 111: 403-409

Postlethwait RW, Musser AW (1976) Changes in the esophagus in 1000 autopsy specimens. J Thorac Cardiovasc Surg 68: 953-956

Preda F, Alloisio M, Lequaglie C, Ongari M, Ravasi G (1986) Leiomyoma of the esophagus. Tumori 72: 503-506

Renigers SA, Michael AS, Bardawil WA, Shapiro DA, Toledo RN, Schmit DJ, Ryva J (1985) Sonographic findings in leiomyomatosis peritonealis disseminata: a case report and literature review. J Ultrasound Med 4: 497-500

Reuter S, Redman H, Miller W, Hoskins P (1970) Gastric angiography. Radiology 94: 271-276

Ribert M, Savinel E, Gosselin B (1973) Leiomyome de l'oesophage d'extension médiastinale. Sem Hop 49: 1265-1267

River L, Silverstein J, Tope JW (1956) Benign neoplasms of the small intestine. Int Abstr Surg 102: 1-38

Rose JD (1936) Myomata of oesophagus. Br J Surg 24: 297-308

Roussel B, Birembau T, Gaillard D, Puchelle JC, D'Albignac G, Pennaforte F, Fandre M (1986) Leiomyomatose oesophagienne familiale associée a un syndrome d'Alport chez un garçon de 9 ans. Helv Paediatr Acta 41: 359-368

Salmela H, Kohler R (1969) Roentgenological characteristics of mesenchymal tumours of the stomach. A retrospective study of 59 patients. Ann Clin Res 1: 57-63

Sasaki K, Gotoh Y, Nakayama Y, Hayasaka H, Ishiyama Y, Miyashita H (1985) Leiomyoma of the rectum. Int Surg 70: 149-152

Scatarige JC, Allen HA, Fishman EK (1987) Computed tomography of the small bowel. Semin Ultrasound CT MR 8: 403-423

Schatzki R, Howes LE (1942) Roentgenological appearance of extramucosal tumors of esophagus. Analysis of intramural extramural lesions of gastrointestinal tract in general. AJR 48: 1-15

Schiebel HM, Cleaver H (1955) Case of multiple leiomyomas of esophagus. Am Surg 21: 1133-1136

Schoembaum SW, Sprayregen S, Kron ES, Siegelman SS (1973) Angiographic demonstration of bleeding gastric leiomyomas. AJR 119: 277-279

Serementis MG, Lyons WS, De Guzman VC, Peabody JW (1976) Leiomyomata of the esophagus. An analysis of 838 cases. Cancer 38: 2166-2177

Shaffer HA (1976) Multiple leiomyomas of the esophagus. Radiology 118: 29-34

Shibata S, Iwasaki N (1970) Angiographic findings in diseases of the stomach. AJR 110: 322-331

Short WF, Young BR (1968) Roentgen demonstration of prolapse of benign polypoid gastric tu-

mors into the duodenum, including a dumbbell-shaped leiomyoma. AJR 103: 317-320

Skandalakis JE, Gray SW, Shepard D (1960) Smooth muscle tumors of the stomach. Int Abstr Surg 110: 209-226

Solomon A, Papo J, Pikielny S, Stern D (1987) Computed tomographic investigation of serosal and intramural gastrointestinal pathology. Gastrointest Radiol 12: 13-17

Solomon MP, Rosenblum H, Rosato FE (1984) Leiomyoma of the esophagus. Ann Surg 199: 246-248

Spaun E, Nielsen L (1986) Leiomyomatosis of the colon and mesentery: report of a case. Am J Gastroenterol 81: 385-388

Standerfer RJ, Paneth M (1982) Recurrent leiomyoma of the oesophagus. Thorax 37: 478-479

Starr GF, Dockerty MB (1955) Leiomyomas and leiomyosarcomas of small intestine. Cancer 8: 101-111

Sweet RH, Soutter L, Tejada C (1956) Muscle wall tumours of oesophagus. J Thorac Surg 91: 3-23

Swinnen E, Meeus L, Pattyn G, Vandevoorde P, Steyaert L (1986) Leiomyoma in Meckel's diverticulum: CT and angiographic studies in one case. J Belge Radiol 69: 355-357

Weinstein EC, Dockerty MB, Waugh JM (1963) Neoplasms of Meckel's diverticulum: collective review. Int Abstr Surg 115: 103-111

Wilson JM, Melvin DB, Gray G, Thorbjarnson B (1975) Benign small bowel tumor. Ann Surg 181: 247-250

Witt JH, Marks MI, Smith EI, Altshuler G, Wilson DA, Humphrey GB (1983) Leiomyoma presenting as prolonged fever, anemia, and thrombocytosis. Cancer 52: 2359-2362

Worton SI (1963) Case n° 194 Mt Sinaï J Hosp 30: 80-84

Yasuda K, Nakajima M, Kawai K (1986) Endoscopic ultrasonography in the diagnosis of submucosal tumor of the upper digestive tract. Scand J Gastroenterol 21 (Suppl 123): 59-67

Zanella FE, Hesse U, Grundmann R (1986) Leiomyom des Dünndarms. Roentgenblätter 39: 255-257

Zollikofer CL, Castaneda-Zuniga WR, Nath PH, Amplatz K (1979) Angiographic appearance of leiomyoma of the small intestine: report of two cases. Cardiovasc Radiol 2: 131-134

4 Lipoma*

Although infrequent, lipomas are the most common non-epithelial benign gastrointestinal tumors after leiomyomas (Weinberg and Feldman 1955). Most gastrointestinal lipomas are asymptomatic and are discovered fortuitously, but they occasionally cause a wide, although nonspecific, spectrum of symptoms and can sometimes even mimic a malignancy (Reichbach and Kobayashi 1970). Until recently, radiologic diagnosis was usually difficult because barium studies could determine the benign nature of the tumor but could not specify the etiology. CT now allows pathognomonic diagnosis by demonstrating the fat density of these tumors (Megibow et al. 1979; Nijssens et al. 1983; Ormson et al. 1985). After a review of general anatomic features, gastrointestinal lipomas are discussed for each gastrointestinal site. The clinical and paraclinical symptoms including barium findings, which suggest the etiology, are discussed before the CT patterns, which are diagnostic.

4.1 General Anatomic Features

Grossly, lipoma presents as a round or ovoid mass with regular or lobulated contours; its yellow coloration is distinctive. The majority of these masses arise within the submucosa, but 5%–10% are subserosal (Ackerman and Chughtai 1975; Agha et al. 1985). Dumbbell tumors, which feature both intraluminal and subserosal components, are less common (Comfort 1931). Multiple lipomas are rare (Deeths et al. 1975; Fawcett et al. 1949; Ormson et al. 1985; Reeder and Hopens 1983). Existence of a collagen capsule, permitting surgical enucleation, distinguishes lipomas from

---

* Written in collaboration with G. Schmutz.

lipomatosis. Surface ulceration is frequent owing to the poor vascularity; however, there is no relation between the size of lipomas and the frequency of ulceration.

Histologically, lipomas are composed of lobules of mature fat cells, similar to normal mature adipose tissue; vascularity is poor. Occasionally, a complex cytologic formula produces a fibrolipoma, a lipofibromyxoma, a lipomyxoma, or an angiolipoma. Cystic transformation is possible (Troisier et al. 1936). By contrast, lipomas have no malignant predisposition. Although Weinberg and Feldman (1955) considered malignant transformation a possibility, no such reports were found in our literature review. Reports of sarcomatous degeneration all concern cutaneous and retroperitoneal lipomas (Celik et al. 1980).

Pathologic associations have been reported, but appear fortuitous (Mayo et al. 1963). For Feldman (1961), however, individuals with lipoma are more likely to have a pancreatic pathology or diabetes.

4.2 Esophagus

These relatively rare entities represent only 1.5% of all gastrointestinal lipomas and 15% of all benign esophageal tumors (Table 4.1). Males are affected more often than females, and diagnosis generally occurs after the age of 50. The site of predilection is the upper third of the esophagus. Esophageal lipomas vary in size; pedunculated tumors can reach 10-15 cm (Elner and Palm 1976; Liliequist and Wiberg 1974; Plachta 1962). There have been no reports of multiple esophageal lipomas (Table 4.2).

Clinical symptomatology is minimal. Esophageal lipomas remain silent for a long period and can thus reach considerable size before

Table 4.1. Frequency of gastrointestinal lipomas

	Esophagus	Stomach	Small intestine	Colon/rectum
Frequency compared to all other gastrointestinal lipomas	1.5%	11.6%	35.8%	51.1%
Frequency compared to other benign tumors (by location)	15%	3%–5%	13%–15%	4%

Table 4.2. General features of gastrointestinal lipomas

	Esophagus[a]	Stomach	Small intestine	Colon/rectum
Mean age	> 50 years	60 years	60 years	60 years
Sex	M > F	1 M/1 F	1 M/1 F	1 M/2 F
Mean diameter	?	5 cm	4 cm	3 cm
Multiple lesions	?	3.1%	< 1%	14%

[a] The low number of cases precludes valid statistical analysis.

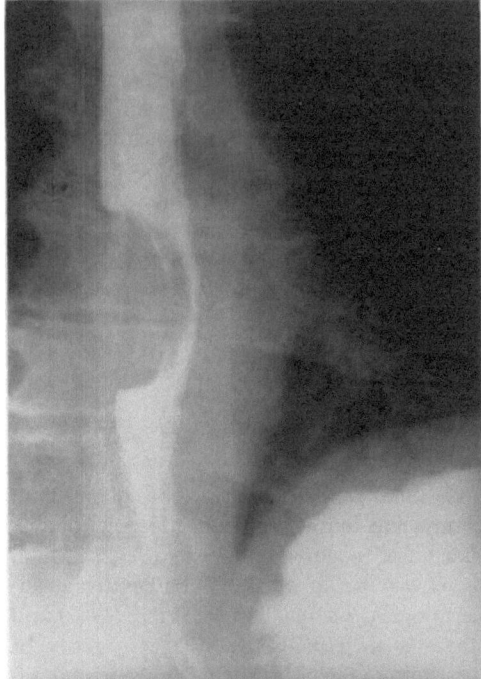

Fig. 4.1. Esophageal lipoma presenting as a nonspecific intramural lesion on barium examination

causing symptoms (Zonderland and Ginai 1984). Dysphagia is the most common presenting complaint. Massive hemorrhage can occur secondary to ulceration (Nora 1964). Regurgitation of a pedunculated lipoma may involve a life-threatening risk of asphyxia (Bernatz et al. 1957).

Barium swallows generally demonstrate a pedunculated, occasionally multilobulated tumor; the esophagus may be dilated above this point (Elner and Palm 1976; Liliequist and Wiberg 1974). Large lipomas are sometimes difficult to distinguish from sarcomas (especially if the surface is irregular and ulcerated), a foreign body, or, if the esophagus is dilated, achalasia. The most common presumptive diagnoses are leiomyoma or a polyp (Fig. 4.1). Endoscopy is not always diagnostic because these tumors are usually covered by normal mucosa (Peiser et al. 1984). Only individuals with considerable clinical symptoms affecting their general condition and patients with hemorrhagic complications require surgery. Owing to the preferential site in the upper third of the esophagus, cervical esophagotomy and resection is often the preferred procedure. Small tumors are best managed by endoscopic resection, and the prognosis is excellent.

4.3 Stomach

Lipomas of the stomach represent 11.6% of all gastrointestinal lipomas discovered during lifetime (Comfort 1931; Weinberg and Feldman 1955) and account for 3%–5% of all benign gastric tumors (Turkington 1965) (Table 4.1). Mean patient age at diagnosis is 60 years; both sexes are equally affected. The antrum is the preferential site of gastric lipomas, which average 5 cm in size and are usually solitary. Multiple gastric lipomas are exceptional (Peabody and Ziskind 1953; Skinner et al. 1983; Troisier et al. 1936).

Although the incidence of clinical latency could not be determined from our review of the literature, the absence of symptoms appears related to tumoral growth within a vast cavity. This would explain the number of incidental discoveries during surgery, on radiologic examinations, and at autopsy. Clinical manifestations of gastric lipomas are a function of their size and location (cardia, antrum). The main clinical symptoms are listed in Table 4.3. Complications prompting diagnosis include bleeding (Agha et al. 1985; Crowe et al. 1986; Giraud et al. 1985; Johnson et al. 1981) and intussusception (20% for Palmer 1951).

Endoscopically, gastric lipomas, like such tumors elsewhere, are covered by normal or ulcerated mucosa (Chu and Clifton 1983; Saviano et al. 1986).

The radiologic diagnosis of lipoma was rarely made prior to the advent of CT, and a benign tumor was often entertained. However, several characteristic signs suggest lipoma on barium studies (Reichbach and Kobayashi 1970): a

Table 4.3. Clinical symptoms of lipomas of the stomach, small intestine, and colon (excluding asymptomatic cases)

	Stomach (68 cases)	Small intestine (75 cases)	Colon/ rectum (45 cases)
Pain	42.7%	53%	55.1%
Nausea/vomiting	33.8%	45.3%	16.5%
Hemorrhage	60.3%	24%	40.6%
Diarrhea and/or obstruction	8%	58%	55.1%
Palpable mass	3%	21.3%	24.8%
Weight loss	13.2%	5%	15%

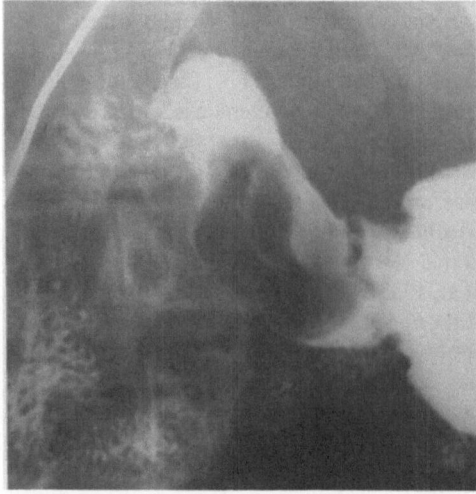

Fig. 4.2. Ulcerated lipoma of the gastric antrum

mass projecting on the gastric region on the plain film, or a rim corresponding to the contrast in density between the lipomatous tissue and the sclerous peritumoral connective tissue.

There are no characteristic signs of lipoma on upper gastrointestinal barium examinations (Figs. 4.2–4.4). Sessile intramural lesions are imaged as smooth, well-circumscribed round filling defects, with pliable edges and normal mucosal folds. The tumor may change shape with external compression; in case of ulceration, a target sign may be seen. Radiologically, large ulcerations may suggest a neoplastic etiology (Agha et al. 1985; Reichbach and Kobayashi 1970).

Lipomas causing intussusception are readily visualized in the distended bulb. Complete central intussusception of the lower portion of the stomach into the duodenum results in opacification of only the upper portion of the stomach and an enormous antral filling defect is observed. In case of complete lateral intussusception, the antral region is laminated, and the upper portion of the bulb is amputated because of displacement by the tumor.

Barium studies of infrequent subserosal lipomas appear normal. The radiologic diagnosis is usually a benign tumor (polyp or benign connective tissue tumor). Arteriograms demonstrate a hypovascular mass, with stretching of the vessels but no malignant features (Agha et al. 1985).

From a therapeutic standpoint, surgery appears indicated only for symptomatic patients (simple resection, antrectomy, or partial gastrectomy for large tumors) (Crowe et al. 1986).

4.4 Small Intestine

Lipomas account for 13%–15% of all benign intestinal tumors (Mayo et al. 1963; Weinberg et al. 1986) and are thus less frequent than leiomyomas in this segment of the gastrointestinal tract. In our literature review, the small bowel was the site of 35.8% of all gastrointestinal lipomas, whereas Hurwitz et al. (1967) and Mayo et al. (1963) cited lower figures of 20%–25% (Table 4.1). There is no sex predominance, and average age at diagnosis is 60 years.

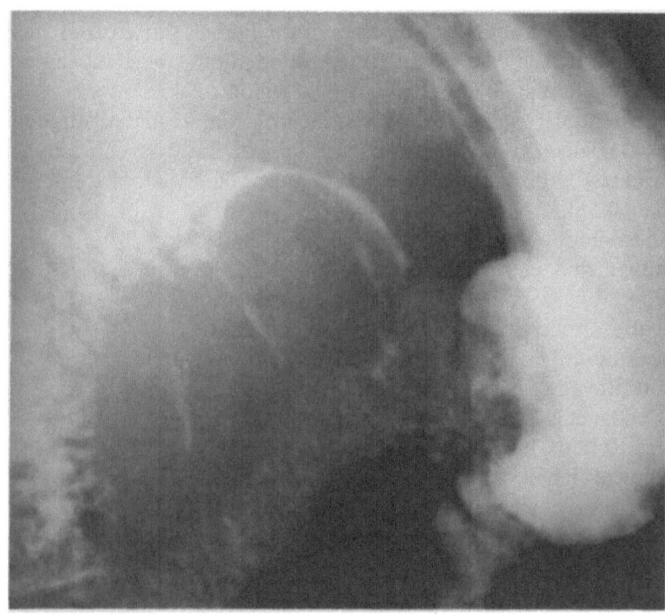

Fig. 4.3. Gastric lipoma that had prolapsed into the duodenal bulb; this lesion was apparently well tolerated functionally because no stasis was observed and the contrast medium opacified the remainder of the duodenum normally

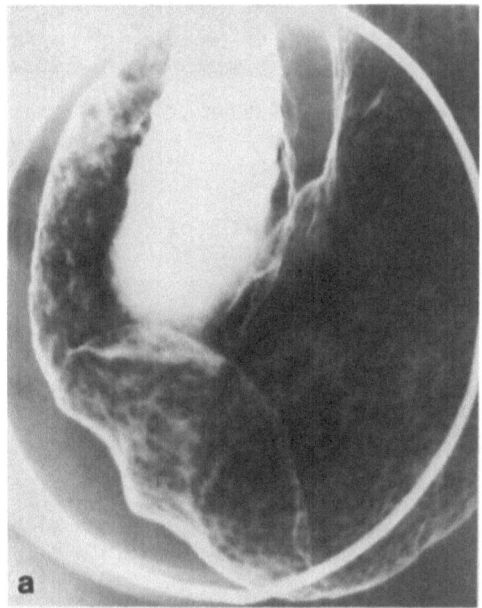

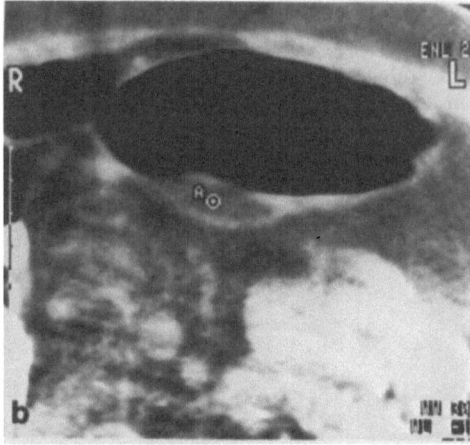

Fig. 4.4a, b. Barium examination (a) and CT study (b). On the barium films the lesion appears intramural and nonspecific. CT scans revealed an average density of -63 HU (A: *cross*), which is pathognomonic for lipoma

The site distribution for 222 cases in the literature managed by surgery included: duodenum 23.4%, jejunum 10.7%, ileum 49.6%, region of the ileocecal valve 16.3% (Bruneton et al. 1984). There are rare reports of lipomas in Meckel's diverticulum (Weinberg and Feldman 1955).

Intestinal lipomas average 4 cm in size, although they can reach up to 30 cm, as in the report by River et al. (1956). While they are nearly almost solitary, multiple lipomas have been described in the same segment (Kirkland and Bayer 1951) and in different segments (Deeths et al. 1975; Fawcett et al. 1949; Haller and Roberts 1963).

Clinical latency occurs in 43% of patients (Bruneton et al. 1984). The main clinical manifestations are summarized in Table 4.3. Lipomas in the terminal ileum or ileocecal valve area can cause symptoms mimicking acute appendicitis (Weinberg and Feldman 1955). A palpable mass often corresponds to intussusception rather than to the tumor itself (Wilson et al. 1975).

Barium studies demonstrate a sessile or pedunculated intramural tumor that changes shape in response to peristaltic activity and on palpation, but only rarely exhibits the translucent appearance particular to lipomas (Carlson and Good 1973) (Figs. 4.5, 4.6). Likewise, in case of hemorrhage, arteriography can reveal the lesion but cannot specify its nature (Sarma et al. 1984; Weiss et al. 1979). Pedunculated duodenal lipomas may be treated endoscopically (Inamura et al. 1983); other cases require enterotomy with complete resection.

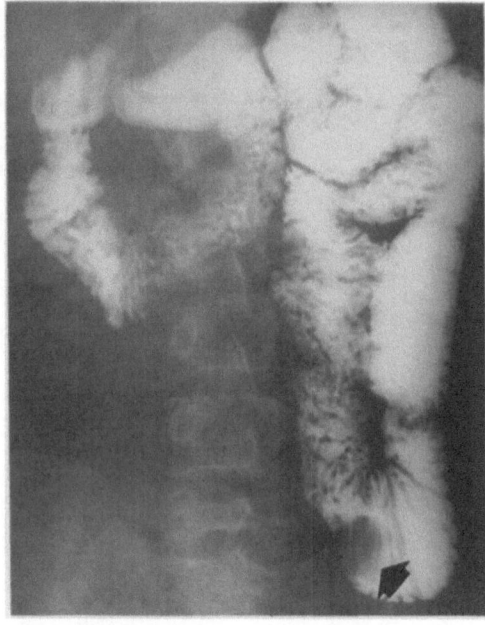

Fig. 4.5. Jejunal lipoma *(arrow)*

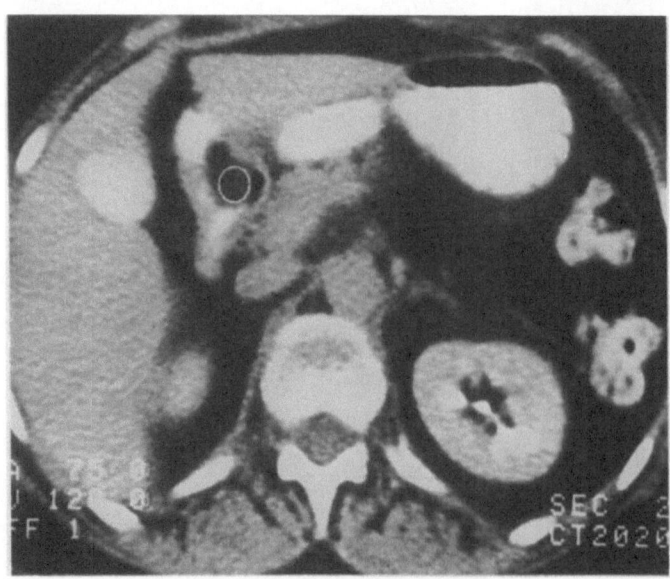

Fig. 4.6. Lipoma of the duodenal bulb: CT study revealed the pathognomonic fat density. (Courtesy of Prof. Baert, Leuven, Belgium)

4.5 Colon and Rectum

For Carlson and Good (1973), lipomas are the most frequent benign colorectal tumor after adenomas and they account for 4% of all benign colon tumors. The colon is also the site with the greatest percentage of gastrointestinal lipomas (51.1% of all cases) (Table 4.1). Most colonic lipomas are discovered in patients aged 50-70 years, and female predominance has been noted.

Frequencies within the colon and rectum are: cecum 29.22%, right colon 20.9%, transverse colon 15.8%, left colon 29.7%, rectum 4.4%. Colonic lipomas are often solitary, but multiple tumors have been found in the same segment (Comfort 1931; Haller and Roberts 1964; Wychulis et al. 1964) and in different segments (Ryberg 1956). Multiple lipomas occur in 13%-14% of patients (Bruneton et al. 1984; Mayo et al. 1963; Weinberg and Feldman 1955). The average size of colonic lipomas is 3 cm.

Clinical latency occurs in 30.3% of all patients. Furthermore, clinical symptoms are not necessarily related to the lipoma itself, which may be an incidental discovery. The frequencies of the main clinical symptoms are summarized in Table 4.3. As with intestinal lipomas, a palpable mass generally corresponds to intussus-ception, the main complication of colorectal lipomas. Less often, the lipoma is expelled spontaneously (Deeths et al. 1975; D'javid 1960) or prolapses through the rectum (Yadoo et al. 1971).

Radiologic diagnosis based on the transparent appearance of lipoma is nearly impossible because of interference by intestinal gas. *Barium enema examination* may demonstrate the characteristic signs of a benign sessile or pedunculated tumor, sometimes accompanied by partial or complete intussusception (Farshi 1980; Margulis and Jovanovich 1960). *Water enema,* advocated by certain authors (Carlson and Good 1973), was reportedly helpful for diagnosis because lipomas have a lower density than water; however, this examination was only performed when lipoma was suspected, and its utility is limited by the fact that not all lipomas are radiolucent. The radiologic appearance rarely suggests a neoplasm (Michowitz et al. 1985). Hall et al. (1985) reported a cecal lipoma revealed by gastrointestinal bleeding; the *angiographic features* suggested angiodysplasia related to intratumoral vascular abnormalities; ulceration led to bleeding.

Colonoscopy can confirm the benign nature of the tumor and may be performed before endoscopic treatment (De Beer and Shinga 1975; Messer and Waye 1982). CT has in fact revolu-

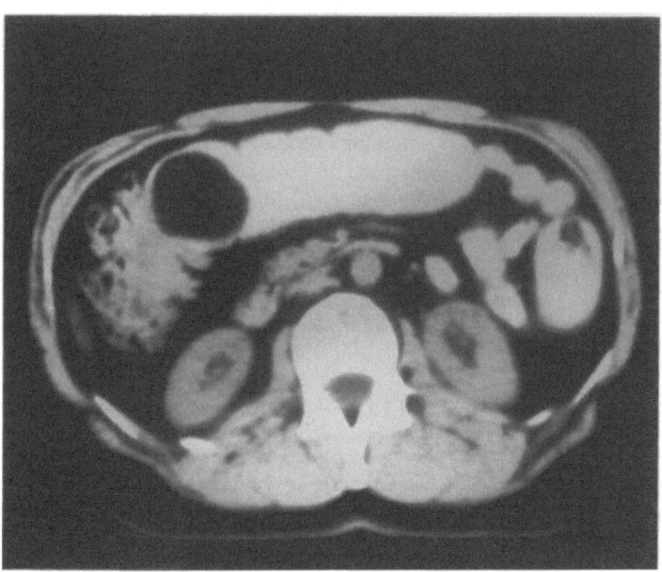

Fig. 4.7. Transverse colon lipoma: CT revealed the fat density of this lesion (comparable to the density of the intra-abdominal fat) and stercoral stasis above the lesion, without signs of obstruction

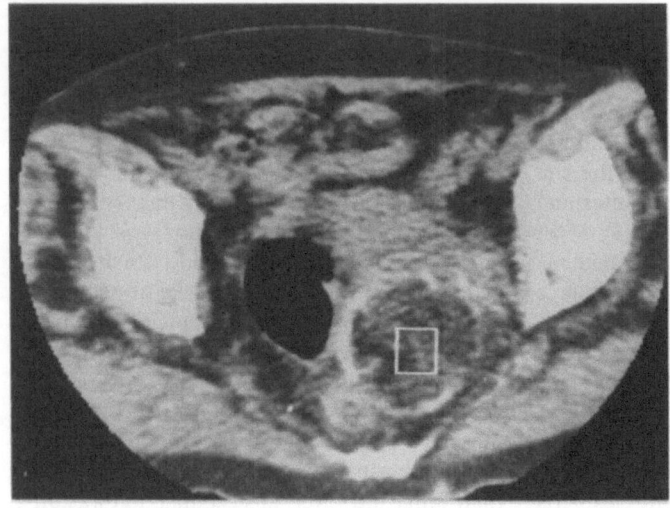

Fig. 4.8. Rectosigmoid lipoma: CT demonstrated the lesion's fat density. (Courtesy of Prof. Solomon, Israel)

tionized the diagnosis of lipomas; CT scans can affirm the diagnosis by demonstrating the fat density of the mass (-90 to -120 Hounsfield units; HU) (Farah et al. 1987; Heiken et al. 1982; Ho et al. 1984; Imoto et al. 1983; Karnel and Pichler 1985; Maderal et al. 1984; Megibow et al. 1979; Nijssens et al. 1983; Olmsted et al. 1987; Ormson et al. 1985; Scatarige et al. 1987; Solomon et al. 1986; Whetstone et al. 1985) (Figs. 4.7, 4.8).

Because endoscopic biopsy is often negative, and because the endoscopic and barium film appearances often suggest a benign tumor, CT is indicated to visualize the subserosal component and analyze tumor density. Once the diagnosis of lipoma has been made, therapy for these constantly benign tumors can be modulated as a function of lesion diameter and location within the gastrointestinal tract, which determine the potential for obstruction.

4.6 References

Ackerman NB, Chughtai SQ (1975) Symptomatic lipomas of the gastrointestinal tract. Surg Gynecol Obstet 141: 565–568

Agha FP, Dent TL, Fiddian-Green RG, Braunstein AH, Nostrant TT (1985) Bleeding lipomas of the upper gastrointestinal tract. A diagnostic challenge. Am Surg 51: 279–285

Bernatz PE, Smith JL, Ellis FH, Andersen HA (1957) Benign pedunculated intraluminal tumors of the esophagus. J Thorac Surg 35: 503–512

Bruneton JN, Quoy AM, Dageville X, Lecomte P (1984) Les lipomes du tube digestif. Revue de la littérature à propos de 5 cas. Ann Gastroenterol Hepatol (Paris) 20: 27–32

Carlson HC, Good CA (1973) Neoplasms of the small bowel. In: Margulis AR, Burhenne HJ (eds) Alimentary tract roentgenology, 2nd edn. Mosby, St Louis, pp 865–902

Celik C, Karakousis CP, Moore R, Holyoke ED (1980) Liposarcomas: prognosis and management. J Surg Oncol 14: 245–249

Chu AG, Clifton JA (1983) Gastric lipoma presenting as peptic ulcer. Case report and review of the literature. Am J Gastroenterol 78: 615–618

Comfort MW (1931) Submucous lipomas of the gastrointestinal tract. Surg Gynecol Obstet 52: 101–118

Crowe JM, Harte P, Dawson K, Power RF (1986) Gastric lipoma as a cause of upper gastrointestinal bleeding. Ir Med J 79: 13–14

De Beer R, Shinga H (1975) Colonic lipomas. Gastrointest Endosc 22: 90–91

Deeths TM, Madden PN, Dodds WJ (1975) Multiple lipomas of the stomach and duodenum. Am J Dig Dis 20: 771–774

D'Javid IF (1960) Lipomas of the large intestine: review of the literature and report of a case. J Int Coll Surg 33: 639–668

Elner A, Palm NG (1976) Pedunculated intraluminal fibrolipoma of the esophagus. Acta Otolaryngol (Stockh) 82: 457–462

Farah MC, Jafri SZH, Schwab RE, Mezwa DG, Francis IR, Noujaim S, Kim C (1987) Duodenal neoplasms: role of CT. Radiology 162: 839-843

Farshi DS (1980) Lipome du côlon. Rapport de trois cas et revue de la littérature. Ann Chir 34: 791-794

Fawcett NW, Bolton VL, Geever EF (1949) Multiple lipomas of the stomach and duodenum. Ann Surg 129: 524-527

Feldman M (1961) An appraisal of associated conditions occurring in autopsied cases of lipomas of the gastrointestinal tract. Am J Gastroenterol 36: 413-416

Giraud F, Garbay M, Chaouat AG (1985) Lipome gastrique: une cause rare d'hémorragie digestive haute. Ann Chir 39: 333-334

Hall PA, Murfitt J, Pollock DJ (1985) Caecal lipomas mimicking colonic angiodysplasia. Br J Radiol 58: 1213-1214

Haller JD, Roberts TW (1963) Lipoma of the colon: a clinicopathologic study of 20 cases. Surgery 55: 773-781

Heiken JP, Forde KA, Gold RP (1982) Computed tomography as a definitive method for diagnosing gastrointestinal lipomas. Radiology 142: 409-414

Ho KJ, Shin MS, Tishler JM (1984) Computed tomographic distinction of submucosal lipoma and adenomatous polyp of the colon. Gastrointest Radiol 9: 77-80

Hurwitz MM, Redleaf PD, Williams HJ, Edwards JE (1967) Lipomas of the gastrointestinal tract; an analysis of seventy-two tumors. AJR 99: 84-89

Inamura K, Fuchigami T, Iida M, Ohgushi H, Omae T, Kimura Y, Iwashita A (1983) Duodenal lipoma. A report of three cases. Gastrointest Endosc 29: 223-234

Imoto T, Nobe T, Koga M, Miyamoto Y, Nakata H (1983) Computed tomography of gastric lipomas. Gastrointest Radiol 8: 129-131

Johnson DC, De Gennaro VA, Pizzi WF, Nealson TF (1981) Gastric lipoma: a rare cause of massive upper gastrointestinal bleeding. Am J Gastroenterol 75: 299-301

Karnel F, Pichler W (1985) Diagnose eines Dickdarmlipoms mittels Computertomographie. Roentgenblatter 38: 231-232

Kirkland WG, Bayer RA (1951) Multiple lipomas of the duodenum: a case report. Gastroenterology 19: 142-147

Liliequist B, Wiberg A (1974) Pedunculated tumors of the esophagus: two cases of lipoma. Acta Radiol [Diagn] (Stockh) 15: 383-392

Maderal F, Hunter F, Fuselier G, Gonzales-Rogue P, Torres O (1984) Gastric lipomas. An update of clinical presentation, diagnosis, and treatment. Am J Gastroenterol 79: 964-967

Margulis AR, Jovanovich A (1960) Roentgen diagnosis of submucous lipomas of the colon. AJR 84: 1114-1119

Mayo CW, Pagtalunan RJG, Brown DJ (1963) Lipoma of the alimentary tract. Surgery 53: 598-603

Megibow AJ, Redmond PE, Bosniak MA, Horowitz L (1979) Diagnosis of gastrointestinal lipomas by CT. AJR 133: 743-745

Messer J, Waye JD (1982) The diagnosis of colonic lipomas. The naked fat sign. Gastrointest Endosc 28: 186-188

Michowitz M, Lazebnik N, Noy S, Lazebnik R (1985) Lipoma of the colon. A report of 22 cases. Am Surg 51: 449-454

Nijssens M, Usewils R, Broeckx J, Ponette E, Baert AL (1983) Lipoma of the duodenal bulb. CT demonstration. Eur J Radiol 3: 39-41

Nora PF (1964) Lipoma of the esophagus. Am J Surg 108: 353-356

Olmsted WW, Ros PR, Hjermstad BM, McCarthy MJ, Dachman AH (1987) Tumors of the small intestine with little or no malignant predisposition: a review of the literature and report of 56 cases. Gastrointest Radiol 12: 231-239

Ormson MJ, Stephens DH, Carlson HC (1985) CT recognition of intestinal lipomatosis. AJR 144: 313-314

Palmer ED (1951) Benign intraluminal tumors of the stomach. A review with special reference to gross pathology. Medicine 30: 108-115

Peabody JW, Ziskind J (1953) Lipomatosis of the stomach. Ann Surg 138: 784-790

Peiser J, Ovnat A, Herz A, Hirsch M, Charuzi I (1984) Lipoma of the esophagus. Isr J Med Sci 20: 1068-1070

Plachta A (1962) Benign tumors of the esophagus: review of the literature and report of 99 cases. Am J Gastroenterol 38: 639-652

Reeder PH, Hopens T (1983) Intestinal lipomatosis. An unusual case. Am J Gastroenterol 78: 185-188

Reichbach E, Kobayashi S (1970) Gastric lipoma mimicking a gastric malignancy. Dig Dis 15: 359-363

River L, Silverstein J, Tope JW (1956) Collective review: benign neoplasms of the small intestine. A critical comprehensive review with reports of 20 new cases. Int Abstr Surg 102: 1-38

Ryberg CH (1956) Lipoma of the colon: report of four cases and review of the literature. Acta Chir Scand 111: 45-53

Sarma DP, Weilbaecher TG, Basavaraj A, Reina RR (1984) Symptomatic lipoma of the duodenum. J Surg Oncol 25: 133-135

Saviano MS, Ricchi E, Pezcoller C, Carriero A (1986) Considerazioni su un caso di lipoma delle stomaco. Minerva Chir 41: 803-807

Scatarige JC, Allen HA, Fishman EK (1987) Computed tomography of the small bowel. Semin Ultrasound CT MR 8: 403-423

Skinner MS, Broadaway RK, Grossman P, Seckinger D (1983) Multiple gastric lipomas. Dig Dis Sci 28: 1147-1149

Solomon A, Michowitz M, Papo J, Yust I (1986) Computed tomographic air enema technique to demonstrate colonic neoplasms. Gastrointest Radiol 11: 194–196

Troisier J, Bariety M, Brouet G (1936) Les lipomes sous-muqueux de l'estomac. Arch Fr Mal Appar Dig 26: 787–807

Turkington RW (1965) Gastric lipomas. Report of a case and review of the literature. Am J Dig Dis 10: 719–726

Weinberg T, Feldman M (1955) Lipomas of the gastrointestinal tract. Am J Clin Pathol 25: 272–281

Weiss A, Mollura JL, Profy A, Cohen R (1979) Two cases of complicated intestinal lipoma: review of small bowel lipomas. Am J Gastroenterol 72: 83–88

Whetstone MR, Zuckerman MJ, Saltzstein EC, Boman D (1985) CT diagnosis of duodenal lipoma. Am J Gastroenterol 80: 251–252

Wilson JM, Melvin DB, Gray G, Thorbjarnarson B (1975) Benign small bowel tumor. Ann Surg 181: 247–250

Wychulis AR, Jackman RJ, Mayo CW (1964) Submucous lipomas of the colon and rectum. Surg Gynecol Obstet 118: 337–340

Yadoo S, Dintsman M, Chaimoff C (1971) Lipomas of the rectum: two case reports. Am J Proctol 22: 120–122

Zonderland HM, Ginai AZ (1984) Lipoma of the esophagus. Diagn Imag Clin Med 53: 265–268

5 Benign Neurogenic Tumors*

Neurogenic tumors of the gastrointestinal tract are rare pathologic entities. Four types with variable frequencies have been identified. The two most common are the schwannoma, which is usually solitary and always encapsulated, and the neurofibroma, which commonly occurs as multiple lesions in von Recklinghausen's disease. Their frequency is undoubtedly overestimated because of problems for histologic differential diagnosis of large lesions from leiomyoma, which is much more common (Wood 1967). Nevertheless, these two neurogenic tumors merit consideration together as far as imaging is concerned because they have no specific differential features. The third form, ganglioneuroma, is exceptional (Wood 1967). The last type, granular cell tumor, has also been referred to as granular cell myoblastoma, an inexact term dating back to when this lesion was thought to derive from muscle. Histochemical studies have since demonstrated the neural origin of this tumor (Aparicio and Lumdsen 1969; Fischer and Wechsler 1962; Lack et al. 1980; Stefansson and Wollmann 1982), which is described in the end of this chapter, after solitary gastric and intestinal neurogenic tumors. Esophageal and colorectal lesions are exceptional.

The gastrointestinal neurogenic tumors encountered in von Recklinghausen's disease are discussed separately because differential diagnosis involves problems which are different from those of solitary tumors. For example, gastrointestinal bleeding in patients with von Recklinghausen's disease can usually be diagnosed macroscopically, and imaging studies are essentially performed to localize the exact site of active bleeding and to detect possible multiple lesions.

---

* Written in collaboration with C. Balu-Maestro.

5.1 Neurogenic Gastric Tumors (Excluding von Recklinghausen's Disease)

5.1.1 General Features

These rare tumors account for only 3% of all benign lesions of the stomach and only 0.3% of all gastric neoplasms (Ming 1973).

Histologically, the *schwannoma* (or neurilemmoma or neurinoma) is a slowly growing, encapsulated tumor composed of Schwann cells in a matrix of collagen. Local tumor growth progressively compresses the nerve, from the periphery inwards. The *neurofibroma* is a nonencapsulated tumor composed mainly of Schwann cells. At the start, tumor growth occurs locally, in the endometrial matrix, and displaces the Schwann cells, which become tortuous and increase in number. As the lesion increases in size, these tumors lose their original characteristics and may be confused with one another or with tumors of muscle origin. Neurogenic gastric tumors develop from the myenteric plexus of Auerbach; cancer arising from Meissner's plexus is much less common (Tate and Furaso 1948). Tumor development may be submucosal, intramural, or dumbbell type (both subserosal and intraluminal components).

The general features of neurogenic gastric tumors were defined by a review of 137 cases in the literature (Beck et al. 1986; Bruneton et al. 1983; Burns et al. 1983; Nardi et al. 1986; Pinto and Novo 1985; Winter et al. 1984). Paragastric lesions, which do not always arise in the stomach, were excluded (Kron 1971; Totterman et al. 1980). Schwannomas are much less frequent than neurofibromas, accounting for less than 10% of the review cases (Beck et al. 1986; Berk et al. 1971; Bucker and Stossel 1961; Gregl et al. 1968; Hecker 1959; Jenett et al. 1983; von Koppenfels 1975; Wissman and Appel 1977). Neurofibromas tend to be solitary rather than a component of von Recklinghausen's disease. For Davis and Berk (1973), a quarter of all patients with von Recklinghausen's disease have one or more gastrointestinal neurofibromas. However, only 15% of all patients with a gastrointestinal neurofibroma also have von Recklinghausen's disease. Regardless of the type, solitary benign neurogenic gastric tumors are rare and are much less common in the stomach than tumors of muscle origin (Grafe et al. 1960; Ochsner and Janetos 1965). Benign neurogenic gastric tumors are four times as common as malignant gastric neoplasms (Hill and Schmitt-Koppler 1972; Leroy et al. 1962).

Outside of von Recklinghausen's disease, multiple lesions are rare (only 4% of the cases reviewed) (Brunet et al. 1971; Cachin et al. 1959; Jurja 1971; Pape and Hackensellner 1952; Peycelon and Replumaz 1958). Fortuitous associations with other lesions include ulcers (Bucker and Stossel 1961; Peycelon and Replumaz 1958) and carcinoma of the stomach (Dupuy et al. 1962). Of the 121 gastric lesions

reviewed, 18.1% involved the upper third, 46.3% the body, and 35.6% the antrum. These lesions are usually smaller than 10 cm in length (Table 15.1). Average patient age at diagnosis of a benign neurogenic tumor of the stomach is 58 years. Discrete female predominance has been observed (56.2% of review cases). The clinical presentation most commonly includes bleeding, generally due to tumoral ulceration. All of the review cases were symptomatic. Tumoral perforation is a rare possibility (Pinto and Novo 1985). There is often a long interval between the onset of vague, nonspecific symptoms and diagnosis (De Oliveira et al. 1986); the long-standing nature of such symptoms is in favor of a benign process. Endoscopy identifies the submucosal nature of these lesions, often visualizes an ulceration, and generally leads to diagnosis of a benign tumor (Hofer 1977). Recurrence is rare after exeresis (Cachin et al. 1959).

5.1.2 Imaging (Figs. 5.1–5.6)

Owing to the frequency of malignant neoplasms and the poorly known risk of degeneration of benign tumors, accurate diagnosis is essential. Gastric endoscopy has supplanted barium studies, but the latter technique remains satisfactory for the detection of benign neurogenic tumors: only 4.1% of the cases reviewed in the literature had a negative barium study (Table 15.1). Although intramural lesions predominate and are difficult to recognize radiologically, association with an ulceration permits identification.

In 51% of cases, barium studies suggest a diagnosis of benign tumor. Although ulceration may be present at gross examination, this is a less frequent barium finding (Brunet et al. 1971; Grosdidier and Guibal 1969). The radiologic features of benign neurogenic gastric tumors are similar to those of leiomyomas, and imaging studies cannot provide a more accurate diagnosis.

Although rarely utilized for this type of tumor, angiography generally demonstrates tumoral hypervascularity. This may explain the massive nature and frequency of hemorrhage (Fujii et al. 1972; Lagadec et al. 1979). Barium studies and angiography have advantageously

Table 5.1. General and radiologic (barium studies) features of benign neurogenic tumors of the stomach and small intestine (excluding von Recklinghausen's disease)

	Stomach	Small intestine
Clinical symptoms	(137 cases)	(102 cases)
Pain	48.2%	45.1%
Upper gastrointestinal bleeding	57.7%	56.8%
Vomiting	10.2%	10.8%
Weight loss	12.4%	1%
Obstruction	–	10.7%
Palpable mass	11%	31.3%
Barium pattern	(95 cases)	(40 cases)
Intraluminal	29.5%	25%
Intramural	55.8%	20%
Subserosal	10.5%	47.5%
Dumbbell	4.2%	7.5%
Ulceration	40%	45%
Radiologic diagnosis	(98 cases)	(42 cases)
False negative	4.5%	14.3%
Benign	51%	35.7%
Malignant	10.2%	16.7%
Inconclusive	34.7%	33.3%
Size	(112 cases)	(50 cases)
<5 cm	48.2%	54%
5–10 cm	37.5%	36%
>10 cm	14.3%	10%

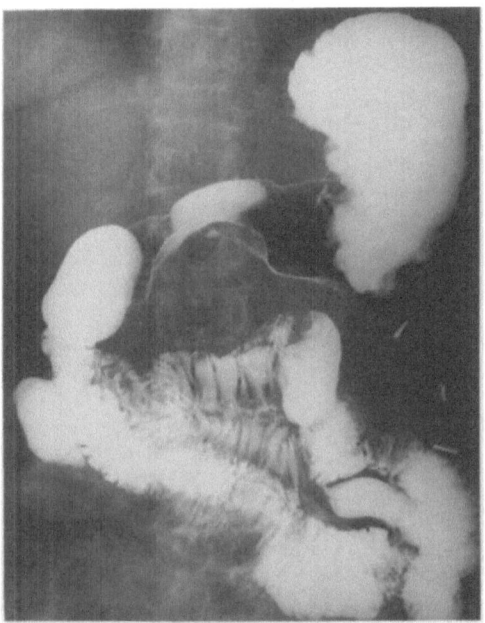 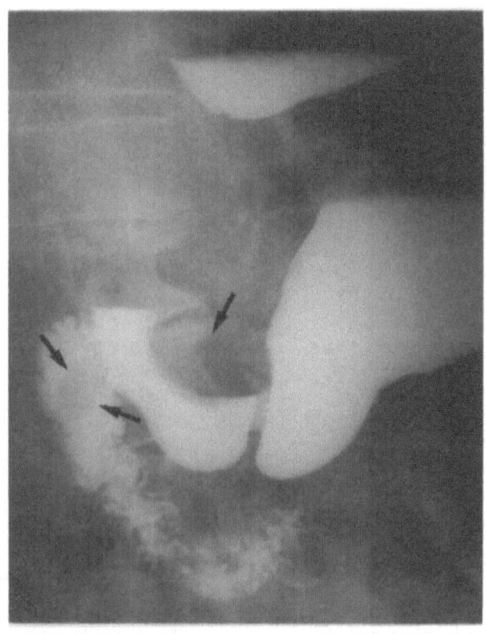

Fig. 5.1. Benign schwannoma in the gastric antrum with a small ulceration

Fig. 5.2. Association of two schwannomas *(arrows)* (stomach, duodenum) in the absence of any signs of von Recklinghausen's neurofibromatosis

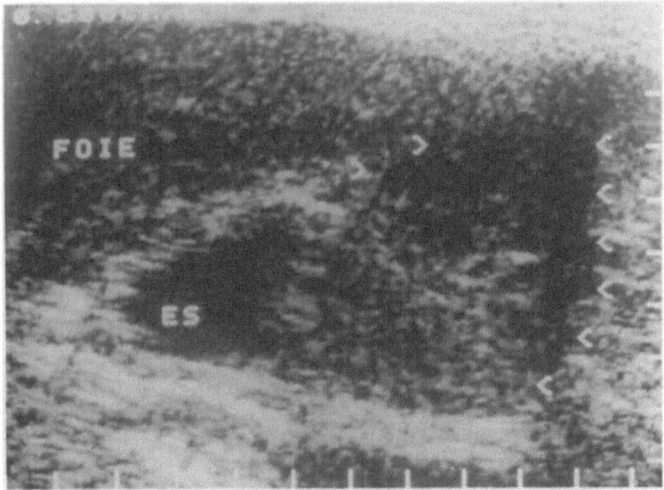

Fig. 5.3. Gastric schwannoma: ultrasonography visualized a solid lesion. Examination was performed after the patient had ingested a sufficient amount of fluid: this technique permits localization of the lesion *(arrows)* with respect to the gastric lumen. *ES*, stomach; *foie*, liver

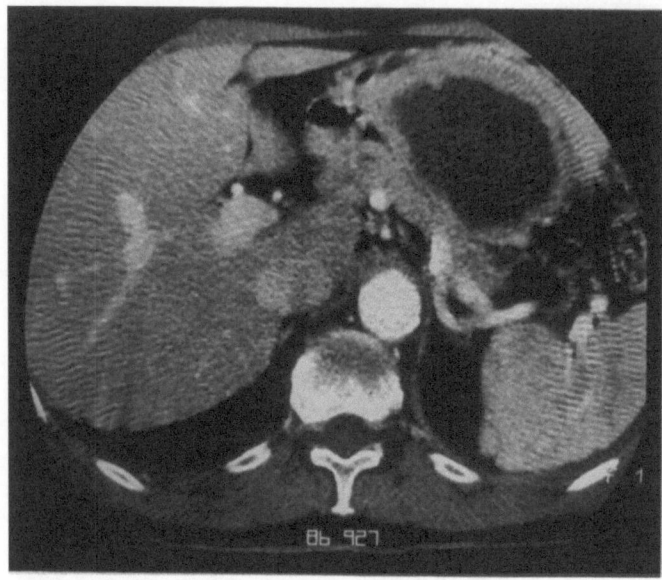

Fig. 5.4. Large subserosal lesion in the stomach, separated from the pancreas by a small rim of fat. This extensively necrotic lesion proved to be a gastric schwannoma

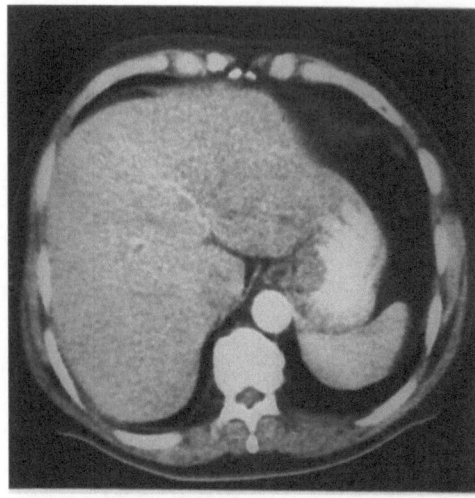

Fig. 5.5. Small schwannoma in the upper stomach, differentiated from the cardia even during examination in dorsal decubitus

been replaced by ultrasonography, sonoendoscopy, and CT.

Two ultrasound patterns have been described: a relatively homogeneous, solid mass and a necrotic lesion (generally corresponding to larger tumors) (Beck et al. 1986; Bruneton

et al. 1984; Jenett et al. 1983; Nardi et al. 1986; Winter et al. 1984). CT demonstrates the subserosal component of this type of lesion (Jenett et al. 1983) and theoretically allows evaluation of tumor hypervascularity after contrast medium injection. The most common diagnosis after radiologic examinations is leiomyoma or a neurogenic tumor.-

5.2 Neurogenic Intestinal Tumors (Excluding von Recklinghausen's Disease)

5.2.1 General Features

As in the stomach, schwannomas are more prevalent than neurofibromas in the small intestine. Solitary neurofibromas represented fewer than 2% of the cases reviewed (Juan et al. 1980; Sobbe and Voelker 1972). Intestinal ganglioneuroma is exceedingly uncommon (Goldman 1968).

Benign neurogenic tumors represent 2.4%–6.4% of all benign intestinal neoplasms (Klepping et al. 1965; Ostermiller et al. 1966; River et al. 1956). They are less common than in the stomach, and, for all authors, they are less frequent than intestinal tumors of muscle origin

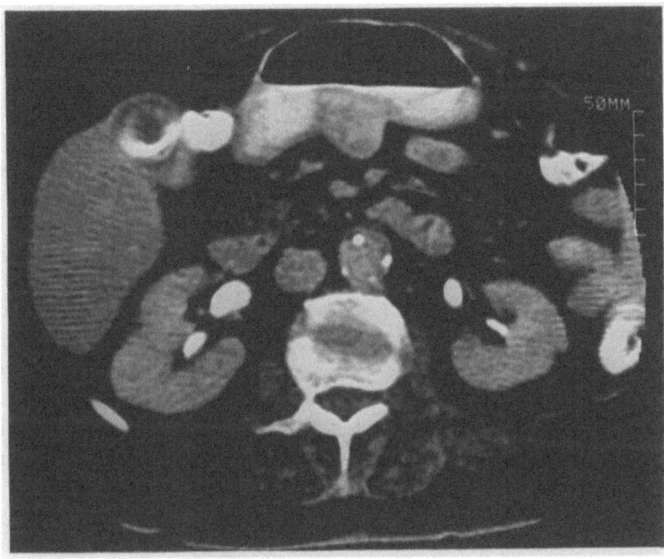

Fig. 5.6. Intramural gastric tumor with both intraluminal and subserosal components. This small mass (3-cm long axis) was a benign schwannoma. Note the presence of a gallstone

(Carlson and Good 1973; River et al. 1956; Wood 1967). Benign tumors account for 60%–85% of all solitary neurogenic intestinal tumors (Bruneton et al. 1984; Nillson and Johnsson 1957). The distribution of 134 benign, solitary intestinal neurogenic tumors reviewed was as follows: duodenum (35.1%), jejunum (50%), ileum (14.9%). Outside of von Recklinghausen's disease, multiple tumors are rare (less than 1.2%), and associations with other lesions appear fortuitous (Bruneton et al. 1984; Jouanneau et al. 1974).

Over 50% of the review cases measured less than 5 cm (Table 15.1). The possibility of subserosal tumors explains why barium studies can be negative. Average age at diagnosis is 47 years; there is no sex predilection (51.9% women in the literature review). Hemorrhage is the main clinical symptom (56.8% of patients), as with solitary gastric neurogenic tumors. This presenting complaint may be long-standing and have gone unexplained for several years (Lifrange 1969). Obstruction was mentioned in 10.7% of the cases reviewed (Table 15.1).

5.2.2 Imaging (Figs. 5.7–5.9)

Benign neurogenic tumors are detected with an acceptable degree of sensitivity by both barium studies and angiography: only 14.3% of the cases reviewed were not identified (Balintffy and Thurzo 1962; Dupuy et al. 1969; Krivine et al. 1964; Lifrange 1969; Popesco-Urlueni 1962). Barium examinations correctly identify intraluminal tumors whereas subserosal lesions, the most common type, are often poorly evaluated. Tumoral calcifications are very rare and suggest malignant degeneration (Cedermak 1949; Lemaître et al. 1976). On arteriograms, these tumors may show homogeneous or non-homogeneous hypervascularity, depending on their size: small lesions tend to be homogeneous whereas larger lesions, whether benign or malignant, appear inhomogeneous, often with a central necrotic zone. The only angiographic feature suggestive of malignancy rather than a benign process is absence of visualization of venous return: this may correspond to thrombosis, which is very rare with benign lesions (Bottger et al. 1973; Brette et al. 1969; Bruneton et al. 1984; Capdeville et al. 1970; Geindre et al. 1969; Gilly 1971; Proff et al. 1972; Will and Hering

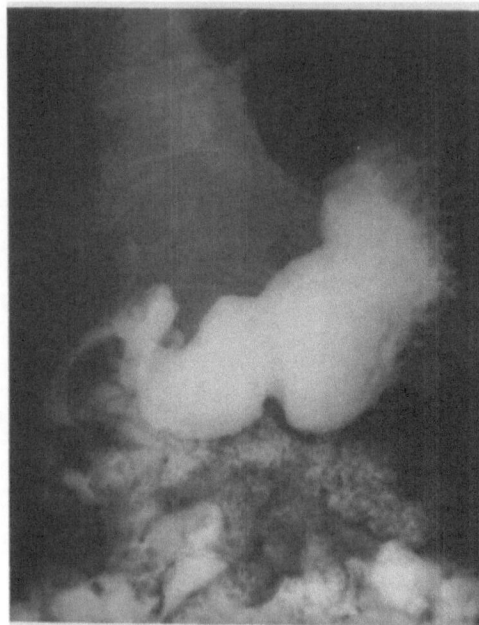

Fig. 5.7. Benign neurogenic tumor of the duodenum

1978). No reports on the ultrasonographic or CT features of these tumors were found in the literature.

5.3 Solitary Benign Neurogenic Tumors of the Esophagus, Colon, and Rectum

5.3.1 Esophagus (Fig. 5.10)

Solitary neurogenic tumors account for only 0.76% of all benign esophageal tumors; all of the cases reported by Plachta (1962) were neurofibromas. Madrid et al. (1986) described a lobulated, intraluminal esophageal lesion that appeared benign at endoscopy (Fig. 5.11).

5.3.2 Colon and Rectum (Fig. 5.12)

Solitary neurogenic colorectal tumors are very infrequent, with colonic sites being particularly rare.

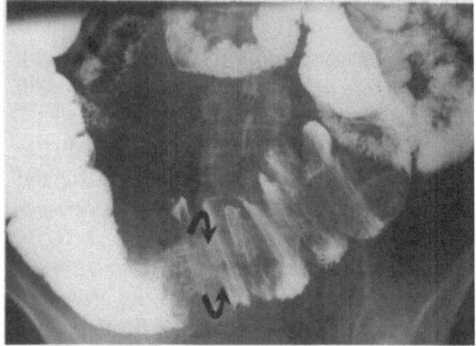

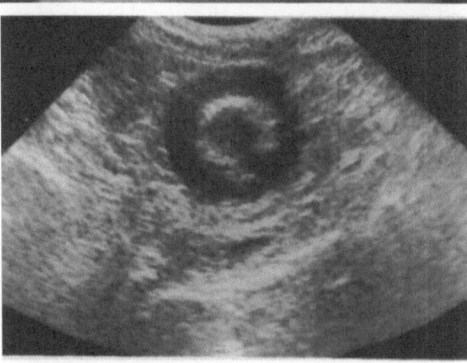

Fig. 5.8a, b. Barium study **(a)** and sonogram **(b)** of an ileal neurofibroma causing intussusception *(arrows).* (Courtesy of Dr. Schmutz, Strasbourg, France)

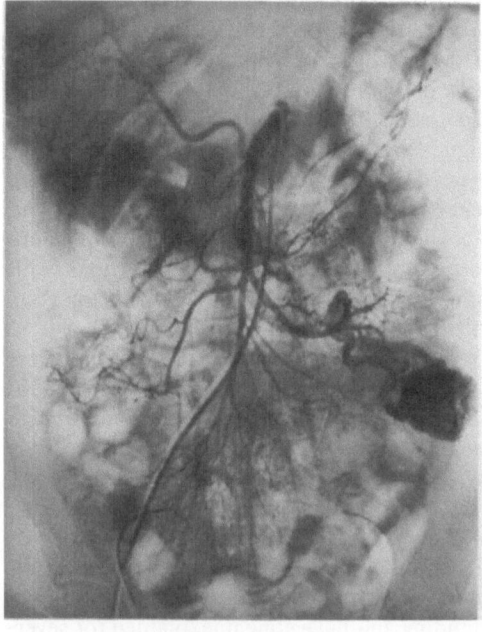

Fig. 5.9. Angiographic study of a duodenal schwannoma: massive tumor hypervascularity with early venous return. However, this pattern cannot be differentiated from that seen with a leiomyoma, for example. Only the small size of the lesion suggests a benign process rather than a malignancy

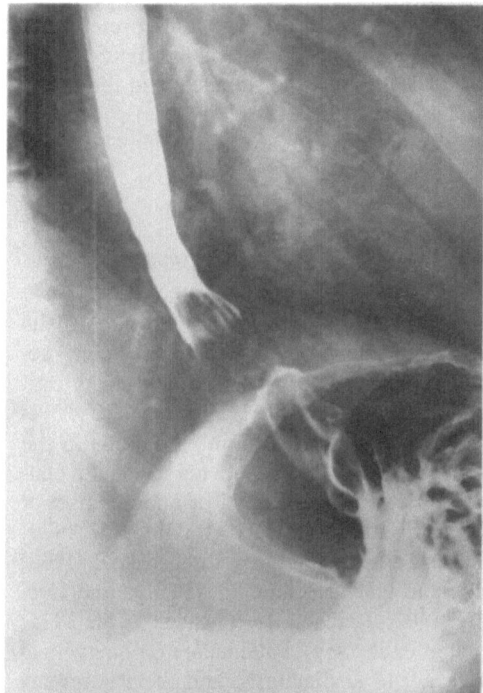

Fig. 5.10. Small lesion in the lower third of the esophagus (neurofibroma)

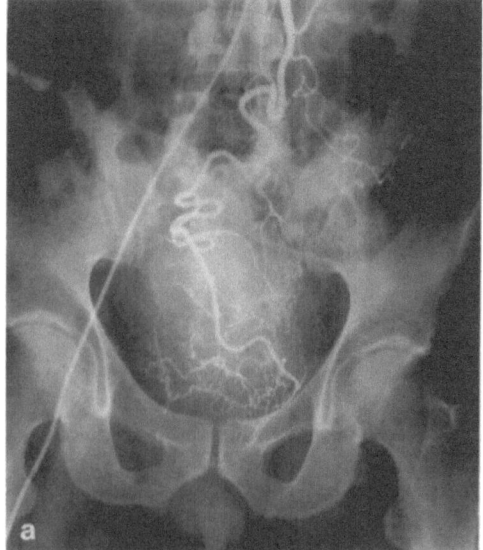

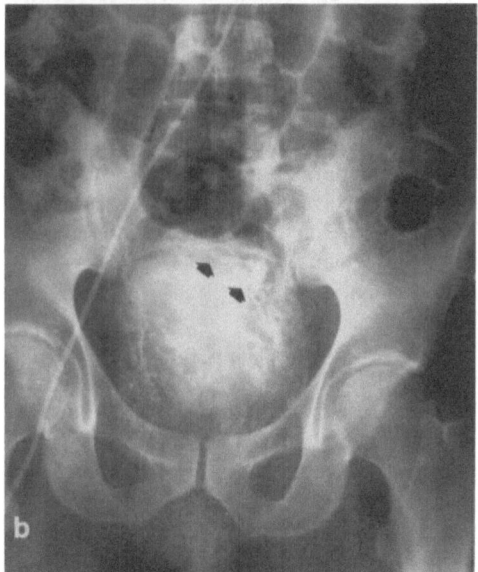

Fig. 5.12a, b. Angiographic study of a rectal neurofibroma. Arterial phase **(a)** increase in the caliber of the inferior mesenteric artery and depiction of abnormal vascularization in the rectum. Peritumoral veins *(arrows)* were rapidly demonstrated along with tumor hypervascularity **(b)**

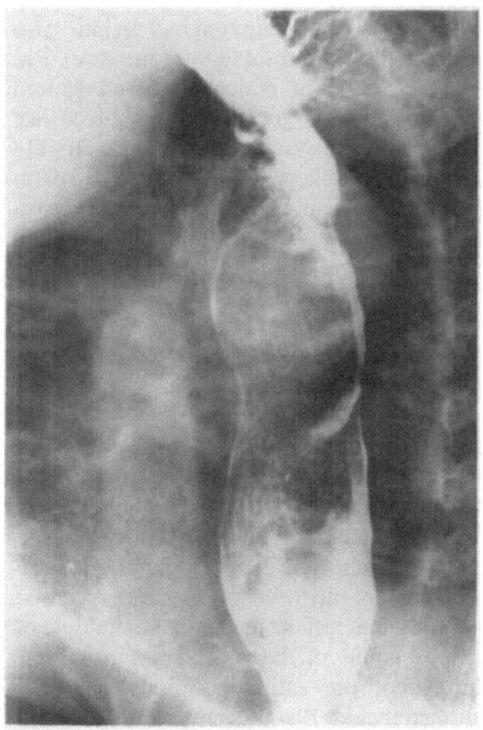

◀ **Fig. 5.11.** Bulky lobulated intraluminal mass in the middle third of the esophagus (neurofibroma). Extensive signs of associated stasis. (Courtesy of Dr. Madrid and Dr. Pardo, Zaragoza, Spain)

In 1963, Weston et al. reviewed 32 anorectal tumors in the literature. Abel et al. (1985) reviewed two cases. In most literature reports, patients were asymptomatic; in particular, no mention was made of the hemorrhagic phenomena described with gastric and small bowel lesions.

5.4 Benign Neurogenic Tumors in von Recklinghausen's Disease

Neurofibromatosis is a congenital, hereditary neuroectodermal dysplasia with diffuse systemic expression. It has an autosomal dominant inheritance pattern, with no sex predilection. The estimated incidence is 1 per 3000 births, with spontaneous mutations being responsible for up to half of all cases (Crowe et al. 1956; Klatte et al. 1976). The classical features of this pathologic entity include cutaneous lesions (*café-au-lait* spots), mental retardation, and congenital skeletal abnormalities. Other manifestations include pheochromocytoma, arterial aneurysms, vascular stenoses, and involvement of the urinary bladder. Overall, approximately 11% of patients with von Recklinghausen's disease have gastrointestinal manifestations (Brasfield and Das Gupta 1972).

The majority of neurogenic tumors in patients with von Recklinghausen's disease are neurofibromas. However, the fortuitous or non-fortuitous existence of a schwannoma (Sivak et al. 1975), a leiomyoma (Lukash et al. 1966), and even a carcinoid tumor (Barber 1976; Hough et al. 1983; Johnson and Weaver 1981) seems to support the hypothesis of Willis (1962), who suggested that neurofibromatosis is not only of neuroectodermal or isodermal origin, but also presents a hamartomous structure characterized by the overgrowth of nerve sheath tissue. Estimates of malignant degeneration are comparable to those for solitary neurogenic tumors (3%–20.8%) (Baldi et al. 1979; Croker and Greenstein 1976; Hochberg et al. 1974). This variation in incidence can be explained by the fact that the percentage of clinically manifest tumors differed in the various series. If all tumors, whether symptomatic or not, are considered together, the frequency of degeneration is probably under 10%.

For Hochberg et al. (1974), the preferential sites, in decreasing order of frequency, were the small intestine, the stomach, and the colon (Finkel et al. 1978; Hassell 1982). Esophageal involvement is quite rare (Reichelt 1973).

5.4.1 Gastric Involvement by von Recklinghausen's Disease

The stomach is not involved as often as the small intestine, and gastric involvement accounts for only 21.3%–24% of all gastrointestinal sites (Vachon et al. 1959). Of 11 cases reviewed, five concerned multiple lesions in the stomach; one-third of patients also had neurofibromatous involvement of another part of the gastrointestinal tract (Baldi et al. 1979; Bucker and Stossel 1961; Lukash et al. 1966; Pape and Hackensellner 1952; Perea and Gregory 1962; Reichelt 1973; Sivak et al. 1975; Vachon et al. 1959). Patients are on an average 51 years old at diagnosis, and there is no sex predilection. As for solitary benign neurogenic tumors, the most common presenting symptoms are gastrointestinal bleeding and abdominal pain. Radiologic features mentioned for ten review cases included an intramural lesion (seven cases), an intraluminal lesion (two cases), and a subserosal lesion (one case). Radiologic studies of patients with recognized neurofibromatosis generally result in correct diagnosis of these neurogenic tumors. Besides confirming the diagnosis, endoscopy can demonstrate the extent of lesions with better sensitivity and may also reveal multiple lesions in the stomach and the duodenum.

5.4.2 Intestinal Involvement by von Recklinghausen's Disease (Fig. 5.13)

The small intestine is the most frequently involved portion of the gastrointestinal tract in patients with von Recklinghausen's disease (approximately 50% of all gastrointestinal lesions) (Vachon et al. 1959). Solitary lesions accounted for only 19% of 24 cases reviewed, and intestinal lesions tended to be multiple (at various points of the small intestine only or throughout the entire gastrointestinal tract) (Bruneton et al. 1984; Debray et al. 1971; Ma-

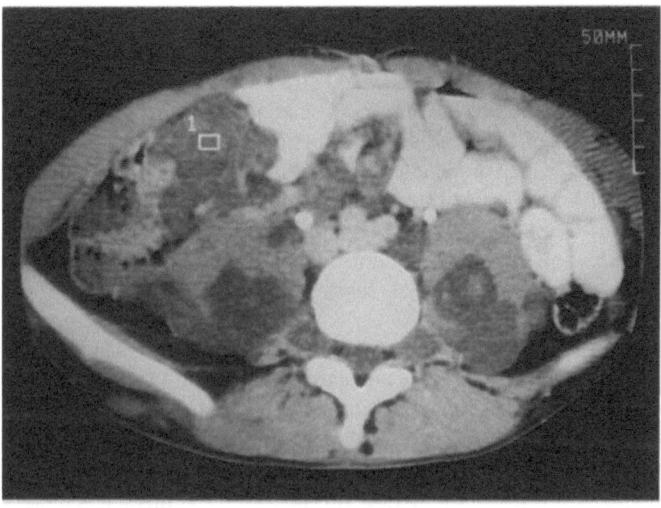

Fig. 5.13. Von Recklinghausen's disease: CT scans demonstrated infiltration of the mesentery and the intestinal wall (*square*, density of 52 HU). A similar lesion was found at the level of the psoas muscle

zare et al. 1968; Rosner et al. 1973; Sivak et al. 1975). Mean patient age at diagnosis is 48 years; there is discrete female predominance (64.3%) (Bruneton et al. 1984).

Hemorrhage was by far the most common presenting symptom (70.8% of cases). Physical examination noted a palpable mass in nearly a third of cases (Bruneton et al. 1984). Barium studies are frequently negative (31.6% of the cases reviewed) because of the lesions' small size and intramural location (45.4% of review cases). Selective superior mesenteric arteriography may suggest the diagnosis by demonstrating one or more hypervascularized tumors (Jouanneau et al. 1974; Lohrmann et al. 1981; Uflacker et al. 1985; Vujic et al. 1983). Owing to the existence of the cutaneous stigmata of neurofibromatosis, a visible lesion is almost always correctly diagnosed as a neurogenic tumor.

CT cannot determine the site of active bleeding in patients with diffuse gastrointestinal lesions. CT scans are primarily obtained to determine the general extent of lesions within the abdominal cavity. Because gastrointestinal neurofibromas in von Recklinghausen's disease are often small, barium studies of the entire tract appear advisable when doubt exists as to the possibility of gastrointestinal involvement. The frequency of multiple lesions in von Recklinghausen's disease underscores the value of this approach before therapy is initiated.

5.5 Granular Cell Tumors

Granular cell tumors are rare pathologic entities that can occur in almost any organ, but show a predilection for the tongue, skin, breast, and gastrointestinal tract. These tumors were formerly incorrectly referred to as myoblastomas because they were thought to be of muscle origin.

5.5.1 General Features

Granular cell tumors are nearly always benign. The exceptional reports of lesions with a malignant course all concerned the esophagus (2%–3.4% of esophageal lesions) (Coutinho et al. 1985; Vuyk et al. 1985). Several cases of multiple lesions have been described and all were associated with involvement of different organs (pharynx, stomach, lungs, skin, genital tract) (Cone and Wetzsel 1982; O'Connell et al. 1978). These tumors originate in the Schwann cells, and nearly all literature reports concern esophageal lesions. Only a few cases of gastric involvement have been published (Schwartz and Gaetz 1965; Strong et al. 1970).

5.5.2 Esophagus

In 1985, Coutinho et al. reviewed 117 cases of esophageal granular cell tumors. The esophagus is the site of 1% of all such tumors (Paskin et al. 1972), which are generally solitary and usually affect the lower third of the esophagus. Multiple esophageal lesions are infrequent (Rubesin et al. 1985); malignant degeneration occurs in less than 3.5% of cases (Coutinho et al. 1985).

There is discrete male predominance, and age at diagnosis is slightly over 40 years. The disease appears more prevalent in blacks than in other races (Coutinho et al. 1985). Owing to their small size, granular cell tumors of the esophagus are often incidental findings (50% of cases for Coutinho et al. 1985). The most common clinical symptom is dysphagia.

Endoscopy reveals most of these lesions (81%) as small, yellowish submucosal nodules raising up the normal-appearing mucosa. On rare occasions, larger lesions are associated with inflammatory reorganization or even tumoral stenosis (Elhadad et al. 1984). The diagnosis is generally made by endoscopic biopsy.

Barium examinations have a sensitivity of 63.4% (Elhadad et al. 1984); filling defects are more common than stenosis, an intraluminal growth, or a subserosal lesion (Johnston and Helwig 1981).

Owing to the rarity of esophageal granular cell tumors and their low malignant potential, endoscopy and barium meals have been advocated for patient follow-up because of the risks associated with surgery. Other authors recommend endoscopic resection (Sandler et al. 1981), although complete surgical resection may be advisable because of the possibility of recurrence (Lack et al. 1980).

5.6 References

Abel ME, Kingsley AEN, Abcarian H, Arlenga P, Barron SS (1985) Anorectal neurilemmomas. Dis Colon Rectum 28: 960–961

Aparicio SR, Lumdsen CE (1969) Light and electron microscope studies on granular cell myoblastoma of the tongue. J Pathol 97: 339–355

Baldi A, Azzario G, Merli G (1979) Le localizzazioni digestive della neurofibromatosi di Recklinghausen. Minerva Chir 34: 363–374

Balintffy J, Thurzo R (1962) A duodenal neurinoma developed around metal foreign bodies. Gastroenterologia (Basel) 98: 354–359

Barber PV (1976) Carcinoid tumor of the ampulla of Vater associated with cutaneous neurofibromatosis. Postgrad Med 52: 514–517

Beck DE, Wheeler RA, Smith MD (1986) Gastric neurofibroma in an adolescent. South Med J 79: 359–361

Berk PN, Scher GS, Bode DF (1971) Unusual tumors of the gastrointestinal tract. AJR 113: 159–170

Bottger E, Dittmar D, Senft KP, Burghard A, Asmar F, Hartmann R (1973) Seltene Duodenaltumoren und ihre Differentialdiagnose. Fortschr Geb Roentgenstr 119: 17–25

Brasfield RD, Das Gupta TK (1972) Von Recklinghausen's disease: a clinicopathological study. Ann Surg 175: 86–104

Brette R, Saubier E, Tissot-Favre A, Gaillard P, Phelip E (1969) Schwannomes duodénaux. A propos de deux observations anatomocliniques dont une avec explorations vasculaires. Arch Fr Mal Appar Dig 58: 359–368

Brunet JP, Bensahel H, Boureau M (1971) Schwannome gastrique chez l'enfant (à propos d'une observation). Ann Chir Infant 12: 297–302

Bruneton JN, Drouillard J, Roux P, Ettore F, Lecomte P (1983) Neurogenic tumors of the stomach. Report of 18 cases and review of the literature. Fortschr Geb Roentgenstr 2: 192–198

Bruneton JN, Drouillard J, Roux P, Ettore F, Aubanel D (1984) Les tumeurs nerveuses de l'intestin grêle. Revue de la littérature à propos de 6 cas personnels. Ann Gastroenterol Hepatol (Paris) 20: 79–84

Bucker J, Stossel HG (1961) Übergutartige Magentumoren. Fortschr Geb Roentgenstr 94: 159–175

Burns DK, Silva FG, Forde KA, Mount PM, Clark HB (1983) Primary melanocytic schwannoma of the stomach. Evidence of dual melanocytic and Schwannian differentiation in an extra-axial site in a patient without neurofibromatosis. Cancer 52: 1432–1471

Cachin M, Pergola F, Terris G, Roques R (1959) Schwannomes multiples du tube digestif. Arch Fr Mal Appar Dig 48: 821–829

Capdeville R, Bennet J, Dubois F, Toulet J (1970) L'artériographie des tumeurs du grêle. A propos de 3 cas de schwannomes. Arch Fr Mal Appar Dig 59: 453–462

Carlson HC, Good CA (1973) Neoplasms of the small intestine. In: Margulis A, Burhenne H (eds) Alimentary tract roentgenology, 2nd edn. Mosby, Saint Louis, pp 865–902

Cedermak J (1949) Neurinomas of the gastrointestinal tract. J Int Coll Surg 12: 5–11

Cone JB, Wetzsel WJ (1982) Esophageal granular cell tumors: report of two multicentric cases with observation on their histories. J Surg Oncol 20: 14–16

Coutinho DS de S, Soga J, Yoshikawa T, Miyashita K, Tanaka O, Sasaki K, Muto T, Shimizu T (1985) Granular cell tumors fo the esophagus: a report of two cases and review of the literature. Am J Gastroenterol 80: 758–762

Croker JR, Greenstein RJ (1976) Malignant schwannosarcoma of the stomach in a patient with von Recklinghausen's disease. Histopathology 3: 79–85

Crowe FW, Shull WJ, Neel JW (1956) A clinical pathological and genetic study of multiple neurofibromatosis. Thomas, Springfield

Davis GB, Berk RN (1973) Intestinal neurofibromas in von Recklinghausen's disease. Am J Gastroenterol 60: 410–414

Debray C, Hardouin JP, Gouin B, Marche C (1971) Les localisations digestives de la maladie de Recklinghausen. Gaz Med Fr 78: 965–974

De Oliveira FJ, Cabral Silveira JM, Martins MI, Marthinho F, Soares F, De Oliveira F (1986) Schwannomas gastricos. A proposito de cinco casos siendo tres malignos. Rev Esp Enferm Apar Dig 69: 124–128

De Schepper A, Hubens A, Van Vooren W, Verbraeken H (1974) Angiography in diagnosis of small bowel tumors. Radiologe 14: 425–430

Dupuy R, Vallin J, Henry JG (1962) Schwannome gastrique associé à un épithélioma glandulaire. Arch Fr Mal Appar Dig 51: 166–169

Dupuy R, Vallin J, Guenin P, Coldefy JM, Bernard J (1969) Invagination intestinale par tumeur bénigne du grêle. Schwannome et histiocytofibrome. Arch Fr Mal Appar Dig 58: 582–583

Elhadad A, Piquet F, Slama JL, Godefroy Y, Paugam B (1984) La tumeur à cellules granuleuses de l'oesophage. Revue de la littérature. A propos de 1 cas. Ann Chir 38: 441–445

Finkel M, Finkel F, Harris A (1978) Von Recklinghausen's disease with involvement of the colon. An endoscopic view. Mt Sinaï J Med 45: 387–389

Fisher ER, Wechsler H (1962) Granular cell myoblastoma: a misnomer. Electron microscopic and histochemical evidence concerning its Schwann cell derivation and nature (granular cell schwannoma). Cancer 15: 936–954

Fujii K, Yamagata S, Suzuki J, Sasaki R, Shoji T, Makabe M, Memezawa H (1972) Angiographic features of submucosal tumours of the stomach. Tohoku J Exp Med 107: 287–299

Geindre M, Coulomb M, Crouzet G, Marty F (1969) Artériographie mésentérique supérieure et tumeurs hémorragiques du grêle. Sem Hop 45: 1634–1639

Gilly G (1971) Neurinom der Pars descendens duodeni. Fortschr Geb Roentgenstr 115: 126–128

Goldman RC (1968) Ganglioneuroma of the duodenum. Relationship to nonchromaffin paraganglioma of the duodenum. Am J Surg 115: 716–719

Good AC (1963) Tumors of the small intestine. Caldwell lecture 1962. AJR 89: 685–705

Grafe W, Thorbjarnarson B, Pearce JM, Beal JM (1960) Benign neoplasms of the stomach. Am J Surg 100: 561–571

Gregl A, Nieman H, Schlachetzki J (1968) Klinische Symptomatik neurogener Magentumoren. Bruns Beitr Klin Chir 216: 640–643

Grosdidier J, Guibal F (1969) Schwannome de l'estomac. Sem Hop 45: 1187–1188

Hassell P (1982) Gastrointestinal manifestations of neurofibromatosis in children. A report of two cases. J Assoc Can Radiol 33: 202–204

Hecker HA (1959) Beitrag zum Neurinom des Magen-Darm-Kanals. Gastroenterologia 91: 266–274

Hill K, Schmitt-Koppler A (1972) Zur Klinik und Histogenese der neurogenen Tumoren des oberen Gastrointestinaltrakts. Dtsch Med (Wochenschr) 97: 899–902

Hochberg FH, Dasilva AB, Galdabini J, Richardson EP (1974) Gastrointestinal involvement in von Recklinghausen's neurofibromatosis. Neurology 24: 1144–1151

Hofer D (1977) Über Neurinome des Magens. Chirurg 48: 185–188

Hough DR, Chan A, Davidson H (1983) Von Recklinghausen's disease associated with gastrointestinal carcinoid tumors. Cancer 51: 2206–2208

Jenett M, Longin F, Ludwig J (1983) Neurinom des Magens. Fortschr Geb Roentgenstr 137: 362–364

Johnson L, Weaver M (1981) Von Recklinghausen's disease and gastrointestinal carcinoids. JAMA 245: 2496

Johnston J, Helwig EB (1981) Granular cell tumors of the gastrointestinal tract and perianal region. Dig Dis Sci 26: 807–816

Jouanneau P, Teniere P, Geffroy Y (1974) Localisations digestives de la maladie de Recklinghausen. A propos d'un cas. Chirurgie 100: 558–565

Juan IK, Sono F, Okada T, Muto M, Furuki A (1980) Neurogenic tumor of small intestine, report of a case with review of literature. Gastroenterol Jpn 15: 112–119

Jurja J (1971) Schwannomes gastriques multiples. J Radiol 52: 387–388

Klatte EC, Franken EA, Smith JA (1976) The radiographic spectrum in neurofibromatosis. Semin Roentgenol 11: 17–33

Klepping C, Cortet P, Michiels R, Dusserre P, Jacquot B, Gaudet M, Michelot M (1965) Les schwannomes de l'intestin grêle (revue de la littérature à propos de deux observations personnelles). J Med Lyon 46: 1607–1632

Krivine JM, Hivet M, Levame M (1964) Les tumeurs apparement bénignes du duodenum. Ann Chir 18: 588–609

Kron B (1971) Schwannome malin de l'épiploon gastrocolique. Sem Hop 47: 2684–2685

Lack EE, Worscham GF, Callihan MD, Crawford BE, Kappenbach S, Rowden GR, Chun B (1980) Granular cell tumor: a clinicopathologic study of 110 patients. J Surg Oncol 13: 301–316

Lagadec B, Blondin G, Van Haecke P (1979) Schwannome exogastrique bénin géant. Artériographie sélective des artères digestives. Med Chir Dig 8: 171-172

Lemaitre G, L'Hermine C, Proye C, Marache P, Ribet M (1976) Aspect radiologique des schwannomes du 2ème duodénum à développement extrinsèque (à propos de 3 observations). Lille Med 21: 827-832

Leroy A, Blanc P, Henry J (1962) Etude analytique des schwannomes digestifs. A propos d'une statistique de 72 cas de schwannomes. J Chir 83: 683-708

Lifrange M (1969) A propos des léiomyomes et des neurinomes de l'intestin grêle. Rev Med Liege 24: 769-772

Lohrmann A, Kottmann F, Donhuijsen K, Goebell H, Weichert HC (1981) Dunndarm-Neurofibrom bei morlans Recklinghausen als Ursache rezidivierender gastrointestinaler Blutungen. Leber Magen Darm 11: 132-135

Lukash WM, Morgan RI, Sennett CO, Nielson OF (1966) Gastrointestinal neoplasms in von Recklinghausen's disease. Arch Surg 92: 905-908

Madrid G, Pardo J, Perez C, Pereda RG, Galbe R, Ros LH, Soler A, Navarro ML, Valero I, Almajano C (1986) The neurofibroma of the oesophagus. Eur J Radiol 6: 67-69

Mazare Y, Champetier J, Micoud M, Verdier JM (1968) Localisation appendiculaire de la neurofibromatose. Rev Lyon Med 17: 601-608

Ming SC (1973) Tumors of the esophagus and stomach. Atlas of tumor pathology, 2nd series, fasc 7. AFIP, Washington

Nardi P, Biagi P, Poggini M, Brettoni A, Bombagli A (1986) Il ruolo dell' ultrasonografia nella diagnosi delle neoplasie non epiteliali dello stomaco. Considerazioni a proposito di due casi. Radiol Med 72: 977-978

Nillson B, Jonsson I (1957) Malignant neurinoma of the duodenum. Report of a case and review of the literature. Acta Chir Scand 113: 357-363

Ochsner SF, Janetos GP (1965) Benign tumors of the stomach. JAMA 191: 881-886

O'Connell DJ, McMahon H, De Meester TR (1978) Multicentric tracheobronchial and esophageal granular cell myoblastoma. Thorax 33: 596-602

Ostermiller W, Joergenson EJ, Weibe L (1966) A clinical review of tumors of the small bowel. Am J Surg 111: 403-409

Pape R, Hackensellner HA (1952) Das röntgenologische Erscheinungsbild der neurogenen Tumoren des Verdauungstrakts. Fortschr Geb Roentgenstr 76: 691-711

Paskin DL, Hull JD, Cookson PS (1972) Granular cell myoblastomas: a comprehensive review of 15-years experience. Ann Surg 175: 501-504

Perea VD, Gregory JL (1962) Neurofibromatosis of the stomach. Report of a case associated with von Recklinghausen's disease and review of the literature. JAMA 182: 259-263

Peycelon R, Replumaz P (1958) A propos des schwannomes gastriques. Arch Fr Mal Appar Dig 47: 465-479

Pinto ADS, Novo JA (1985) Gastric neurilemmoma: case report. Mt Sinaï J Med 52: 647-649

Plachta A (1962) Benign tumors of the esophagus. Review of literature and report of 99 cases. Am J Gastroenterol 38: 639-652

Popesco-Urlueni M (1962) A propos des schwannomes de l'intestin grêle. Arch Fr Mal Appar Dig 51: 1120-1131

Proff E, Hill K, Schmitt-Koppler A (1972) Zur Klinik und Histogenese der neurogenen Tumoren des oberen Gastrointestinaltraktes. Dtsch Med Wochenschr 97: 899-902

Reichelt H (1973) Ein aussergewöhnlicher Fall einer Neurofibromatosis von Recklinghausen mit Röntgenologischem Nachweis von Krankheitsmanifestationen an Thorax, Mediastinum, Schädel, Osophagus, Magen und Kolon. Rontgenblatter 26: 361-366

River L, Silverstein J, Tope JW (1956) Collective review: benign neoplasms of small intestine. A critical comprehensive with reports of 20 new cases. Int Abstr Surg 102: 1-38

Rosner D, Hivet M, Lagadec B, Conte J (1973) Schwannomes multiples à localisation digestive (maladie de von Recklinghausen). A propos d'un cas familial. Med Chir Dig 2: 39-44

Sandler RS, Wood DR, Bozymski EM (1981) Endoscopic removal of a granular cell tumor of the esophagus. Gastroenterol Endosc 27: 70-72

Schwartz DT, Gaetz HP (1965) Multiple granular cell myoblastomas of the stomach. Am J Clin Pathol 44: 453-457

Sivak MV, Sullivan BH, Farmer RG (1975) Neurogenic tumor of the small intestine. Review of the literature and report of a case with endoscopic removal. Gastroenterology 68: 374-380

Sobbe A, Voelker D (1972) Das Neurofibrom des Dünndarms. Fortschr Geb. Roentgenstr 116: 572-574

Stefansson K, Wollmann RL (1982) S-100 protein in granular cell tumors (granular cell myoblastomas). Cancer 49: 1834-1838

Strong EW, Mc Divitt RW, Brasfield RD (1970) Granular cell myoblastoma. Cancer 25: 415-422

Tate RW, Furaso WJ (1948) Neurofibroma of the stomach. Am J Surg 75: 607-613

Totterman S, Lindfors O, Nickels J (1980) A schwannoma of the lesser omentum. Fortschr Geb Roentgenstr 132: 585-586

Uflacker R, Alves MA, Diehl JC (1985) Gastrointestinal involvement in neurofibromatosis: angiographic presentation. Gastrointest Radiol 10: 163-165

Vachon A, Chattot R, Pasquier J, Aimard G (1959) Nouvelle observation de schwannomes digestifs associés à une maladie de Recklinghausen. Arch Fr Mal Appar Dig 48: 836-838

Von Koppenfels R (1975) Neurome und Myome des Magens. Fortschr Geb Roentgenstr 122: 164-166

Vujic I, Sbrocchi RD, Standley JH, Seymour EQ (1983) Angiographic demonstration of gastrointestinal neurofibromas in von Recklinghausen's disease. Gastrointest Radiol 8: 283-284

Vuyk HD, Snow GB, Tiwari RM, Van Velsen D, Veldhuizen RW (1985) Granular cell tumor of the proximal esophagus. A rare disease. Cancer 55: 445-449

Weston SD, Marren M, Cohan MH, Schlachter IS (1963) Neurofibroma of the rectum and colon. J Int Coll Surg 40: 285-293

Will C, Hering K (1978) Neurinom des Dunndarms. Fortschr Roengenstr 129: 646-647

Willis RA (1962) The borderland of embryology and pathology. 2nd edn. Butterworths, Washington

Winter J, Schubert GE, Greiner L, Prohm P (1984) Das Magenneurinom. Leber Magen Darm 14: 164-168

Wissmann C, Appel W (1977) Exulzeriertes Neurofibrom des Magens. Fortschr Geb Roentgenstr 127: 77-78

Wood DA (1967) Tumors of the intestines. Atlas of tumor pathology, sect 6, fasc 22. AFIP, Washington

6 Benign Vascular Tumors*

Benign vascular gastrointestinal tumors are rare, often asymptomatic lesions that involve considerable diagnostic problems. In addition to lymphangiomas, which can be considered congenital malformations, they include several types of hemangioma: cavernous hemangioma, capillary hemangioma, glomus tumor, hemangiomatosis, and multiple phlebectasia. Owing to their rarity, the general features of these different lesions are all discussed together; individual gastrointestinal sites are described thereafter. Lymphangioma is discussed last because of its usual clinical latency and the absence of any hemorrhagic risk, which differentiates such lesions from hemangioma.

6.1 General Features

For practical purposes, benign vascular gastrointestinal tumors can be divided into hemangiomas and lymphangiomas. Hemangiopericytomas, which have an indeterminate natural course, are discussed separately (see Chap. 24).

Several more or less complex classifications have been proposed for hemangiomas, which include several benign tumors (Gentry et al. 1949; Kaijser 1941; Wood 1967). The four types described by Kaijser (1941) include cavernous hemangioma (diffuse infiltrating, polypoid, or circumscribed), capillary hemangioma, angiomatosis, and multiple phlebectasia. The very rare glomus tumor, or glomangioma, must also be cited (Ambrosius 1955). It is not always easy to determine the origin of a hemangioma or decide whether it is really a tumoral process rather than a pseudotumoral mass (Crawford 1976).

Clinical symptoms may include cutaneous lesions. Imaging studies of these small, often soft tumors are frequently inconclusive, making diagnosis difficult. The elevated risk of hemorrhage is responsible for a non-negligible mortality rate, which only 40 years ago was as high as 40%–50% (Bancroft 1931; Gentry et al. 1949). The previously constant fatal outcome of uncontrollable bleeding has improved recently, more because of the increased efficacy of reanimation and surgical procedures than because of any real improvement in diagnosis. These lesions apparently have no malignant propensity.

Cavernous hemangiomas represent one-quarter of all hemangiomas. Solitary and multiple lesions are equally common. Intraluminal growth of solitary, often polypoid lesions can cause obstruction; they range in size from several millimeters to several centimeters and are usually asymptomatic. Multiple cavernous hemangiomas, which can be considered a malformation rather than a tumoral process, may be larger than solitary tumors (up to 20 cm). Although multiple cavernous hemangiomas may occur in all layers of the gastrointestinal wall, the mucosa and the muscularis muscosa are most commonly involved. Owing to their possibly large size, diffuse cavernous hemangiomas can cause massive hemorrhage.

Capillary hemangiomas, which represent fewer than 10% of all hemangiomas (Gentry et al. 1949; Hansen 1948), are usually solitary, well-circumscribed intraluminal growths around 1 cm in diameter.

The *glomus tumor* is an exceedingly rare small lesion that can develop either intramurally or intraluminally (Ambrosius 1955).

Hemangiomatosis is often associated with another, extragastrointestinal hemangioma. It ac-

---

* Written in collaboration with A. Geoffray, A. Rogopoulos, C. Balu-Maestro.

counts for 2%–12% of all hemangiomas and cannot be differentiated grossly from diffuse cavernous hemangioma.

Multiple phlebectasia represents 40%–60% of all gastrointestinal hemangiomas. These 1–5 mm lesions usually involve the submucosa, but on rare occasions have been found in the muscularis propria and the subserosa. Two types have been identified: an autosomal dominant form occurring in Osler-Rendu-Weber disease and a non-hereditary type. Both types involve a significant risk of hemorrhage.

Lymphangiomas correspond more to malformations than to true neoplasms, even though they are classified as angiomas (Wood 1967). From a histopathogenic standpoint, gastrointestinal lymphangiomas are similar to cystic hygromas of the neck. Composed of multiple lymphatic channels surrounded by endothelial cells with a benign appearance, gastrointestinal lymphangiomas have been classified as simple, cellular (cystic), and cavernous (the most frequent form) (Watson and McCarthy 1940).

6.2 Gastrointestinal Hemangiomas

6.2.1 Esophagus

Esophageal hemangiomas are infrequent lesions that account for only 2.1% of all benign tumors of the esophagus (Plachta 1962). Some of the 56 cases reviewed by Govoni in 1982 were actually hemangioendotheliomas. The lower third of the esophagus is involved most often in literature reports; the middle and upper thirds are involved only rarely (Govoni 1982; Plachta 1962). These lesions are usually smaller than 5 cm; giant forms are exceptional (Feist et al. 1976). Esophageal hemangiomas tend to be asymptomatic, especially when small. Hemorrhage and dysphagia are infrequently reported (Vinson et al. 1926). Endoscopically, these are submucosal lesions.

Barium studies reveal the submucosal nature of these lesions, which sometimes develop intraluminally. Giant forms may suggest a tumoral process (Feist et al. 1976). Endoscopic resection is the standard treatment whenever possible.

6.2.2 Stomach

Hemangiomas represent 1.2% of all benign gastric tumors (Ming 1973; Ochsner and Janetos 1965; Plachta and Speer 1957). There is no preferential site within the stomach. Most gastric hemangiomas are smaller than 1 cm; larger lesions suggest a vascular malformation rather than a tumor (Kerekes 1964). One-quarter of all cases are diagnosed in patients under the age of 30 (Ming 1973). As for hemangiomas in other gastrointestinal sites, these lesions are usually asymptomatic. In the absence of an ulcer, bleeding in a young individual should suggest the possibility of hemangioma.

Preoperative radiologic diagnosis is possible in those rare instances when phleboliths are visualized (Flannery and Caster 1957; Kerekes 1964; Simms 1985). In the absence of this very inconstant pathognomonic sign, gastric hemangiomas may be either intramural or intraluminal.

6.2.3 Small Intestine (Figs. 6.1, 6.2)

The majority of hemangiomas occur in the small intestine. For Carlson and Good (1973), two-thirds of all gastrointestinal hemangiomas affect the small intestine, and hemangiomas account for 13.1% of all intestinal tumors (Carlson and Good 1973). The site of predilection is the jejunum, followed by the ileum;

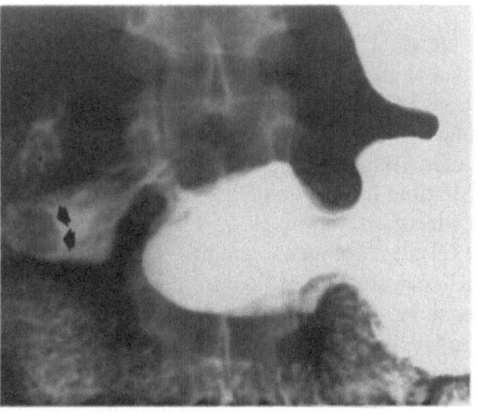

Fig. 6.1. Small duodenal bulb hemangioma *(arrows)*

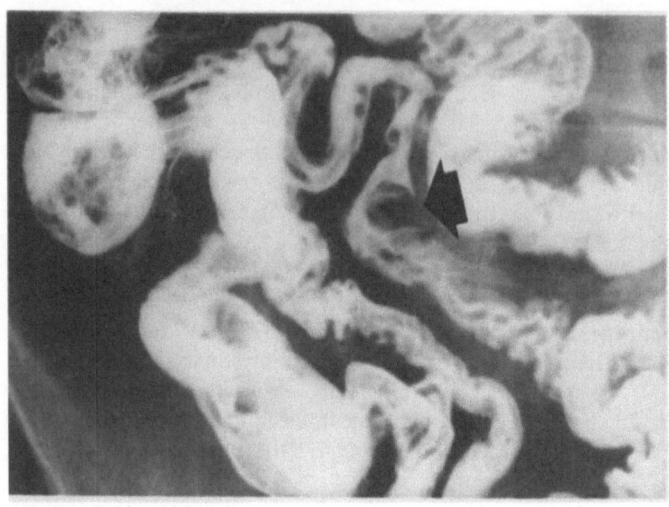

Fig. 6.2. Ileal hemangioma *(arrow)*

duodenal hemangiomas are very uncommon (2%) (Carlson and Good 1973). Multiple intestinal hemangiomas (spider telangectasias or multiple nodular angiomas) suggest Osler-Rendu-Weber syndrome (Gentry et al. 1949). Intestinal hemangiomas are usually asymptomatic. Bleeding is the major clinical symptom. Three radiologic patterns have been described:

- Often multiple, intraluminal filling defects.
- Nodular-appearing, segmental mucosal abnormalities.
- Phleboliths associated with either of the above patterns.

6.2.4 Colon and Rectum (Fig. 6.3)

Colorectal hemangiomas are rare, as Dachman et al. (1988) were able to review only 200 cases in the literature. The rectum is the site of one-half of all cases, followed by the sigmoid colon (Bancroft 1931; Dachman et al. 1988). Multiple lesions involving the majority of the entire gastrointestinal tract are rare (Mellish 1971), as are hemangiomas associated with Klippel-Trénaunay syndrome (Ghahremani et al. 1976).

Today, 75% of all colorectal hemangiomas are diagnosed before the age of 30 years (Godlust et al. 1971). The patient's age, along with the generally painless and recurrent nature of rec-

tal bleeding, may suggest the correct diagnosis and prompt further investigation by endoscopy and imaging techniques, even if the initial workup is inconclusive (Perez et al. 1987). Intussusception is rare (Ghahremani et al. 1976).

Endoscopically, extramucosal nodular deformities may or may not be identified as dilated veins. The mucosa is often congestive and edematous. Even if doubt persists following endoscopy, biopsy should be avoided because of the major risk of hemorrhage.

Radiologically, plain films may suggest the diagnosis for a tumoral mass or when phleboliths are visualized (50% of cases) (Dachman et al. 1988; Grieco and Bartone 1967; Lyon and Mantia 1984; Stening and Heptinstall 1970). Phleboliths are of unquestionable diagnostic value for several reasons:

- Because they are rarely seen in patients younger than 40 years; multiple phleboliths in a young subject suggest the diagnosis of colorectal hemangioma.
- The central distribution of these phleboliths on frontal views suggests the diagnosis (Davy-Miallou et al. 1987).
- These phleboliths tend to lie posteriorly, in the presacral space, on lateral radiographs (Marine and Lattomus 1958).

Barium studies image colorectal hemangiomas as solitary or multiple intraluminal lesions which cause scalloping of the intestinal wall.

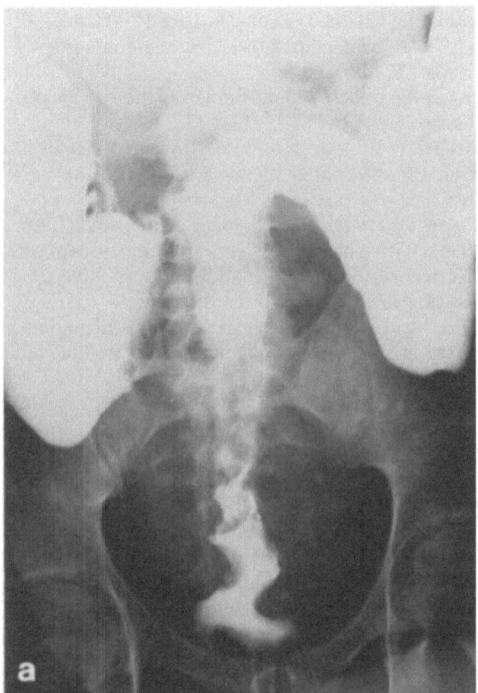

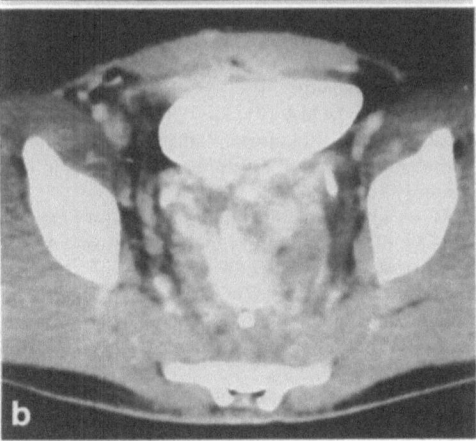

Fig. 6.3a, b. Rectal hemangioma: barium **(a)** and CT studies **(b).** Note the small intratumoral calcifications. (Courtesy of Dr. Perez, Barcelona, Spain)

A soft or rigid mass effect may be seen on post-evacuation views. Solitary, intraluminal polypoid lesions are infrequent. Circumferential lesions are fairly common in the rectum. The differential diagnoses include colitis cystica profunda, endometriosis, polypoid ulcerative colitis, and lymphoma. Angiographic studies have described both hyper- and hypo-

vascular lesions; hypovascularity is related to intratumoral thrombosis (Dachman et al. 1988; Lyon and Mantia 1984). Precontrast CT scans may demonstrate a mass containing phleboliths; subtle, non-homogeneous enhancement is noted after contrast medium injection (Perez et al. 1987). A constellation of the above findings generally allows the correct diagnosis of colorectal hemangioma.

6.3 Lymphangiomas

Gastrointestinal lymphangiomas are two times less common than hemangiomas and must be differentiated from lymphatic cysts and intestinal lymphangiectasia. Lymphatic cysts are always smaller than 1 cm and asymptomatic (Davis et al. 1987). Occasionally, an extensive lymphangioma can be distinguished from lymphangiectasia only on the basis of associated symptoms. Primary lymphangiectasia is associated with idiopathic hypoproteinemia and protein-losing enteropathy (Waldmann et al. 1961). Secondary lymphangiectasia occurs in numerous disorders, including sarcoidosis, intestinal lymphoma, carcinoma, and constrictive pericarditis.

Esophageal sites are exceedingly rare (Watson-Williams 1934). Likewise, these lesions represent only 0.5% of all benign tumors of the stomach (Ming 1973). Gastric lymphangioma presents as submucosal masses corresponding to dilated lymphatic vessels: this actually corresponds to polypoid-like lymphangiectasia (Chodack and Hurwitz 1964).

Most of the 39 cases of intestinal lymphangioma reviewed by Davis et al. (1987) occurred in the jejunum and the ileum; only eight concerned the duodenum. These often multiple, lobulated tumors are commonly responsible for obstruction. Intestinal lymphangioma associated with hemangioma may be seen in Maffucci's syndrome. As for gastric and esophageal lymphangiomas, only large intestinal lesions are symptomatic, the most common symptom being obstruction. By contrast, the risk of hemorrhage is nil (Agha et al. 1983). These intramural tumors have no radiologic features that distinguish them from other benign intestinal tumors. Intraluminal development has occasionally been reported (Davis et al. 1987).

Twenty-one cases of colonic lymphangioma were reviewed in 1983 by Agha et al. The gross, clinical, and radiologic features were similar to lymphangiomas in other parts of the gastrointestinal tract, and there were no preferential sites within the colon or rectum (Arnett and Friedman 1956; Mortensen and Anthony 1981).

6.4 References

Agha FP, Francis IR, Simms SM (1983) Cystic lymphangioma of the colon. AJR 141: 709-710

Ambrosius K (1955) Tumores primarios del intestino delgado. Rev Invest Clin 7: 503-511

Arnett NL, Friedman PS (1956) Lymphangiomas of the colon: roentgen aspects. A case report. Radiology 67: 882-885

Bancroft FW (1931) Hemangioma of the sigmoid and colon. Ann Surg 94: 828-838

Carlson HC, Good CA (1973) Neoplasms of the small bowel. In: Margulis AR, Burhenne HJ (eds). Alimentary tract radiology, 2nd edn, vol 2. Mosby, Saint Louis, pp 865-902

Chodack P, Hurwitz A (1964) Lymphangectasis of stomach simulating polypoid neoplasm. Arch Intern Med 113: 225-229

Crawford T (1976) Arteries, veins and lymphatics. In: St Clair Simmers W (ed) Systemic pathology, vol 1, 2nd edn. Churchill Livingstone, London, pp 161-162

Dachman AH, Ros PR, Shekitka KM, Buck JL, Olmsted WW, Hinton CB (1988) Colorectal hemangioma: radiologic findings. Radiology 167: 31-34

Davis M, Fenoglio-Preiser C, Haque AK (1987) Cavernous lymphangioma of the duodenum: case report and review of the literature. Gastrointest Radiol 12: 10-12

Davy-Miallou C, Legrand I, Curet P, Bellin MF, Bousquet JC, Grellet J (1987) Hemangiome rectosigmoïdien: valeur d'orientation des phlébolithes associés. A propos d'un cas. J Radiol 68: 545-548

Feist OH, Siconolfi EP, Gilman E (1976) Giant cavernous hemangioma of the esophagus. JAMA 235: 1146-1147

Flannery MG, Caster MP (1957) Hemangioma of the stomach with a roentgenologic diagnostic point. AJR 77: 38-39

Gentry RW, Dockerty MB, Clagett OT (1949) Collective review: vascular malformations and vascular tumors of the gastrointestinal tract. Int Abstr Surg 88: 281-323

Ghahremani GG, Kangarloo H, Volberg F, Meyers M (1976) Diffuse cavernous hemangioma of the colon in the Klippel-Trenaunay syndrome. Radiology 118: 673-678

Godlust D, Chalut J, Rault JJ, Bigot R, Monnier JP (1971) L'hémangiomatose rectosigmoïdienne. J Radiol 52: 108-111

Govoni AF (1982) Hemangiomas of the esophagus. Gastrointest Radiol 7: 113-117

Grieco RV, Bartone NF (1967) Roentgen visualization of phleboliths in hemangioma of the gastrointestinal tract. AJR 101: 406-408

Hansen PS (1948) Hemangioma of the small intestine. With special reference to intussusception. Review of the literature and report of three new cases. Am J Clin Pathol 18: 14-42

Kaijser R (1941) Diagnosis of cavernous hemangiomas in the digestive tract. Acta Radiol 22: 665-686

Kerekes ES (1964) Gastric hemangioma: a case report. Radiology 82: 468-469

Lyon DT, Mantia AG (1984) Large-bowel hemangiomas. Dis Colon Rectum 27: 404-414

Marine R, Lattomus WW (1958) Cavernous hemangioma of the gastrointestinal tract: report of a case and review. Radiology 70: 860-863

Mellish RWP (1971) Multiple hemangiomas of the gastrointestinal tract in children. Am J Surg 121: 412-417

Ming SC (1973) Tumors of the esophagus and stomach. Atlas of tumor pathology, 2nd series, fasc 7. AFIP, Washington

Mortensen NJM, Anthony PP (1981) Lymphangioma of the caecum. Endoscopy 13: 254-255

Ochsner SF, Janetos GP (1965) Benign tumors of the stomach. JAMA 191: 881-887

Perez C, Andreu J, Llauger J, Valls J (1987) Hemangioma of the rectum: CT appearance. Gastrointest Radiol 12: 347-349

Plachta A (1962) Benign tumors of the esophagus. Review of literature and report of 99 cases. Am J Gastroenterol 38: 639-652

Plachta A, Speer FD (1957) Gastric polyps and their relationship to carcinoma of the stomach: review of literature and report of 65 cases. Am J Gastroenterol 28: 160-175

Simms SM (1985) Gastric hemangioma associated with phleboliths. Gastrointest Radiol 10: 51-53

Stening SG, Heptinstall DP (1970) Diffuse cavernous hemangioma of the rectum and sigmoid colon. Br J Surg 57: 186-189

Vinson PP, Moore AB, Bowing HH (1926) Hemangioma of the esophagus. Report of a case. Am J Med Sci 172: 416-418

Waldmann TA, Steinfeld JL, Dutcher T, Davidson JD, Gordon RS (1961) The role of the gastrointestinal system in "idiopathic hypoproteinemia". Gastroenterology 41: 197-207

Watson WL, McCarthy WD (1940) Blood and lymph vessel tumors: a report of 1,056 cases. Surg Gynecol Obstet 71: 569-588

Watson-Williams E (1934) Specimen lymphangioma of the oesophagus. Proc Roy Soc Med 27: 1288

Wood DA (1967) Tumors of the intestines. Atlas of tumor pathology, fasc 22. AFIP, Washington

7 Benign Fibrous Tumor Tissues*

Benign fibrous tumors are rare pathologic entities occurring essentially in the esophag⸱⸱⸱ and small intestine. Extraesophageal lesions particular are easily confused with leiomy mas (Rankin and Newell 1933). Resection curati re owing to the absence of recurrence.

7.1 Esophagus (Fig. 7.1)

Fibrovascular polyps (also referred to as fibr ma, angiofibrolipomà, or fibrolipoma, c pending on the presence of certain tissue represent 21% of all benign tumors of t esophagus (Ming 1973; Plachta 1962; Schmi et al. 1961). They are the most common beni esophageal tumors after leiomyoma. In litei ture reports, the site of predilection within t esophagus is variable. For Plachta (1962) ai Schmidt et al. (1961), lesions of the lower thi of the esophagus predominate, whereas i Totten et al. (1953), the upper third is the me common site. While these polyps vary in si from 1 to 20 cm, most measure under 5 c Giant forms are encountered in the proxin third, where these pedunculated lesions rea considerable dimensions before causing clinical symptoms (Brun et al. 1986; Ming 1973). Histologically, fibrovascular polyps are sub-mucosal proliferations of mature fibrous tissue, with variable degrees of vascularization and fatty infiltration, and myxomatous modification. Inflammation is minor, and ulceration is rare (Stout and Lattes 1957). Multiple polyps are uncommon (Ming 1973), but associations with eosinophilic leukocyte infiltration (corresponding to an eosinophilic granuloma) have been reported (Leand 1968). Malignant

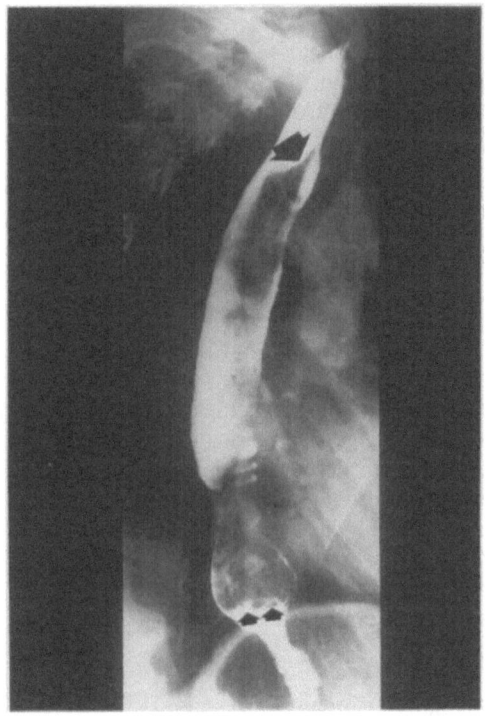

upper third *(large arrow);* the lower tip lay just above the end of the esophagus *(small arrows).* (Courtesy of Dr. Schmutz, Strasbourg, France)

degeneration is exceptional (Marcial-Rojas and Suau 1959; Stout and Lattes 1957).

Marked male predominance (72%) has been reported by Carter and Kulkarni (1984). Clinical symptoms include obstruction, dysphagia, and vomiting (Totten et al. 1953). Bleeding and painful ulceration are rare. Several older reports mention expulsion of giant lesions.

On *endoscopic examination,* these benign-appearing, pedunculated tumors may be inflam-

---

* Written in collaboration with A. Geoffray, A. Rogopoulos, and C. Balu-Maestro.

matory and ulcerated, whereas the mucosa above and below the lesion appears normal (Brun et al. 1986).

Barium studies demonstrate centrally located, more or less rounded, relatively large intraluminal lesions with well-defined limits. The contours of the esophagus are smooth and regular. The base of the tumor is not always visible. The differential diagnoses include pedunculated papilloma, intraluminal pedunculated leiomyoma, hamartoma, pedunculated angioma, pedunculated hematoma, carcinosarcoma, polypoid carcinoma, and angiosarcoma (Dieter 1970; Feldman 1939; Hinderleider et al. 1979; Lallemant et al. 1980; Shah 1975).

Endoscopic resection is indicated whenever possible for high lesions; thoracotomy is mandatory in other cases (Brun et al. 1986).

7.2 Stomach

Fibromas and fibromyxomas are both rare benign fibrous gastric tumors. Gastric fibromyxomas, which occur essentially in the antrum, are ulcerated, submucosal tumors which may attain 8 cm in diameter (Shockman and Rosen 1965). Gastric fibromas are also submucosal, but can affect any part of the stomach; they are also often ulcerated (Palmer 1951).

7.3 Small Intestine

Of all benign intestinal tumors, 3.4%–7.8% are of fibrous origin (Carlson and Good 1973; Wood 1967). These sessile or pedunculated lesions may be either intramural or intraluminal. Intraluminal lesions can cause obstruction that may prompt diagnosis. Ulceration is infrequent, but can cause bleeding. Small lesions are asymptomatic. The differential diagnosis is leiomyoma. Transitional forms between the two tumors (leiomyofibroma) are possible; pure fibromas are very rare (Rankin and Newell 1933).

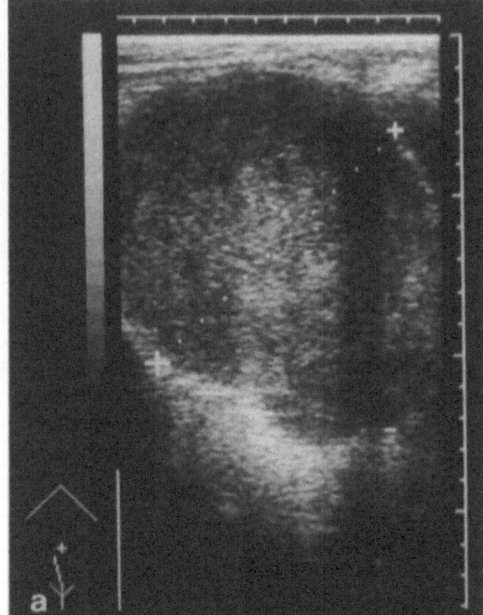

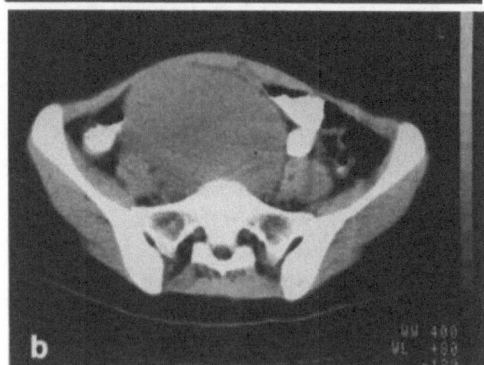

Fig. 7.2a,b. Cecal fibroma. Ultrasonography **(a)** demonstrated a solid, homogeneous mass (11 cm between the *two crosses*). CT **(b)** visualized a solid presacral mass. (Courtesy of Prof. Hoeffel, Toul, France)

7.4 Colon and Rectum (Figs. 7.2, 7.3)

Benign fibrous colorectal tumors are also very infrequent. In published reports, the left colon appears affected more often than the right colon. Only three cases of colonic fibroma of the right colon were mentioned in 45 cases reviewed by Clifton and Landry (1927). These lesions may spread either intraluminally or into the subserosa (Hoeffel et al. 1986; Rose 1972).

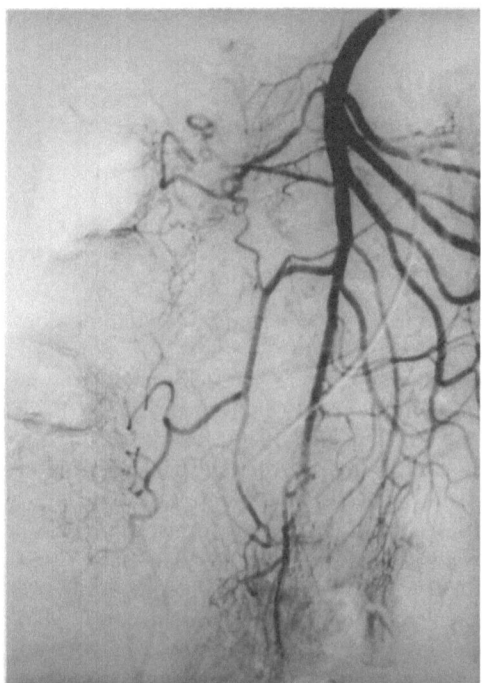

Fig. 7.3. Right colon fibroma. After opacification of the superior mesenteric artery, angiography demonstrated a lesion occupying the entire right colon, without any true hypervascularity. (Courtesy of Prof. Drouillard and Prof. Tavernier, Bordeaux, France)

7.5 Conclusion

Aside from fibrovascular polyps, benign fibrous lesions of the gastrointestinal tract have no features which permit accurate diagnosis of these rare entities prior to surgery. The most common preoperative diagnosis is leiomyoma or, for small lesions, a benign neurogenic tumor.

7.6 References

Brun JG, Maitre F, Koskas F, Celerier M, Bitoun A, Vasset M, Dubost C (1986) Polype fibrovasculaire de l'oesophage. Presse Med 15: 189–191

Carlson HC, Good CA (1973) Neoplasms of the small bowel. In: Margulis AR, Burhenne HJ (eds) Alimentary tract radiology, 2nd edn, vol 2. Mosby, Saint Louis, pp 865–902

Carter MM, Kulkarni MV (1984) Giant fibrovascular polyp of the esophagus. Gastrointest Radiol 9: 301–303

Clifton HC, Landry BB (1927) Fibromata of the intestines. Report of a case and review of the literature. Boston Med Surg J 197: 8–19

Dieter RA (1970) Pedunculated esophageal hematoma in a child. J Thorac Cardiovasc Surg 59: 851–854

Feldman M (1939) Adenocarcinomatous pedunculated polyp of the esophagus. Report of a case. Am J Dig Dis 6: 453

Hinderleider CD, Aguam AS, Wilder JR (1979) Carcinosarcoma of the esophagus. A case report and review of the literature. Int Surg 64: 13–19

Hoeffel JC, Weryha B, Dally P, Aymard B (1986) Aspects scanographiques des tumeurs du côlon à développement extra-muqueux périphérique. J Radiol 67: 137–140

Lallemant Y, Gehanno P, Cornet A (1980) Benign angiomatous pediculated tumor of the esophagus. Ann Otolaryngol Chir Cervicofac 97: 917–922

Leand PM, Murray GF, Zuidema GD, Shelley WM (1968) Obstructing esophageal polyp with eosinophilic infiltration. So-called eosinophilic granuloma. Am J Surg 116: 93–96

Marcial-Rojas RA, Suau P (1959) Epidermoid carcinoma in mucosa overlying a pedunculated lipoma of the esophagus. J Thorac Cardiovasc Surg 37: 427–434

Ming SC (1973) Tumors of esophagus and stomach. Atlas of tumor pathology, 2nd series, fasc 7. AFIP, Washington

Palmer ED (1951) Benign intramural tumors of the stomach: a review with special reference to gross pathology. Medicine 30: 81–181

Plachta A (1962) Benign tumors of the oesophagus. Review of literature and report of 99 cases. Am J Gastroenterol 38: 639–652

Rankin FN, Newell CE (1933) Benign tumors of the small intestine. Report of twenty-four cases. Surg Gynecol Obstet 57: 501–507

Rose TF (1972) True fibroma of the caecum. Med J Aust 1: 532–533

Schmidt HW, Clagett OT, Harrisson EG (1961) Benign tumors and cysts of the esophagus. J Thorac Cardiovasc Surg 41: 717–732

Shah B (1975) Hamartomatous polyp of the esophagus. Arch Surg 110: 326–328

Shockman AT, Rosen JH (1965) Fibromyxoma of the stomach. Del Med J 37: 225–228

Stout AP, Lattes R (1957) Tumors of the esophagus. Atlas of tumor pathology, fasc 20, AFIP, Washington

Totten RS, Stout AP, Humphreys GH III, Moore RL (1953) Benign tumors and cysts of the esophagus. J Thorac Cardiovasc Surg 25: 606–622

Wood DA (1967) Tumors of the intestines. Atlas of tumor pathology, fasc 22. AFIP, Washington

8 Aberrant Pancreas*

Aberrant pancreas, or pancreatic heterotopia, refers to pancreatic tissue without anatomic, vascular or neurogenic connections with the main gland (Ashikari et al. 1967; Gaspar Fuentes et al. 1973). Despite their heterotopic character, these intramural lesions are included in the part on benign tumors because of their frequency and neoplastic radiographic appearance. Furthermore, a small percentage of these lesions undergo malignant degeneration comparable to that which can be observed in the pancreas itself.

8.1 General Features

The general features discussed hereafter were defined from a review of 573 cases in the literature (Lai and Tompkins 1986; Nicolau et al. 1983). Although not uncommon, pancreatic heterotopia is often an incidental finding; the frequency in autopsy series is 0.5%–5.6% (Ashikari et al. 1967; Barbosa et al. 1946; Barrocas et al. 1973; Pearson 1951). For Feldman and Weinberg (1952), the incidence is higher in the duodenum, and especially in children (up to 15% of cases). In surgical series, the frequency of aberrant pancreas varies from 0.2% to 0.8% (Barbosa et al. 1946; Busard and Walter 1950; Nakao et al. 1980).

Compared to other benign gastrointestinal tumors, aberrant pancreas is relatively rare. This is particularly true in the stomach, where it accounts for only 15% of benign gastric tumors (Debray et al. 1978; Potet and Duclert 1970) and is thus less common than gastric adenoma or leiomyoma (Ochsner and Janetos 1965). In the duodenum, aberrant pancreas is the most

common benign tumor after adenoma (Albot et al. 1959).

Heterotopic pancreas is usually small, ranging in size from 0.1 to 5 cm (Barrocas et al. 1973; Lai and Tompkins 1986); gastric lesions are usually the largest. Aberrant pancreatic tissue causing clinical symptoms appears to be larger in size than asymptomatic forms. Of 136 cases reviewed, 79.4% were smaller than 2 cm, 17.6% were between 2 and 4 cm, and only 3% were larger than 4 cm (Nicolau et al. 1983). There is generally a single focus of aberrant pancreas; double and triple lesions are exceptional (Debord et al. 1981; Feldman and Weinberg 1952).

Approximately 70% of all cases of aberrant pancreas occur in the gastrointestinal tract (Frank et al. 1968). The bile ducts, and in particular the gallbladder, are the most common extragastrointestinal sites (Dolan et al. 1974; Leger et al 1979); involvement of the main bile duct is less common (Sabini et al. 1970). The liver (Mobini et al. 1974), the hilus of the spleen, and the pancreatico-splenic omentum may also harbor heterotopic pancreas (Dolan et al. 1974). Other sites are exceptional, especially in the thorax (Beskin 1961; Tilson and Touloukian 1972).

The most frequent gastrointestinal sites are the stomach and the duodenum. In our literature review of 528 cases, site frequencies were as follows: stomach (56.7%), duodenum (27.7%), jejunum (9.7%), Meckel's diverticulum (4.3%) (Lai and Tompkins 1986; Witczak and Badowski 1979), ileum (0.2%) (Anseline et al. 1981), esogastric junction (0.6%), esophagus (0.2%) (Razi 1966). These figures correspond to earlier studies in which the stomach and the duodenum represented over 60% of all cases in the gastrointestinal tract (Krieg 1940; Poppi 1935). In the stomach, involvement of the antrum accounts for 90.8% of cases; the midsto-

---

* Written in collaboration with A. Geoffray, A. Rogopoulos, and C. Balu-Maestro.

mach is affected in only 9.2% of cases. In the duodenum, aberrant pancreas has a predilection for the second segment (60% of cases), followed by the duodenal bulb and the first segment (34.5%), and the third duodenum (5.5%) (Nicolau et al. 1983). These figures correspond to earlier literature reviews that dealt essentially with antropyloric and second duodenum lesions (Feldman and Weinberg 1952; Palmer 1951).

Heterotopic pancreatic tissue may occur in all layers of the gastrointestinal tract wall, but the majority are found in the submucosa (57% of cases), followed by the muscularis (28%), the subserosa (10%), and the mucosa (5%) (Nicolau et al. 1983).

A four-stage histologic classification has been proposed (Jochimsen et al. 1981):

Type I   Complete, containing all of the usual components of pancreatic tissue
Type II Pancreatic exocrine tumors, without islet cells
Type III Pancreatic endocrine tumors, with islet cells and excretory ducts
Type IV Pure ductal tumors, containing only excretory ducts, which have a tendency for cystic degeneration (Leger et al. 1974)

Owing to the frequency of asymptomatic lesions, complications related to aberrant pancreas are hard to quantify (adenomatous transformation, cystic dystrophy, cystadenoma, or carcinoma). Adenomatous transformation generally involves development of a non-insulin-secreting islet cell adenoma responsible for Zollinger-Ellison syndrome; this complication was especially well studied by Hivet et al. (1971).

Accurate diagnosis of the small ectopic nodule as an ulcerogenic tumor conditions the therapeutic approach, because aberrant pancreas can be managed by simple resection with only partial gastrectomy.

Insulin-secreting islet cell adenoma is less common and produces a hypoglycemic syndrome (Leger et al. 1979). This heterotopia is usually small, often lying outside the gastrointestinal tract (retroperitoneum, splenic hilus, omentum).

Cystic degeneration, a complication investigated by Leger et al. (1974), occurs only in ductal

structures. These lesions can attain considerable dimensions which are responsible for bile duct compression. Duodenal sites are most prevalent (Leger et al. 1974; Murat et al. 1971; Potet and Duclert 1970).

Cystadenomatous transformation of aberrant pancreas is exceptional (Fresnel et al. 1971), but the large dimensions of such lesions may cause gastrointestinal stenosis.

Non-insulin-secreting islet cell carcinoma is very rare (Andretta and Cirri 1967; Barbosa et al. 1946; Barrocas et al. 1973; Hickman et al. 1981). Pancreatic heterotopia appears to have no malignant potential (Barrocas et al. 1973), even though malignant degeneration of an aberrant pancreas has been entertained as a possibility in connection with glandular gastric carcinoma (Barrocas et al. 1973; Debray et al. 1978).

Aberrant pancreas is discovered in men more often than in women (sex ratio 2:1). Diagnosis is most often made in individuals aged 30–50 years. Clinically asymptomatic forms are very common (65.6% for Dolan et al. 1974), and heterotopic pancreas is often discovered fortuitously at diagnosis of another lesion. Determination of the respective role of each lesion in the clinical symptomatology can thus be difficult.

Table 8.1 summarizes the clinical symptoms reported for 146 review cases, with solitary symptomatic aberrant pancreas having been differentiated from heterotopia associated with another lesion. Despite the absence of pathognomonic signs, 16.1% of all symptomatic cases mentioned bleeding. Biliary obstruction may be caused by a juxta-ampullary lesion (Berenguer et al. 1972; Hivet et al. 1971; Krivine et al. 1964) or a complication, such as cystic dystrophy of an aberrant pancreas in the second duodenum (Leger et al. 1974; Potet and Duclert 1970; Prandi et al. 1972). Hypoglycemia (Leger et al. 1979), Zollinger-Ellison syndrome, and upper gastrointestinal tract stenosis (Matsumoto et al. 1975) have also been reported occasionally.

Endoscopically, aberrant pancreas manifests as a firm, regular chamois yellow nodule with duct-like structures in its center. Endoscopy can visualize 80% of cases and correctly identifies the lesion as a benign tumor or even aberrant pancreas (if typical features are pre-

Table 8.1. Clinical symptoms at diagnosis of aberrant pancreas (146 patients, excluding asymptomatic cases)

Symptom	Overall frequency (146 cases)	Sympto-matic, solitary aberrant pancreas (93 cases)	Aberrant pancreas associated with another gastrointesti-nal lesion (53 cases)
Abdominal pain	60.2%	60.2%	60.3%
Nausea/vomiting	19.2%	18.2%	20.7%
Hemorrhage (clinical or occult)	18.5%	16.1%	22.6%
Biliary obstruction	7.5%	10.8%	0.2%
Upper gastrointestinal stenosis	4.8%	7.5%	–
Deterioration in general condition	4.8%	6.5%	0.2%

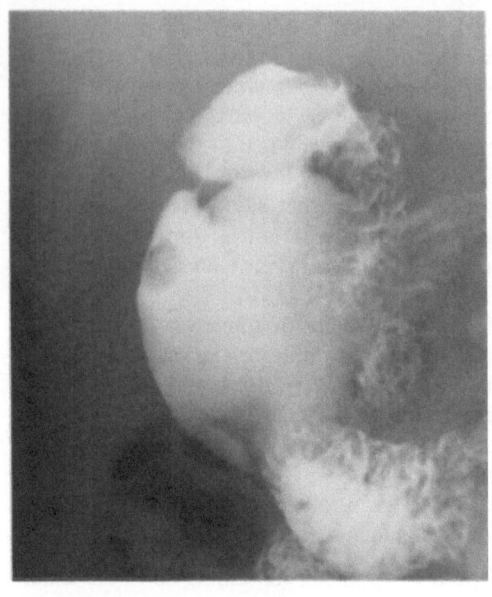

Fig. 8.1. Small lesion in the gastric antrum (aberrant pancreas)

sent) 50% of the time (Lai and Tompkins 1986; Lagache et al 1980; Lukash et al. 1970; Rose et al. 1980; Stone et al. 1971).

Therapeutic approaches for aberrant pancreas depend on radiologic and endoscopic findings. Owing to the potential risk of malignant degeneration, most authors recommend simple resection (Dupuy et al. 1963; Frank et al. 1968; Leger et al. 1979). Complicated forms may require more radical procedures, and possibly even duodenopancreatectomy. However, Hickman et al. (1981) recommend that all lesions under 3 cm merely be monitored by radiology and endoscopy; these authors reserve surgery for larger lesions or those for which modification is visualized on serial studies.

8.2 Imaging (Figs. 8.1–8.3)

Barium examinations were negative in 23.7% of the cases reviewed (Nicolau et al. 1983). A lesion with the typical appearance (a small, well-defined intramural mass with a central umbilication) can be accurately diagnosed as a benign tumor or even aberrant pancreas. Failure to correctly diagnose aberrant pancreas can have several causes:

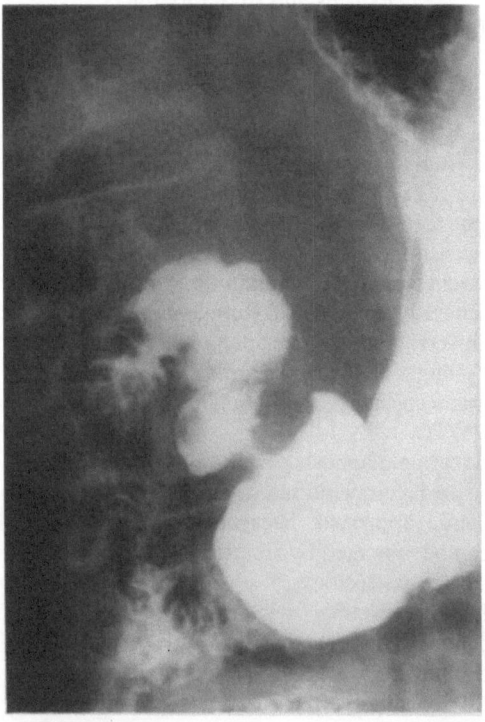

Fig. 8.2. Aberrant pancreas in the prepyloric region of the gastric antrum

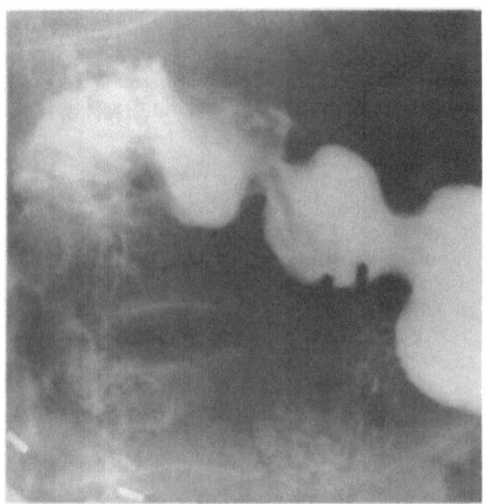

Fig. 8.3. Aberrant pancreas in the duodenal bulb

- Rare pedunculated lesions (Hivet et al. 1971); subserosal lesion responsible for pseudo-extrinsic compression.
- A hemorrhagic complication preventing satisfactory radiologic study, causing the lesion to be overlooked
- Misinterpretation of radiologic films because a concurrent ulcerating or tumoral lesion susceptible to explain clinical symptomatology is clearly seen.
- Above all, complication by cystic dystrophy, producing atypical radiologic images such as stenosis.

Non-complicated aberrant pancreas has occasionally been explored by angiography (Fujii et al. 1972), but detection of moderate hypervascularization did not allow diagnosis.

8.3 Conclusion

Aberrant pancreas is a rare, usually asymptomatic tumor discovered fortuitously. Endoscopy and radiologic examinations generally permit diagnosis. Radioendoscopic surveillance can be proposed for small lesions in the stomach or duodenum; surgery can be reserved for lesions likely to create complications because of their location (ampullary region) or large dimensions.

8.4 References

Albot G, Poilleux F, Cherigie E, Berthet G, Saint-Quen C (1959) Hémorragies par tumeurs bénignes de la deuxième portion du duodénum. Tumeurs de la papille exceptées. Arch Fr Mal Appar Dig 48: 129-152

Andretta O, Cirri GP (1967) Sul pancreas aberrante del canale alimentare e sulla sua transformazione neoplastica. Arch De Vecchi Anat Pathol 49: 959-982

Anseline P, Grundfest S, Carrey W, Weiss R (1981) Pancreatic heterotopia. A rare cause of bowel obstruction. Surgery 90: 110-113

Ashikari R, Roberts M, Dreiling DA (1967) Duodenal ulcer in aberrant pancreas: case report and review of literature. J Mt Sinaï Hosp 34: 111-115

Barbosa JJ, Dockerty MB, Waugh JM (1946) Pancreatic heterotopia: review of the literature and report of 41 authenticated surgical cases, of which 25 were clinically significant. Surg Gynecol Obstet 82: 527-542

Barrocas A, Fontenelle LJ, Williams MJ (1973) Gastric heterotopic pancreas: a case report and review of literature. Am Surg 39: 361-365

Berenguer J, Sala T, Carrasquer J, Rodrigo M, Garrido G, Pertejo V (1972) Pancreas aberrante duodenal, causa exceptional ictericia obstructiva. A proposito de una observacion. Rev Esp Enferm Apar Dig 36: 567-571

Beskin CA (1961) Intralobar enteric sequestration of the lung containing aberrant pancreas. J Thorac Cardiovasc 41: 314-317

Busard JM, Walter W (1950) Heterotopic pancreatic tissue: report of a case presenting symptoms of ulcer and review of the recent literature. Arch Surg 60: 674-682

Debord JR, Majarakis JD, Nyhus LM (1978) An unusual case of heterotopic pancreas of the stomach. Am J Surg 141: 269-273

Debray CH, Leymarios J, Benhamou G, Marche C (1978) Triple lésion antrale: double néoplasme (dont un développé sur une cicatrice ulcéreuse) et pancréas aberrant. Sem Hop 54: 163-167

Dolan RV, Remine WH, Dockerty MB (1974) The fate of heterotopic pancreatic tissue. A study of 212 cases. Arch Surg 109: 762-765

Dupuy R, Vallin J, D'Oblonsky A, Pagniez G (1963) Pancréas aberrant. Rev Int Hepatol 13: 439-454

Feldman M, Weinberg T (1952) Aberrant pancreas: a cause of duodenal syndrome. JAMA 148: 893-898

Frank P, Blum H, Eisenbeth R, Philippe E (1968) Les pancréas aberrants intragastriques (à propos de 4 cas). Bull Assoc Nord Loth Gastroenterol 19: 399-403

Fresnel P, Sibilly A, Foucher G, Fresnel PL (1971) Cystadénome pancréatique ectopique. Presse Med 79: 2496

Fujii K, Yamagata S, Suzuki J, Sasaki R, Shoji T, Makabe M, Memezawa H (1972) Angiographic features of submucosal tumours of the stomach. Toheku J Exp Med 107: 287-299

Gaspar Fuentes A, Campos Tarrech JM, Fernandez Burgui JL, Castellis Tejon E, Ruiz Rossello J, Gomez Perez J, Armengol Miro J (1973) Ectopias pancreaticas. Rev Esp Enferm Apar Dig 39: 255-268

Hickman DM, Frey CF, Carson JW (1981) Adenocarcinoma arising in gastric heterotopic pancreas. West J Med 135: 57-62

Hivet M, Moinet PH, Lagadec B, Vivier J, Poilleux J (1971) Le syndrome de Zollinger-Ellison sur pancréas aberrants duodénaux. Tumeurs ulcérogènes du duodénum (à propos de 5 observations). Ann Chir 25: 883-894

Jochimsen PR, Shirazi SS, Lewis JW (1981) Symptomatic ectopic pancreas relieved by surgical excision. Surg Gynecol Obstet 153: 49-52

King EG (1940) Heterotopic pancreatic tissue producing pyloric obstruction. Ann Surg 113: 364-370

Krivine JM, Hivet M, Levame M (1964) Les tumeurs apparemment bénignes du duodénum. Ann Chir 18: 588-600

Lagache G, Combemale B, Triboulet JP (1980) Les pancréas aberrants gastriques. Neuf observations. Ann Chir 34: 44-47

Lai ECS, Tompkins RK (1986) Heterotopic pancreas. Review of a 26 year experience. Am J Surg 151: 697-700

Leger L, Lemaigre G, Lenriot JP (1974) Kystes sur hétérotopies pancréatiques de la paroi duodénale. Nouv Presse Med 3: 2309-2314

Léger L, Louvel A, Chiche B, Michali P (1979) Les hétérotopies pancréatiques. A propos de 8 nouveaux cas. J Chir 116: 553-560

Lukash WM, Johnson RB, Bishop RP (1970) Aberrant pancreas in the stomach: radiographic and gastroscopic findings. Gastrointest Endoscop 16: 148-150

Matsumoto Y, Kawai Y, Kimura K (1975) Aberrant pancreas causing pyloric obstruction. Surgery 76: 827-829

Mobini J, Krouse TB, Cooper DR (1974) Intrahepatic pancreatic heterotopia: review and report of a case presenting as an abdominal mass. Am J Dig Dis 19: 64-70

Murat J, Gignoux M, Lesbros F (1971) Dystrophie kystique sur pancréas aberrant du bulbe duodénal (un cas avec symptomatologie clinique). Ann Chir 25: 1203-1208

Nakao T, Yanoh K, Itoh A (1980) Aberrant pancreas in Japan. Review of the literature and report of 12 surgical cases. Med J Osaka Univ 30: 57-63

Nicolau A, Bruneton JN, Balu C, Aubanel D, Roux P (1983) Etude radiologique du pancréas aberrant de topographie gastroduodénale. A propos de 11 observations. J Radiol 64: 319-324

Ochsner SF, Janetos GP (1965) Benign tumors of the stomach. JAMA 191: 881-889

Palmer ED (1951) Benign intramural tumors of the stomach: a review with special reference to gross pathology. Medicine 30: 81-181

Pearson S (1951) Aberrant pancreas. Review of the literature and report of three cases, one of which produced common and pancreatic duct obstruction. Arch Surg 63: 168-184

Poppi A (1935) Sui pancreas aberranti. Arch Ital Mal Appar Dig 4: 534-579

Potet F, Duclert N (1970) Dystophie kystique sur pancréas aberrant de la paroi abdominale. Arch Fr Mal Appar Dig 59: 223-238

Prandi D, Maillard JN, Potet F (1972) Traitement chirurgical de la dystrophie kystique sur pancréas aberrant de la paroi duodénale (à propos de 3 cas). Arch Fr Mal Appar Dig 61: 193-198

Razi MD (1966) Ectopic pancreatic tissue of oesophagus with massive upper gastrointestinal bleeding. Arch Surg 92: 101-104

Rose C, Kessaram RA, Lind JF (1980) Ectopic gastric-pancreas: a review and report of 4 cases. Diagn Imag 49: 214-218

Sabini AM, Baden JP, Norman JD, Martin JR (1970) Heterotopic pancreatic tissue in the common bile duct or ampulla of Vater. Am Surg 36: 662-666

Stone DD, Riddervold HO, Keats TE (1971) An unusual case of aberrant pancreas in the stomach. A roentgenographic and gastrophotographic demonstration. AJR 113: 125-128

Tilson MD, Touloukian RJ (1972) Mediastinal enteric sequestration with aberrant pancreas: a formes frustres of the intralobar sequestration. Ann Surg 176: 669-671

Witczak W, Badowski A (1979) Przypadek heterotopii trzustki w uchylku meckela. Wiad Lek 32: 33-35

9 Endometriosis*

Intestinal endometriosis is defined as the presence of functional or non-functional endometrial tissue in the intestinal wall. It is generally associated with genital endometriosis.

9.1 General Features

Although hard to determine, the frequency of gastrointestinal endometriosis has been estimated at between 1% and 11% (MacCaffee and Friedmann 1960; Tedeschi and Massand 1971). This variation in frequency may be related to the different definitions used for intestinal endometriosis. Certain authors include all cases of endometriosis of the abdominal cavity that are accompanied by gastrointestinal manifestations, whereas others reserve the term for lesions that infiltrate the intestinal wall, i.e., endometriomas (Caligaris et al. 1982).

Two anatomic types have been described:

- Solitary gastrointestinal endometriosis: the extensive associated fibrosis is responsible for stenotic phenomena. Differentiation of benign endometrioma from a malignant lesion requires surgery.
- Intestinal endometriosis, which may be accompanied by genital endometriosis: this pathology may present as disseminated minimal lesions or as extensive infiltration of the entire posterior stage of the pelvis. Histologically, glandular endometrial tubes are evident. These heterotopic foci (hemorrhagic and microcystic) are surrounded by a double barrier (histocytomacrophagic cells and fibrous collagen) which reorganizes the intestinal wall, creating adherences. The possibility of carcinoma can usually be ruled out because the intestinal mucosa is intact, but mucosal ulcerations may be present (Henson 1964). Malignant transformation, although possible (Brooks and Wheeler 1977), is exceptional, and it is even rarer than ovarian endometriosis, which accounts for only 1% of all cases (Brooks and Wheeler 1977).

Sites of involvement in the gastrointestinal tract reported by Tedeschi and Massand (1971), in decreasing order of frequency, were: rectosigmoid (72%), rectum (13.5%), terminal ileum (7%), cecum (3.6%), and appendix (3%).

Three mechanisms have been implicated to explain the development of endometriosis in such diverse sites as the gastrointestinal tract, the genital organs, the integuments, and the lungs: tubal propagation, propagation through the lymphatics, and venous propagation (Caligaris et al. 1982; Ranney 1980). A hereditary factor has also been described (Ranney 1980).

Women are affected while genitally active and most commonly around 40 years of age. The associated or promoting factors are the same as for genital endometriosis (primary sterility, genital lesions such as uterine fibroma, follicular ovarian cyst, endometrial hyperplasia).

Clinical manifestations suggest an intestinal pathology in less than one-third of cases. In the remaining two-thirds, intestinal endometriosis is asymptomatic and is an incidental finding at coelioscopy or at gynecologic surgery. Even when present, abdominal pain, rectal bleeding, diarrhea, and chronic obstruction are not always cyclic or correlated with menstruation. Acute complications and intussusception are rare (Swann 1962). Functional gynecologic signs exist in fewer than 25% of

---

* Written in collaboration with A. Geoffray, A. Rogopoulos, and C. Balu-Maestro.

patients (bleeding, dyspareunia, dysmenor-
rhea). Rectal endometriosis may be detected
by digital rectal examination (Ponka et al.
1973).

Endoscopy may identify a non-ulcerated submucosal swelling or diffuse, small submucosal
nodules. In other cases, narrowing may be
demonstrated, in particular at the rectosigmoid junction, with a folded and congestive
mucosa. Coelioscopy is the must effective
technique for confirmation of genital endometriosis and demonstration of spread towards the rectosigmoid (Ponka et al. 1973).

Medical treatment consists in administration
of steroid hormones to atrophy the endometri-
um; an anti-gonatropic steroid with a low an-
drogenic activity is currently used (Lauersen
et al. 1975). Fibrous stenosis rarely responds to
medical therapy and is an indication for surgical resection.

9.2 Imaging

Barium studies and ultrasonography are the
two imaging techniques of choice. Abnormalities demonstrated on barium films include:

– More or less long, pliable sections of eccentric stenosis with smooth borders.
– Polypoid or sessile appearance, with intact
  mucosa.
– Mucosal folds lying close together (Culver
  et al. 1958; Lilja and Probst 1966).

These images have no specificity, and the clinical context may suggest carcinosis rather than
a primary malignant tumor. On lateral films,
deformation of the anterior wall at the level of
the rectosigmoid junction is usually diagnosed
as carcinosis. Polypoid lesions have been observed in the cecum (Figs. 9.1-9.3.)

Pelvic ultrasonography may suggest the diagnosis when cystic lesions are visualized. Sonograms of infiltrating lesions may appear normal, but hysterography will demonstrate pathognomonic diverticular images in the uterus.

Owing to its rarity, gastrointestinal endometriosis is rarely diagnosed radiologically. Infiltrating lesions without any associated clinical
gynecologic symptoms may be diagnosed as
carcinosis. Endometriomas sometimes occur

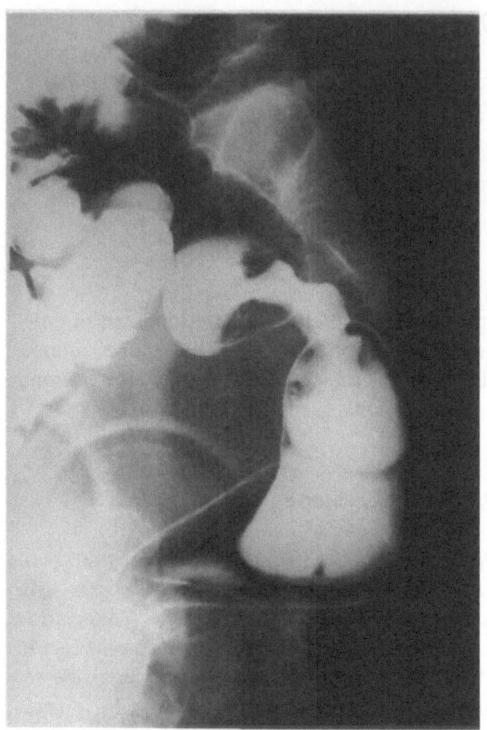

Fig. 9.1. Colorectal stenosis caused by endometriosis. (Courtesy of Dr. Schmutz, Strasbourg, France)

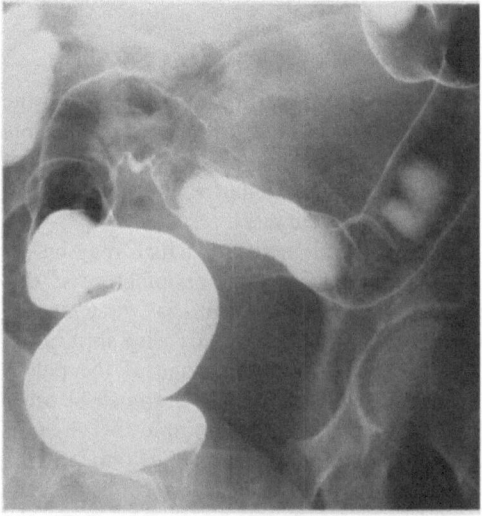

Fig. 9.2. Moderate stenosis of the sigmoid caused
by pelvic endometriosis

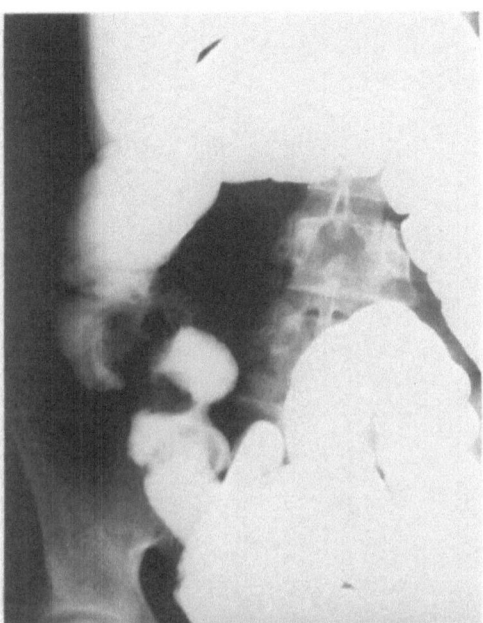

Fig. 9.3. Ileocecal stenosis caused by pelvic endometriosis

in relatively elderly patients and may cause partial obstruction that prompts investigation and diagnosis. The only finding which goes against diagnosis of a primary malignant tumor is the fact that the mucosa usually appears intact, both radiologically and endoscopically.

9.3 References

Brooks JJ, Wheeler JE (1977) Malignancy arising in extragonadal endometriosis. A case report and summary of the world literature. Cancer 40: 3065-3073

Caligaris P, Ducassou MJ, Masselot R, Maurin B, Cardon JM, Bricot R (1982) L'endométriose digestive. Conceptions actuelles. J Chir (Paris) 119: 693-698

Culver GJ, Pereira RM, Seibel R (1958) Radiographic features of rectosigmoid endometriosis. Am J Obstet Gynecol 76: 1176-1184

Henson SW (1964) Endometrioma of the rectum simulating carcinoma. JAMA 187: 1026-1027

Lauersen NH, Wilson KH, Birnbaum S (1975) Danazol: an antigonatropic agent in the treatment of pelvic endometriosis. Am J Obstet Gynecol 123: 742-747

Lilja B, Probst F (1966) Intestinal endometriosis. Acta Radiol [Diagn] 4: 545-556

MacCaffee HG, Friedmann AI (1960) Intestinal endometriosis. Obstet Gynecol Br Emp 67: 549-555

Ponka JL, Brush BE, Hodgkinson CP (1973) Colorectal endometriosis. Dis Colon Rectum 16: 490-499

Ranney B (1980) Etiology, prevention, and inhibition of endometriosis. Clin Obstet Gynecol 23: 875-883

Swann M (1962) An endometrioma of the caecum causing an intussusception. Br J Surg 50: 199-202

Tedeschi LG, Massand GD (1971) Endometriosis of the intestine: a report of seven cases. Dis Colon Rectum 14: 360-365

Malignant Tumors

10 Carcinoma of the Esophagus*

Despite the wide variation in the frequency of esophageal cancer from one country to another, the prognosis is constantly poor, although high-risk patients may benefit from endoscopy and barium studies. Certain esophageal conditions and a number of dietary and environmental factors are known to promote this type of cancer. Modern imaging techniques, and CT in particular, have acquired diagnostic value because they can determine "resectability". A tumor can be considered operable when complete, potentially curative surgical resection appears possible. In addition to their role in disease staging, imaging studies are indicated for post-therapy follow-up and detection of metastatic disease. Imaging data are also used to select palliative procedures aimed at improving the quality of patient survival. Epidermoid cancers, which account for 90% of all esophageal malignancies, must be differentiated from adenocarcinoma, a much rarer pathology associated with particular circumstances warranting separate discussion.

10.1 Pathology

10.1.1 Epidemiology

In the United States, cancer of the esophagus accounts for 1% of all cancers and 7% of all gastrointestinal tract malignancies (Thompson 1983, 1985). The incidence varies by geographic region from 10 to 260 per 100 000 population. Esophageal carcinoma reaches endemic proportions in Asia, in a zone extending along the northern and eastern shores of Iran, the Caspian sea, and into Kazakhstan, Uzbekistan and China. The incidence in northern

Iran is particularly high: 174 in 100 000 (Rosenberg et al. 1982). Endemic clusters have also been found in France and South Africa (Silber 1985).

Male predominance occurs worldwide, except in Iran. However, male predilection appears more important for adenocarcinoma than for epidermoid lesions (Sjogren and Johnson 1983; Wang et al. 1986). A certain racial predominance has also been noted, particularly in the United States, where esophageal cancer is much more common among blacks and Porto Ricans than in whites.

Mean patient age at diagnosis is between 40 and 60 years. Esophageal cancer is exceptional in childhood (Moore 1958), although adenocarcinoma tends to affect younger patients than epidermoid lesions.

10.1.2 Pathogenesis

Implicated etiologic agents include dietary and environmental factors, pre-existing chronic esophageal lesions, genetic factors, and certain associated tumors.

10.1.2.1 Dietary and Environmental Factors

Smoking and alcohol consumption are the prime risk factors. Alcohol intake appears especially linked to lesions of the middle third of the esophagus (Kuylenstierna and Munck-Wickland 1985). The role of tobacco abuse and alcohol appears to be more important for the development of adenocarcinoma than for epidermoid carcinoma (Wang et al 1986; Weisburger et al. 1982). Other factors implicated in certain regions include boiling-hot tea, silicone fibers, and mycotoxin-contaminated food. Associations with dietary deficiencies in

---

* Written in collaboration with P. J. Valette.

vitamin C, riboflavin, vitamin E, magnesium, zinc, and molybdenum have also been reported (Correa 1982; Schottenfeld 1984). The role of vitamin A remains controversial. Esophageal cancer tends to occur in individuals whose diet is poor in fats and animal proteins and rich in carbohydrates. The exact etiologic agents and mechanism of carcinogenesis remain unclear, even though several substances (i.e., nitrosomines) have been found to cause experimental cancers in animals (Schottenfeld 1984).

10.1.2.2 Pre-existing Chronic Esophageal Lesions

Esophageal cancer develops with an inhabitual frequency in certain chronic conditions:

- Scar tissue formation after lye strictures (Hopkins and Postlewait 1981) or, exceptionally, after thoracic irradiation for a benign tumor or malignancy such as lung carcinoma, breast cancer, or Hodgkin's disease (Goffman et al. 1983; Jones et al. 1985; O'Connell et al. 1984; Scherrill et al. 1984). Maeta et al. (1986) cited anterior gastrectomy as a promoting factor for esophageal cancer. Scar tissue formation can lead to an epithelioma (usually squamous cell) which may remain clinically silent for long intervals (10–50 years).
- Inflammatory lesions: esophageal tumors that develop from megaesophagus (approximately 8% of all esophageal cancers) are similar to the lesions which develop on scar tissue: they tend to be epidermoid and evolve over relatively long periods (20 years).
- Peptic esophagitis: patients in whom peptic esophagitis is complicated by brachyesophagus or stenosis may ultimately develop cancer. The frequency has been put at around 2.3%–9% in individuals with endobrachyesophagus(Kuylenstierna and Munck-Wickland 1985). Most of these tumors are adenocarcinomas situated in the lower third of the esophagus (Halpert et al. 1983; Wang et al. 1986).
- Other chronic lesions: Plummer-Vinson syndrome, on rare occasions, a tumor which develops from a diverticulum (Saldana et al. 1982) or degeneration of a benign tumor.

Chronic esophagitis favored by stasis or reflux is a common feature of these long-standing esophageal lesions. In many instances, the malignancy is promoted by factors such as alcohol and smoking. Other mechanisms can intervene in the lower esophagus. Carcinogenesis of complicated reflux esophagitis appears related to cylindrical metaplastic epithelialization of the peptic ulcers. This process is accompanied by dysplasia, which is especially severe when the Barrett epithelium acquires the mucosal features of the gastric cardia.

10.1.2.3 Genetic Factors

An association of esophageal cancer and tylosis is the only known genetic link, and 70% of all patients with tylosis develop esophageal cancer. Familial clusters have, however, been reported on the shores of the Caspian Sea (Ghadirian 1985).

10.1.2.4 Associated Tumors

The similarity of the squamous cell epithelial lining and exposure to the same aggressive agents (alcohol, tobacco) explain the frequent association with a head and neck malignancy. One percent of all head and neck cancers are associated with a synchronous or metachronous esophageal lesion (Thompson et al. 1978). Discovery of an esophageal tumor or a head and neck cancer should systematically prompt searches for other disease foci in these regions, it being remembered that such lesions are often latent.

10.2 Anatomic Features

10.2.1 Macroscopic Features

The three most commonly encountered tumoral forms, in order of decreasing frequency, are polypoid lesions, ulcerations, and infiltrative cancer. Associations of these three types occur in 22% of cases. Superficially spreading lesions are rare.

10.2.2 Location

Both French and American series cite the middle third of the esophagus as the most common location (50% of cases), followed by the lower third (30%) and the upper third (15%) (Thompson 1983).

10.2.3 Histology

Epidermoid lesions, which account for 90% of all esophageal cancers (Postlethwait 1978; Rosenberg et al. 1982), include a variety of malignant epithelial tumors (Rosenberg et al. 1982)·

- Squamous cell carcinoma (well, moderately, or poorly differentiated).
- Variants of squamous cell carcinoma (spindle cell carcinoma, pseudosarcoma, verrucous carcinoma , carcinoma in situ).
- Adenocarcinoma, adenocanthoma.
- Adenoid cystic carcinoma (cylindroma).
- Mucoepidermoid carcinoma.
- Adenosquamous carcinoma.
- Undifferentiated carcinoma.
- Oat cell carcinoma.

Epidermoid cancer clearly predominates in the upper and middle thirds of the esophagus. Adenocarcinoma, which represents 60% of all cancers of the lower third (Wang et al. 1986), must be differentiated from epithelioma of the gastric cardia that has spread to the distal esophagus.

Examination of the esophagectomy specimen may reveal a second disease focus (often more distal than proximal) and/or an intraepithelial cancer near, or at some distance from the main lesion. Multiple lesions are present in 3.1%-10.6% of all cases (Parisot et al. 1985; Reboud et al. 1983).

10.2.4 Patterns of Spread

10.2.4.1 Review of the Vascularization of the Esophagus

The cervical esophagus is irrigated by the lower thyroid artery, the thoracic segment by the bronchial arteries, and the lower portion by the gastric artery and the left inferior diaphragmatic branches of the abdominal aorta. The cervical esophagus is drained by the lower thyroid veins; the thoracic portion is drained by the azygos vein, the hemi-azygos vein, and the accessory hemi-azygos vein. The abdominal esophagus drains into both the azygos vein and the left gastric vein, which is a branch of the portal venous system. The lymphatic drainage network of the esophagus corresponds to the arterial irrigation. The lymphatic channels draining the cervical esophagus empty into the deep cervical nodes, either directly or indirectly through the retropharyngeal or paratracheal nodes. The lymphatics of the thoracic esophagus empty into the posterior mediastinal nodes; the lymphatics of the abdominal esophagus empty into the left gastric nodes. The rich lymphatic networks of the mucosa, submucosa, and muscularis can extend for several centimeters both above and below a region. Because of the longitudinal nature of this extensive nodal system, esophageal tumors tend to spread into the submucosa while leaving the mucosa intact. This complex lymphatic network is also responsible for the frequency of extensive nodal metastases in patients with esophageal cancer.

10.2.4.2 Local Extension

The laxity of the esophageal submucosa and the rich blood-lymphatic network explain the development of intraepithelial disease sites at a distance from the primary tumor; such lesions must be distinguished from multifocal neoplasms. Absence of a serosa in the esophagus permits direct, early tumoral extension, thus explaining the poor prognosis of even small lesions (Soga et al. 1982).

Distant Spread. Owing to the nature of the lymphatic vascularization and drainage of the esophagus, lymphatic involvement cannot be predicted as a function of the site of the cancer. For example, the subdiaphragmatic nodes are invaded in an average of 59% of patients regardless of the location of the primary tumor (32% in patients with a cancer of the upper third; 40% for cancers of the middle third; 70% for cancers of the lower third) (Akiyama et al. 1981). The mode and unpredictable character of tumoral spread make complete thoracoabdominal CT scans essential for the workup of patients with esophageal cancer.

Mediastinal invasion, in order of frequency, concerns the pleura, trachea and bronchi, the lungs, aorta, pericardium, azygos vein, diaphragm, and pulmonary veins (Mandard et al. 1981).

Metastases are common at the time of diagnosis and occur essentially in the lungs and the liver. Metastasis to the adrenal glands, peritoneum, kidneys, brain, and skeletal system is less frequent (Rosenberg et al. 1982).

10.2.5 Evolution

Local evolution of an esophageal cancer can result in perforation (mediastinum, lungs, pleura) and subsequent infectious complications or a fistula between the esophagus and the respiratory tract (trachea, bronchi). Massive hemorrhage may occur after invasion of a large vessel. Pneumopathies secondary to regurgitation are especially common.

10.2.6 TNM Classification

Various staging systems have been developed for esophageal cancers. Table 10.1 gives the TNM classification (Hermanek and Sabin 1987). Other systems are based on tumor size rather than the degree of esophageal wall infiltration: for example, a T1 lesion has a diameter less than or equal to 5 cm; a T2 is a lesion with a diameter over 5 cm, and T3 lesions extend into the adjacent structures (American Joint Committee Staging of Cancer of the Esophagus 1978). Other classifications have been developed with practical aims in mind. The four-category Van Andel et al. system (1979) defines operable-curable cancer; operable-incurable cancer; inoperable-curable cancer; and inoperable-incurable cancer. Moss et al. (1981) devised a CT staging system in which stages I and II are resectable while stages III and IV are unresectable. Stage I corresponds to an intraluminal esophageal mass with no abnormality of the esophageal wall. Stage II corresponds to tumoral wall thickening without any mediastinal abnormality; stage III is associated with direct local invasion, and stage IV corresponds to disease with distant metastases. This classification is based on the TNM system (Hermanek and Sobin 1987) (Table 10.2).

Table 10.1. TNM clinical classification of esophageal cancer. (From Hermanek and Sobin 1987)

T – Primary tumor

TX	Primary tumor cannot be assessed
T0	No evidence of primary tumor
Tis	Carcinoma in situ
T1	Tumor invades lamina propria or submucosa
T2	Tumor invades muscularis propria
T3	Tumor invades adventitia
T4	Tumor invades adjacent structures

N – Regional lymph nodes

NX	Regional lymph nodes cannot be assessed
N0	No regional lymph node metastasis
N1	Regional lymph node metastasis

M – Distant metastasis

MX	Presence of distant metastasis cannot be assessed
M0	No distant metastasis
M1	Distant metastasis

Table 10.2. Staging of esophageal cancer. (From Hermanek and Sobin 1987)

Stage 0	Tis	N0	M0
Stage I	T1	N0	M0
Stage IIA	T2	N0	M0
	T3	N0	M0
Stage IIB	T1	N1	M0
	T2	N1	M0
Stage III	T3	N1	M0
	T4	Any N	M0
Stage IV	Any T	Any N	M1

10.3 Clinical Symptoms and Endoscopy

10.3.1 Clinical Symptoms

The typical patient is a 60-year-old man who complains of recent-onset dysphagia that has rapidly become severe. The patient often indicates a site high in the esophagus which may not correspond to the true location of the lesion. Dysphagia, which is present in 96% of all cases for Barajas-Martinez et al. (1986), is usually associated with weight loss (81%); regurgitation and retrosternal pain are less common (approximately 33% of cases). The average interval between the first symptom and diagnosis of esophageal cancer is 3.6 months (Barajas-Martinez et al.1986). Other presenting symptoms (dysphonia, hepatic or osseous tumors, enlarged supraclavicular nodes, respiratory manifestations) generally reflect disease extension. However, early esophageal cancers may bs associated with only minimal clinical symptoms such as pain during meals or a tickling sensation (Endo et al. 1986). Asymptomatic early cancer may be diagnosed fortuitously during endoscopic workups for a chronic esophageal or gastric condition.

10.3.2 Endoscopy

Fibroscopy can accurately measure the distance of a tumor from the mouth and can identify the macroscopic features of the tumor (polypoid lesion, ulceration, or stenosis) and the normal or irregular appearance of the esophageal mucosa. Along with allowing thorough examination of that portion of the esophagus above the lesion, fibroscopy is especially helpful for guiding biopsies. *Endosonography* is discussed in the section on imaging techniques (Sect. 10.4). *Staining with 2% toluidine blue and 3% Lugol's solution* are helpful for detection of small mucosal lesions, but they cannot identify submucosal disease sites. *Abrasive cytology* can also demonstrate early cancers (Tsang et al. 1987). Systematic *exfoliative cytology* is advised for individuals at high risk for esophageal cancer (chronic esophageal condition or head and neck cancer).

The endoscopic features of early esophageal cancer (Endo et al. 1986) include polypoid, plateau-like, erosive, ulcerative, mixed, multiple, and unclassified lesions. These endoscopic findings have a prognostic value for small cancers, because adenopathies are rare with erosive or flat lesions, but frequent with polypoid and plateau-like lesions (Endo et al.

1986). Endoscopic data can also serve as the basis for therapeutic decisions and for monitoring response to local therapy in patients who do not undergo surgery.

10.4 Diagnostic Imaging

Chest X-rays, barium studies, and CT are the three indispensable staging examinations for esophageal cancer. The data provided by endosonography will probably make this technique indispensable once it becomes more widespread (although the high frequency of stenosing lesions sometimes precludes satisfactory exploration). Transtracheal lymphography, azygos venography, and radionuclide studies no longer have any indications. Magnetic resonance imaging (MRI) is currently under assessment.

10.4.1 Standard Chest X-rays

Although chest X-rays will undoubtedly be replaced in the future by a good quality scout view taken at the start of CT scanning, chest radiographs are an inexpensive staging technique which can detect an associated bronchial cancer (Norton et al. 1980) or an abnormality related to esophageal cancer: mediastinal widening, tracheal deviation, abnormal azygoesophageal line, tracheoesophageal line or retroesophageal stripe (Daffner et al. 1978).

10.4.2 Barium Esophagography
(Figs. 10.1–10.9)

Both conventional and double-contrast barium esophagograms can be used. Double-contrast studies can detect early and superficial tumors, but neither technique can identify in situ lesions. The prognostic value of detecting early superficial tumors less than 3.5 cm long by double-contrast examination remains controversial (Suzuki et al. 1972; Zornoza and Lindell 1980). Early cancers may or may not exhibit certain features that are occasionally visible only on double-contrast films (Cozzi et al. 1987; Levine et al. 1986; Sato et al. 1986). These infiltrative, polypoid, stenosing, or su-

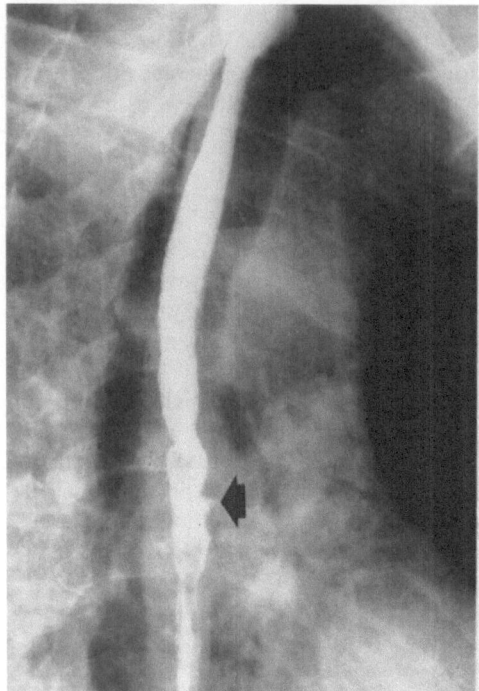

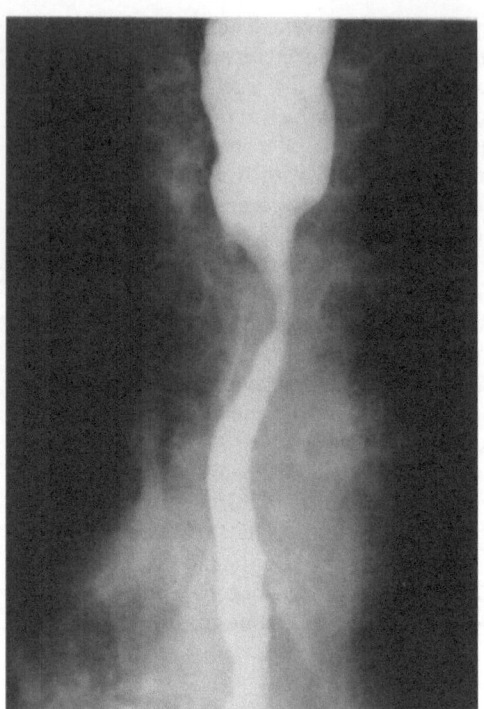

Fig. 10.1. Ulcerated cancer in the lower third of the esophagus *(arrow)*

Fig. 10.2. Stenosing cancer of the middle third of the esophagus

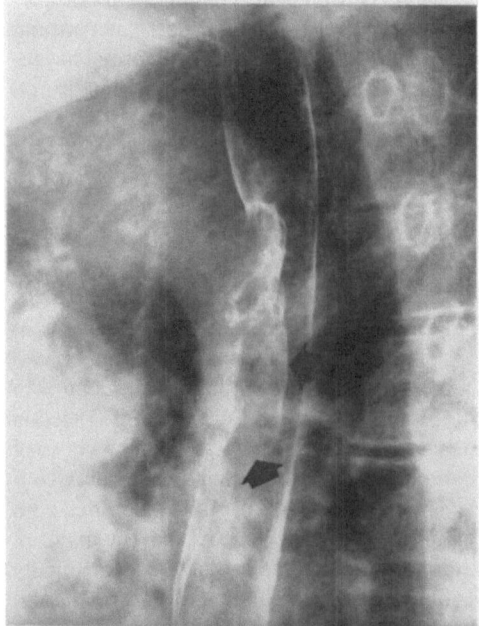

Fig. 10.3. Polypoid cancer of the esophagus *(arrows)*

perficially spreading lesions all measure less than 2.5 cm. Polypoid tumors manifest as sessile, endoluminal lesions with an irregular lobulated surface, with or without moderate signs of esophageal wall infiltration (Levine et al. 1986). Infiltrative tumors may cause retraction and parietal rigidity. Stenosing forms are often concentric. Superficial tumors have a granular appearance (Levine et al. 1986) or a feathered, flat mucosa with tiny nodulations and barium poolings (Sato et al. 1986). The differential diagnoses for nodular or granular images include reflux esophagitis, herpetic esophagitis, candidal esophagitis, eosinophilic esophagitis, cystic esophagitis, acanthosis nigricans, and glycogenic acanthosis (Graziani et al. 1985).

The typical esophageal tumor is often an advanced cancer with one or more of the following appearances: polypoid growth, ulceration, circumferential lesion. Infiltration and varicoid patterns are less common. Images suggestive of varices, achalasia, or a local inflammatory lesion are even rarer (Lawson and Dodds 1976).

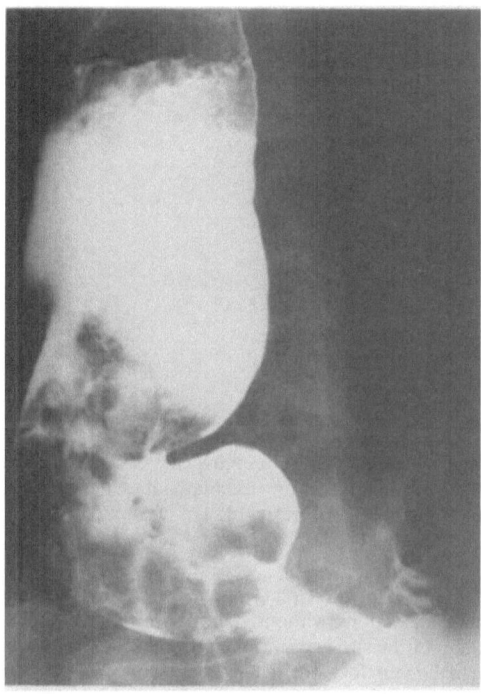

Fig. 10.4. Differential diagnosis: epitheliosarcoma of the esophagus

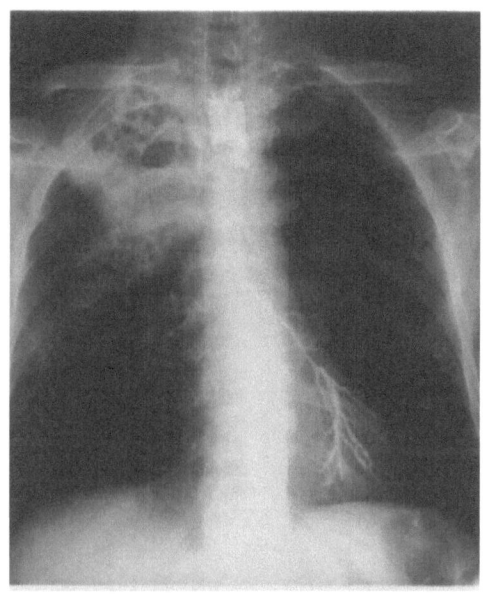

Fig. 10.5. Esophageal cancer causing complete stenosis at the junction of the upper and middle thirds. Presence of an abscess in the right lung secondary to aspiration. Radiologic examination revealed the site of the tumoral lesion and a false channel (left bronchial opacification).

Fig. 10.6. Superficial spreading of an early esopha- ▶ geal cancer. (Courtesy of Dr. Schmutz, Strasbourg, France)

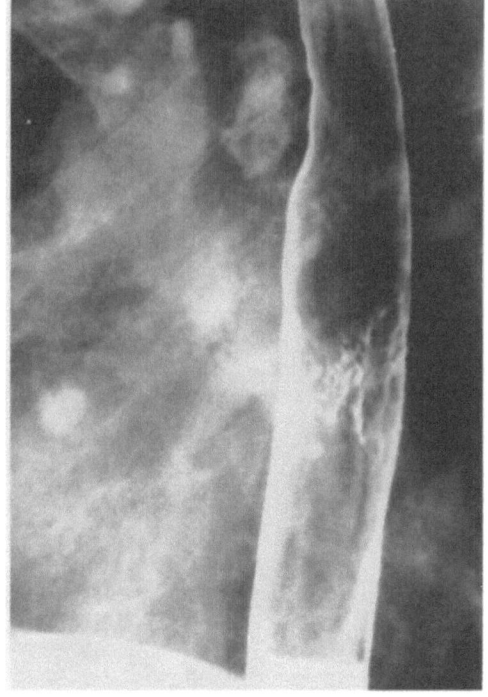

Barium swallows can evaluate the degree of intraluminal involvement, but generally cannot assess the exact length of a tumoral lesion within the esophagus. Akiyama (1980) reported that single-contrast studies in all planes allow evaluation of the axis of the esophagus. Esophageal tortuosity, angulation, or displacement correspond to mediastinal invasion, although the false-negative rate is 10%–16%, and there are 8% false-positive errors (Akiyama 1980; Akiyama et al. 1981; Mori et al. 1979). Double-contrast barium esophagrams are actually better suited for screening for early esophageal cancer rather than for the workup of mediastinal extension, which is best handled by other techniques (endosonography and/or CT). However, esophageal barium studies remain indispensable for the workup

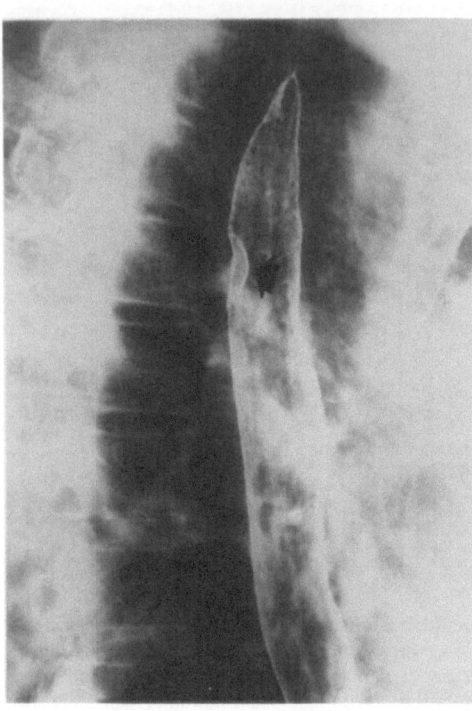

◀ **Fig. 10.7.** Sessile endoluminal lesion corresponding to an early esophageal cancer *(arrow)*. (Courtesy of Dr. Schmutz, Strasbourg, France)

▼ **Fig. 10.8** *(left)*. Early esophageal cancer under 2.5 cm presenting as an irregular, lobulated sessile lesion *(arrow)*. (Courtesy of Dr. Schmutz, Strasbourg, France)

Fig. 10.9 *(right)*. Esophageal cancer manifesting as small ulcerations without stenosis *(arrows)*. Examination of the surgical specimen revealed several other malignant foci not demonstrated by the barium examination

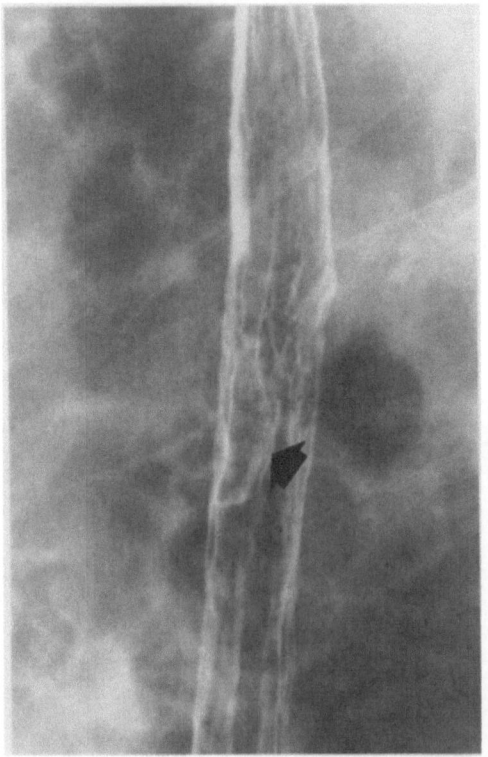

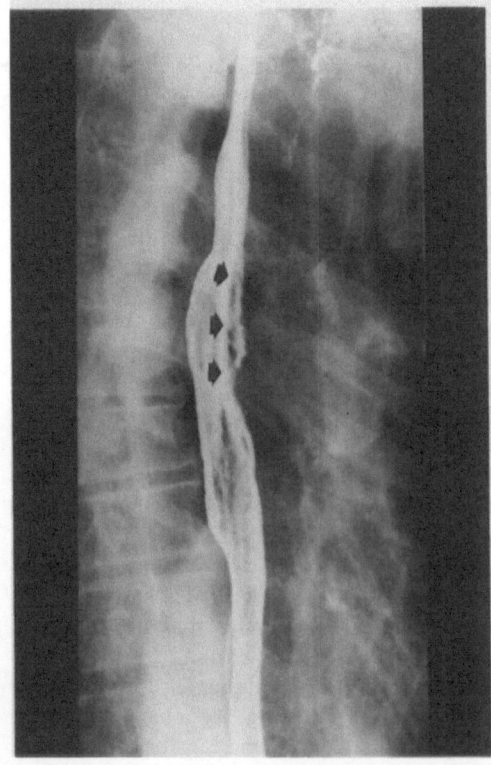

of several pathologies, including head and neck cancers and lung cancer, and for individuals who have suffered lye stricture or have reflux esophagitis (Thompson 1983). The use of barium esophagography for post-therapy patient follow-up is discussed in the section on the imaging of complications and response to therapy (Sect. 10.7).

10.4.3 Computed Tomography

Pretherapy CT of patients with esophageal cancer is used to define three categories: resectable tumors, non-resectable lesions, and indeterminate lesions. Accurate definition of operability is essential to reduce the morbidity in individuals with a very poor prognosis. The value of CT for posttherapy follow-up is discussed in a later section (Sect. 10.7).

10.4.3.1 CT Technique

CT scanning of esophageal cancers requires exploration of the chest and upper abdomen. The neck region must also be explored in patients with involvement of the cervical esophagus (Marx and Balfe 1987). Oral administration of a low-contrast product permits visualization of the esophageal lumen, except in patients with severe obstruction. Oral contrast is especially useful for exploration of the gastroesophageal junction and gastric wall. Oral contrast using effervescent crystals is particularly indicated for examination of the gastroesophageal junction in the left lateral decubitus position; such studies are indispensable for cancers of the lower third of the esophagus. Examination in the left lateral decubitus position combined with esophageal opacification permits differentiation of a tumoral process from normal prominent soft tissue of the gastroesophageal junction. The dorsal decubitus position is used for all other examinations. Halvorsen and Thompson (1987) emphasized the value of scans taken in maximum inspiration, which moves the esophagus away from the posterior edge of the trachea. Intravenous injection of iodinated contrast material is required for investigation of the abdomen (search for liver metastases) and is helpful when examining the thorax of thin subjects with scant body fat. Contiguous 1-cm thick slices are taken.

10.4.3.2 CT Features of Primary Esophageal Cancer (Figs. 10.10–10.14)

Opacification allows evaluation of the esophageal wall, which is normally 3–5 mm thick (Halvorsen and Thompson 1987). Esophageal cancer typically presents as irregular, concentric wall thickening with irregular narrowing of the lumen (Marx and Balfe 1987). Dilatation is common above sites of stenosis. Less common CT findings include focal wall thickening, symmetric circumferential involvement, or an intraluminal mass. Very small cancers may not be detected by CT scans.

Esophageal tumors have a homogeneous soft tissue density. Calcification, like the presence of intraluminal air (corresponding to a large ulceration or a tracheobronchial fistula), is rare at diagnosis. The homogeneous tissue density precludes differentiation from esophagitis, a benign tumor, or metastases. Esophageal varices usually cause more symmetric thickening. Tumor length is an important factor, but CT tends to overestimate rather than underestimate this parameter (Marx and Balfe 1987). The depth of penetration has both diagnostic and prognostic importance. Paraesophageal involvement, corresponding to a T3 tumor (stage III), manifests as increased paraesophageal density because of direct tumoral spread into the adjacent structures, without the interposition of fat. This analysis is difficult in cachetic patients. Evaluation of local disease extension involves several problems (Coulomb et al. 1981; Schneekloth et al. 1983):

- A paucity of fat in the subject can hinder evaluation of tumoral spread.
- Adherence between the esophageal cancer and the mediastinal structures is possible even in the absence of invasion.
- Transmural extension of an esophageal cancer into the mediastinum creates the same CT images as a tumor which merely causes wall thickening.

Endosonography is indicated whenever possible to solve these diagnostic problems.

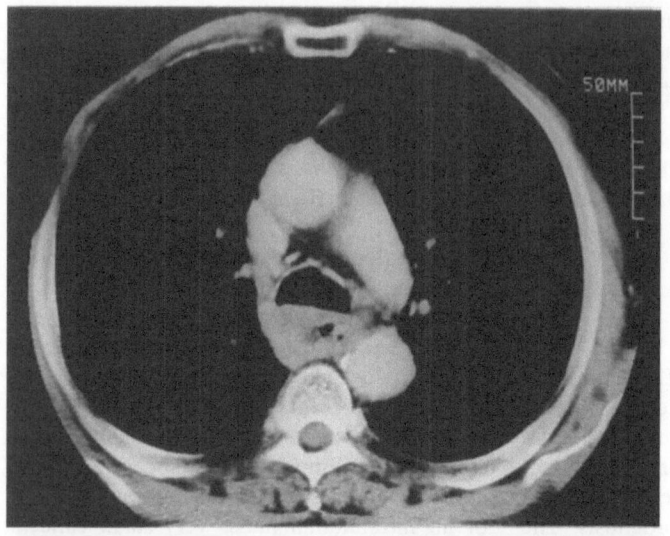

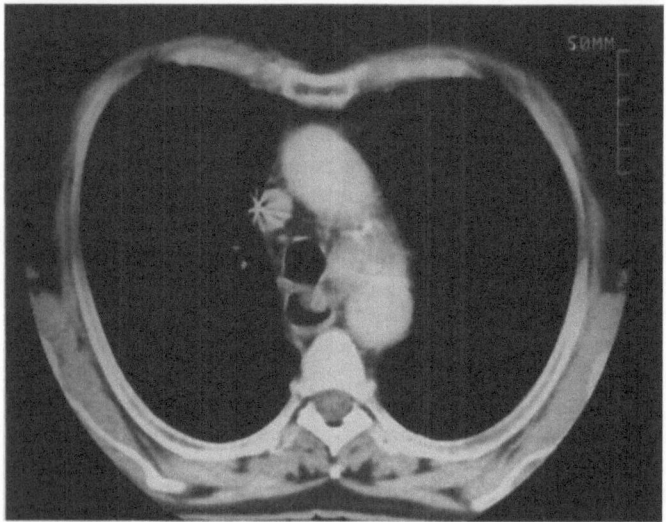

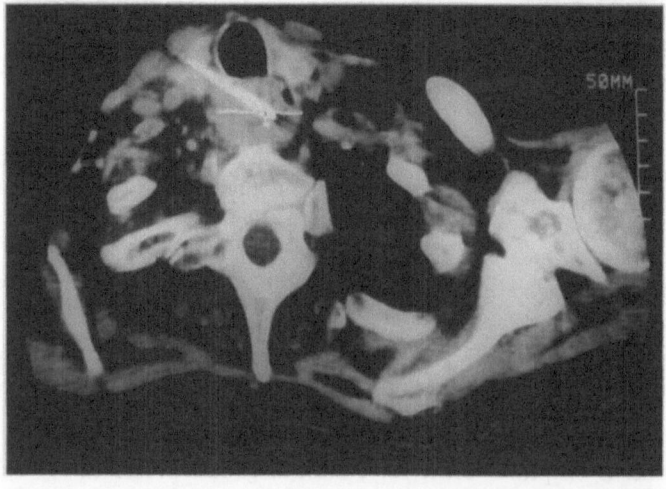

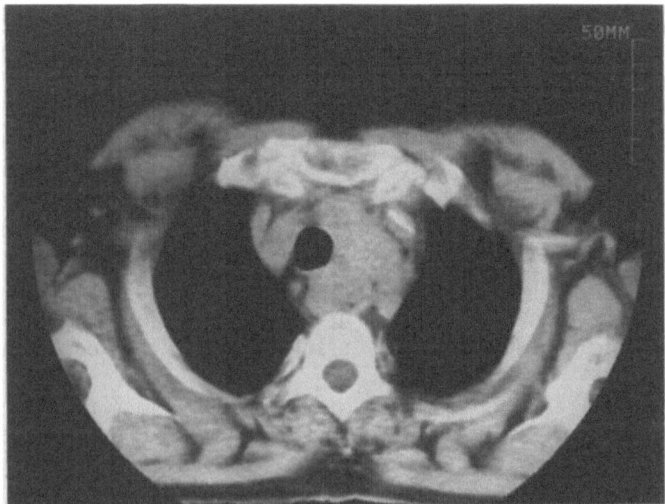

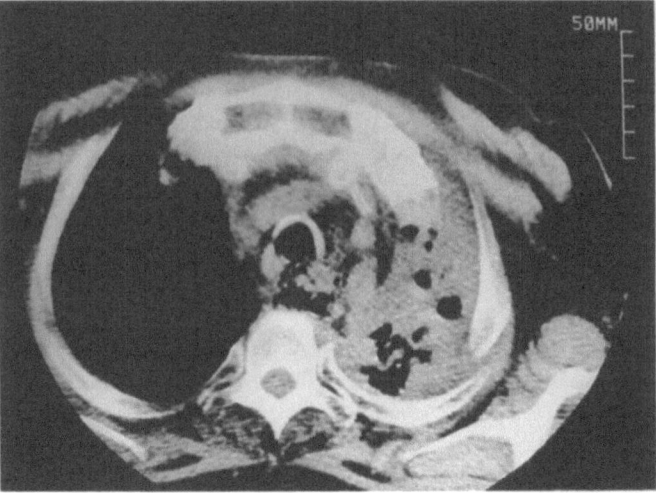

◄ **Fig. 10.10** *(above).* Esophageal cancer: CT demonstrated parietal thickening with stenosis of the lumen. This lesion caused moderate mediastinal infiltration behind the left pulmonary artery

Fig. 10.11 *(middle).* Small esophageal cancer demonstrated as an endoluminal lesion without mediastinal extension by CT

Fig. 10.12 *(below).* Cancer of the upper third of the esophagus displacing the lumen to the left. Endoscopy was not diagnostic for cancer; diagnosis was obtained by CT-guided percutaneous biopsy. The long axis of this lesion measured 3.5 cm

Fig. 10.13 *(above).* Tumor in the upper third of the esophagus causing anterosuperior mediastinal extension. Presence of a left subclavicular catheter

Fig. 10.14 *(below).* Ulcerated esophageal cancer creating a tracheoesophageal fistula, which led to infectious complications in the upper left lobe

10.4.3.3 Mediastinal Spread to Viscera
(Figs. 10.15, 10.16)

Invasion of the respiratory tract can cause both displacement and indentation of the airway; these two signs have a predictive value of 93%–100% (Becker et al. 1986; Halvorsen and Thompson 1987). Indentation is never visible on scans of the normal esophagus taken in deep inspiration. For Halvorsen and Thompson (1987), invasion manifests as inward bowing of the posterior wall of the tracheobron-

chial tract and usually reflects invasion of the distal trachea and the left mainstem bronchus. CT workup of a patient with esophageal cancer may, on rare occasions, reveal a tracheoesophageal fistula as a communication between the two structures.

Extensively analyzed by Picus et al. (1983), aortic invasion by esophageal cancer corresponds to contact between the esophagus and the aorta, with intact fat planes above and below the area of contact. Contact over more than one-quarter of the circumference of the

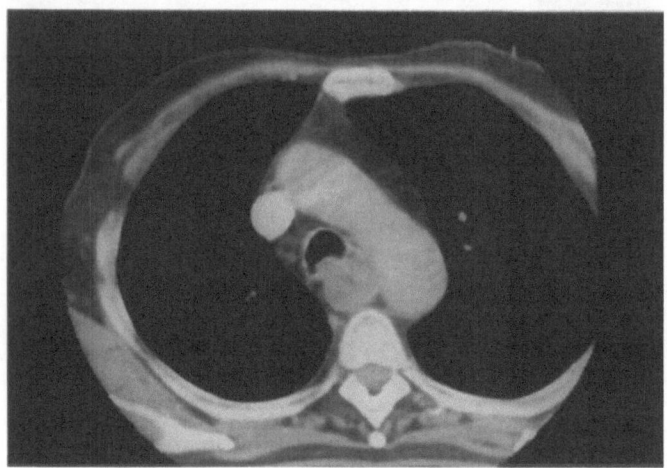

Fig. 10.15. Esophageal cancer invading the trachea

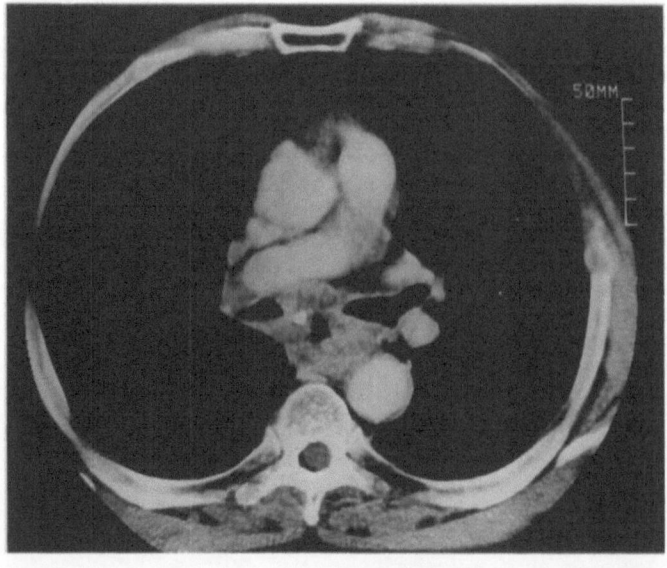

Fig. 10.16. Bulky esophageal cancer infiltrating the tracheobronchial region

aorta is considered indicative of invasion; this sign has a predictive value of 80–95%. By contrast, contact limited to less than one-eighth of the circumference (less than 45°) probably means an absence of aortic invasion. When contact is between 45° and 90°, the possibility of aortic involvement cannot be accurately assessed. When fat is absent between the esophagus and the aorta, as in cachetic individuals, evaluation can be difficult. False-positive errors can occur in individuals with postradiation fibrosis or inflammation. For Marx and Balfe (1987), however, radiotherapy does not alter the appearance of the mediastinal fat.

Pericardial involvement can be suspected when contact is visualized between the esophagus and the pericardium, and the fat planes above and below are intact. The pericardium of the left atrium is most often involved by esophageal cancer. *Bone* involvement is readily visualized by CT as osseous destruction in continuity with the esophageal tumor. Detection of early bone involvement requires examination with bone windows. Sufficient distention of the stomach is necessary to assess possible *gastric* involvement, otherwise there is a risk of false-positive error. CT diagnosis of invasion of the *pleura* and the diaphragmatic crura is generally difficult (Becker et al. 1986). Overall, CT workups for detection of mediastinal extension of esophageal cancer to viscera should concentrate on exploration of the respiratory tree and the aorta.

10.4.3.4 Nodal Extension (Figs. 10.17, 10.18)

Potential nodal invasion must be assessed in both the mediastinum and abdomen; the neck must also be thoroughly examined in patients with a cancer of the upper third of the esophagus. Mediastinal adenopathies are often not detectable by CT because of confluence with the tumor mass. The paratracheal, para-aortic, pericardial, and subcarinal regions must all be explored. For Marx and Balfe (1987), enlarged nodes measuring 6 mm or more in diameter can be considered metastatic. For Coulomb et al. (1981) and Glazer et al. (1985), adenopathies can be considered metastatic when their small axis measures at least 10 mm. CT cannot analyze nodal architecture, and even the size data it provides are no safeguard against false-negative and false-positive errors. Some metastatic nodes are normal in size (Columb et al. 1981) while non-metastatic hypertrophic nodes may reach 6–10 mm, in particular in patients with a history of inflammation. CT underevaluation of mediastinal node invasion does not obligatorily affect clinical therapeutic options, but does worsen the prognosis. In patients with cancer of the upper third of the esophagus, extramediastinal adenopathies must be searched for in the cervical region. Exploration of the abdomen is important regardless of the site of the esophageal cancer. The gastrohepatic ligament must be investigated to detect left gastric adenopathies. Other

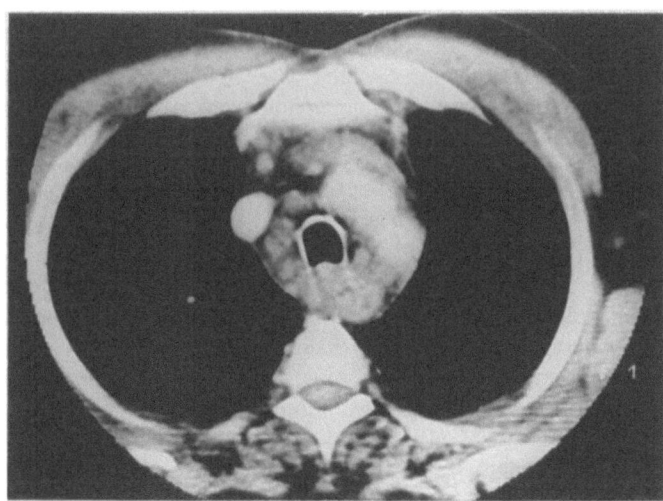

Fig. 10.17. Esophageal cancer with metastatic mediastinal lymph nodes

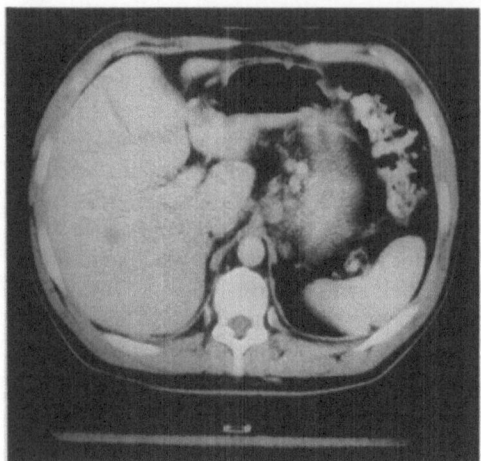

Fig. 10.18. Celiac adenopathies and hepatic metastases of a cancer of the lower esophagus (not visible on this scan)

potential disease sites include the celiac, portal, and splenic regions. If nodes with a small axis of 8 mm or more on scans are considered metastatic, CT can be considered to have adequate sensitivity, but its specificity remains low (43% for Balfe et al. 1984) owing to the possibility of normal-sized metastatic nodes.

10.4.3.5 Metastatic Disease

CT plays an essential role for the workup of metastases (Salonen et al. 1987). Lung metastases may be either solitary or multiple; solitary nodules should be punctured under CT guidance. Hepatic metastases have a variable appearance before and after intravenous contrast medium injection. Necrotic and calcified lesions are rare.

10.4.3.6 Overall Value of CT

Local exploration of esophageal tumors is relatively unsatisfactory with CT (Salonen et al. 1987). Thompson (1983), reviewing both his personal cases and those of Coulomb et al. (1981), Daffner et al. (1979), and Moss et al. (1981), reported 5%–6% false-positive and false-negative errors for CT diagnosis of me-

diastinal involvement. For Halvorsen and Thompson (1987), CT had accuracy rates of 96% for diagnosis of tracheobronchial involvement, 98% for detection of hepatic metastases, and 92% for aortic invasion, but was only 65% accurate for diagnosis of mediastinal adenopathies and 87% accurate for metastatic abdominal nodes.

Overall, CT can determine the surgical curability in 85%–90% of cases, especially for cancers of the upper and middle thirds of the esophagus. The value of CT is much lower for defining the resectability of cancers of the lower third of the esophagus and the gastroesophageal junction (only 41% for cancer of the gastroesophageal junction) (Thompson et al. 1983). For Rousset et al. (1986), CT has an elevated positive predictive value, but a low negative predictive value (66%) for diagnosis of mediastinal invasion and adenopathies. Although authors disagree as to the exact value of CT for locoregional staging of esophageal cancers (Quint et al. 1985b), fairly accurate identification of three tumor categories (resectable, unresectable, indeterminate) appears possible through reduction of the number of indeterminate cases (Taylor 1986). Patients with tracheobronchial, aortic, or bone involvement are not candidates for surgery, and such lesions are readily evidenced by CT. Certain patients with gastric, pleural, pericardial, or diaphragmatic involvement may nevertheless benefit from curative surgery (Becker et al. 1986; Samuelsson et al. 1984; Thompson et al. 1983). Total transthoracic esophagectomy (TTE) may be feasible even in patients with periesophageal adenopathies or infiltration of the mediastinal periesophageal fat (en bloc resection of the tumor mass and surrounding tissues); this is not possible with transhiatal esophagectomy (THE). For Kron et al. (1984), CT demonstration of these elements can be used to determine eligibility for TTE or THE.

10.4.4 Ultrasonography (Figs. 10.19–10.23)

Conventional abdominal ultrasonography is indicated for detection of hepatic metastases and nodal invasion. Ultrasound-guided biopsy is helpful for evaluating solitary hepatic nodules.

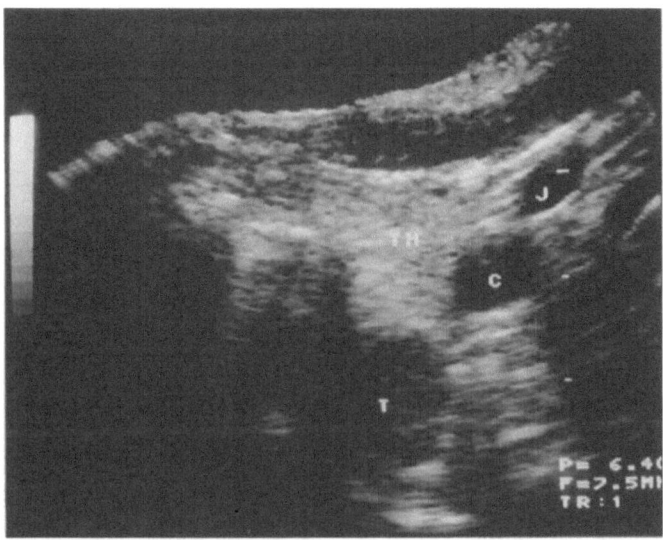

Fig. 10.19. Cervical sonogram of a cancer of the upper third of the esophagus *(T)*. This hypoechoic lesion lies posterior to the left lobe of the thyroid gland *(Th)*, between the primary carotid artery (C) and the left internal jugular vein *(J)*

The value of *endosonography* cannot yet be quantified because series to date are less extensive than comparable CT studies. The normal esophageal wall measures 3–4 mm on ultrasound scans. Dancygier and Classen (1986) devised a practical system that divides the esophageal wall into three layers, from inside to out: a hyperechoic layer; a thicker, hypoechoic layer which corresponds to the muscularis propria; and a hyperechoic layer. Along with analyzing local involvement with a very good degree of accuracy, ultrasonography can determine the length of tumoral spread and detect secondary disease sites. Mediastinal nodes can be investigated, but, as with CT, normal and metastatic nodes cannot be differentiated on the basis of size alone.

False-positive errors can result from images of pseudoinvasion subsequent to tumor compression by the water-filled balloon (Tio et al. 1986). The main difficulties encountered with endosonography concern stenosing tumors; 25% of such lesions cannot be satisfactorily investigated with ultrasound for Takemoto et al. (1986). Despite this reserve, endosonography will undoubtedly rapidly acquire an essential role in local disease workups of esophageal cancer. Owing to its value for detection of sec-

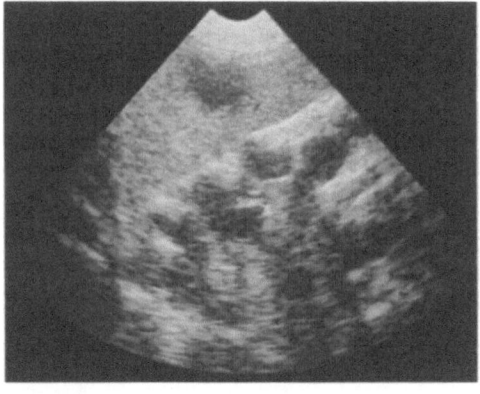

Fig. 10.20. Cancer of the middle third of the esophagus: abdominal ultrasonography revealed multiple lymph node nodules and liver metastases

ond disease sites and assessment of both tumoral and paraesophageal extension, ultrasound can be considered complementary to CT.

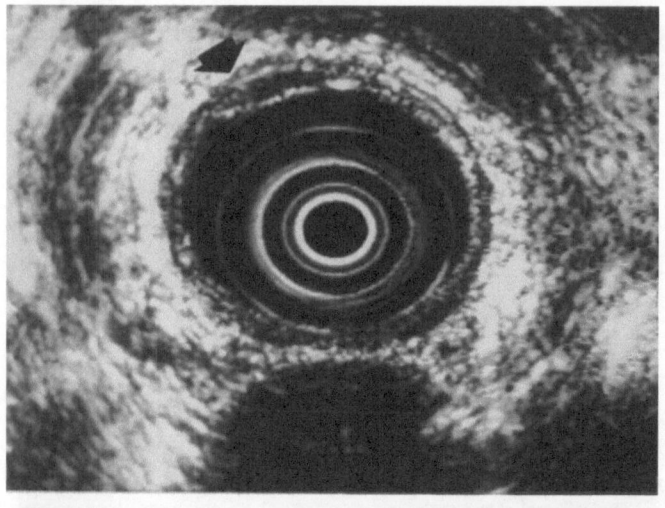

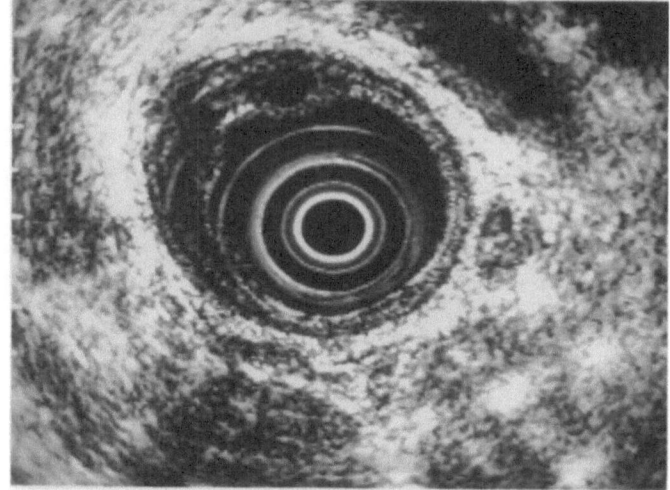

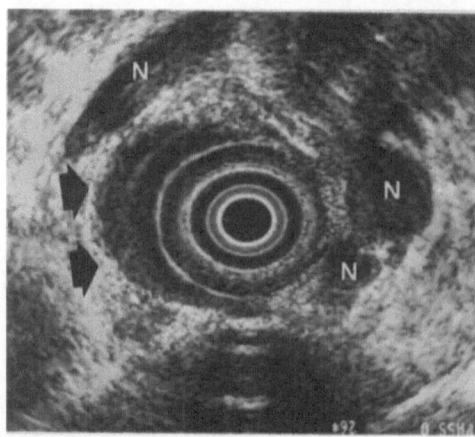

▲ **Fig. 10.21** *(above).* Endosonography of the esophagus demonstrating a superficial cancer: the continuous hypoechoic line around the neoplastic lesion indicates that the submucosa is still intact *(arrow)*

Fig. 10.22 *(below).* Endosonography of the esophagus: this superficial polypoid cancer did not invade the submucosa

◄ **Fig. 10.23.** Endosonography of the esophagus: esophageal cancer *(arrows)*; satellite adenopathies *(N)*

10.4.5 Other Techniques

To date, preliminary studies have failed to demonstrate *MRI* as being more valuable for the workup of esophageal cancer than CT (Quint et al. 1985a) (Figs. 10.24-10.27). *Azygos venography* is valuable only when positive and in such cases always corresponds to an unresectable tumor (Crummy et al. 1968; Mori et al. 1979). This invasive technique has been abandoned in favor of CT. *Transtracheal lymphography*, using films obtained 24 h and 3-7 days after injection, can visualize small metastatic nodes from 6 to 16 mm (Sugimachi et al. 1982) and neoplastic filling defects. However, this technique does not appear to have been used by other teams to improve the score of imaging techniques for detection of metastatic mediastinal nodes. Kondo et al. (1982) demonstrated that routine *gallium 67* scans are not justified for staging esophageal cancers.

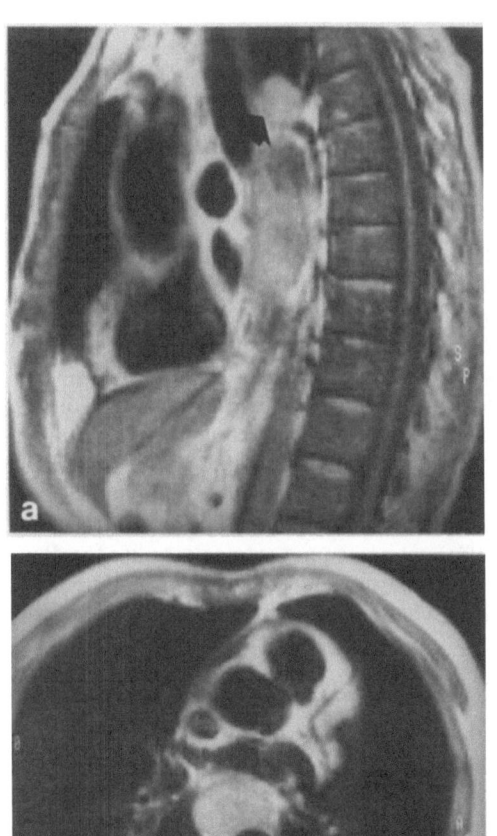

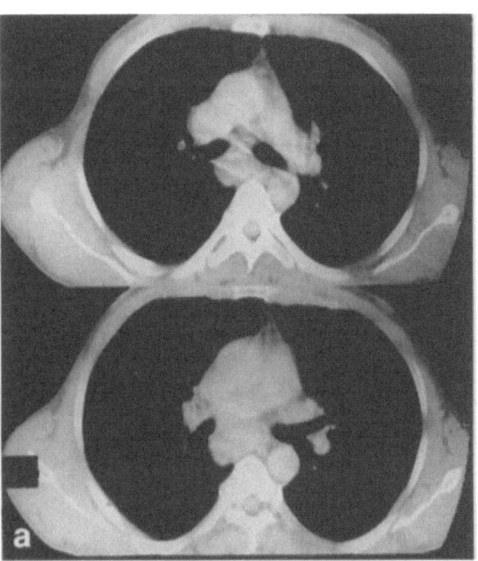

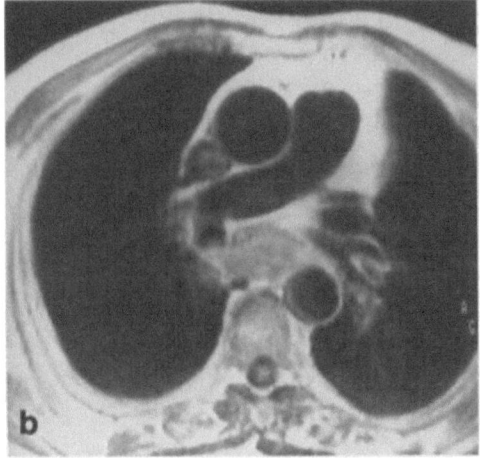

Fig. 10.24a, b. MRI of an esophageal cancer: sagittal scanning **(a)** demonstrated a metastatic lymph node *(arrow)* above the arch of the azygos vein. Transverse scans **(b)** confirmed that the bronchial structures and the aorta were not invaded by the tumor

Fig. 10.25a, b. CT and MRI studies of an esophageal cancer. Differentiation between the tumor and the bronchial structures in particular was difficult with CT **(a)** whereas MRI **(b)** demonstrated the integrity of the vascular and bronchial structures, which were not invaded by this esophageal cancer

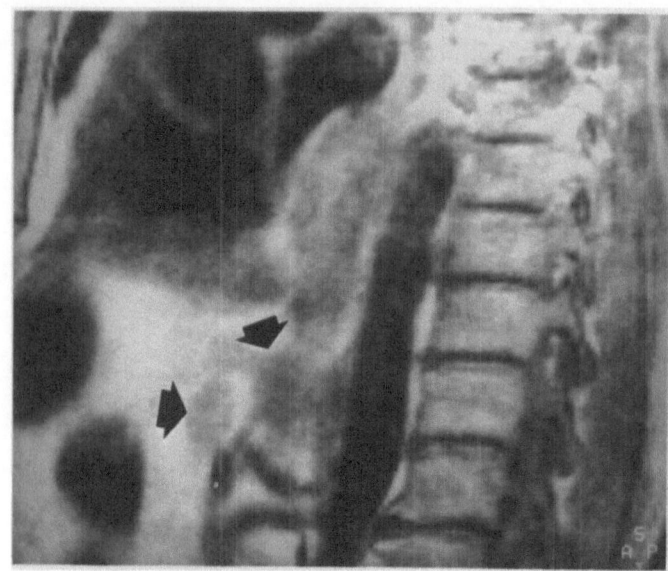

Fig. 10.26. Cancer of the lower third of the esophagus, with metastatic lymph nodes *(arrows)* above the origin of the celiac trunk

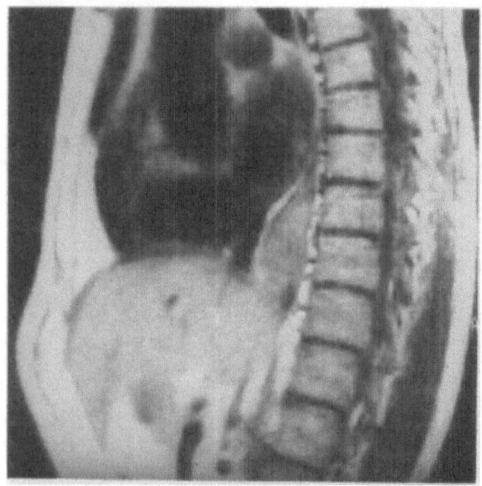

Fig. 10.27. Cancer of the lower third of the esophagus: no invasion of the anterior or posterior mediastinal structures

10.5 Prognostic Factors

Aside from the patient's general condition (respiratory status in particular) and existence of an associated tumor, the depth of tumor penetration and the presence of adenopathies are the two main factors associated with a poor prognosis (Skinner et al. 1982; Skinner et al. 1986). Depth of penetration actually appears more important than the length of tumoral spread; furthermore, the length of a lesion is not always correlated with the degree of penetration (Sato et al. 1986). However, 75% of all lesions over 5 cm are associated with a risk of metastases (Rosenberg et al. 1982). The prognosis for in situ tumors (35%-90% at 5 years) reflects the existence of infraradiological and sometimes infraendoscopic lesions (Huang 1981), which require cytology studies for diagnosis (Akiyama 1980; Gua-Qing 1981; Huang 1981). Significant differences thus appear to exist among the prognoses of T1, T2, and T3 tumors (Beatty et al. 1979; Galandiuk et al. 1986). In addition to tumor-dependent parameters, the presence of adenopathies plays an important prognostic role. For Rosenberg et al. (1982), patients without nodal involvement have a prognosis of 20%-30% at 5 years, whereas the presence of adenopathies reduces the prognosis at 5 years to below 10%. Average survival for patients with CT-proven invasion of the subdiaphragmatic nodes is only 3 months (Halvorsen et al. 1986).

Other tumor-dependent prognostic factors include:

- Tumor location in the esophagus: Rosenberg et al. (1982) and Thompson (1985) emphasized the very poor prognosis of cancers of the cervical esophagus (0% at 5 years). Other authors cite a somewhat better 5-year prognosis of 9.6%–27% (Collin and Spiro 1984; Kakegawa et al. 1985).

- Histologic form: adenocarcinoma has a worse prognosis than epidermoid cancer.
- Existence of solitary or associated invasion of the aorta, trachea, pericardium, liver, or abdominal nodes (Halvorsen and Thompson 1987).

10.6 Therapeutic Options

Surgery, the only potentially curative treatment for esophageal cancer at present, may be completed or replaced by radiotherapy. Other techniques [bouginage, endoscopic laser therapy, bipolar electrocoagulation therapy (BICAP), balloon dilation, intubation] can provide symptomatic palliation, in particular by reducing dysphagia. Multiagent chemotherapy has given rather variable results to date and is currently the field of ongoing research (Campbell et al. 1985; Kelsen 1982).

10.6.1 Surgery

Total or subtotal esophagectomy with reconstruction of gastrointestinal continuity is possible for 39%–85% of patients (Earlam and Cunha-Melo 1980a; Van Andel et al. 1986; Wong 1987). Intestinal continuity is usually obtained by mobilizing the stomach into the thorax and creating an esogastric anastomosis. Interposition of a segment from the small intestine or colon between the esophagus and stomach is performed when necessary. Two techniques have been developed: TTE by a right thoracotomy or a left thoraco-abdominal incision allows direct visualization of the cancer or invasion. THE with blind dissection by cervical and abdominal incisions and esophagogastrostomy does not allow direct visualization of the tumor and thus precludes wide resection of the tissues. Total and subtotal esophagectomy can both relieve clinical symptoms and improve the quality of patient survival (Sugimachi et al. 1986).

Even for patients with unresectable tumors, mediastinal involvement does not automatically contraindicate esogastrostomy-type surgery for palliation of clinical symptoms. However, the morbidity and mortality rates are generally high in patients in poor general and local condition. This underscores the importance of the presurgery workup, and especially pulmonary examinations to detect chronic respiratory insufficiency or an associated tumor (lung cancer or head and neck malignancy) (Parisot et al. 1985; Reboud et al. 1983).

Postoperative mortality has decreased over the past 15 years, thanks to improvement in reanimation techniques, and now stands at between 5% and 6.8% (Larson et al. 1985; Tam et al. 1987). In the series of Van Andel et al. (1986), 85% of all of esophageal cancers were resectable, and the postoperative mortality was 20%.

Recurrent disease for cancers treated less than 5 years previously usually affects the lymph nodes. The causes of death in patients treated between 5 and 10 years earlier include both relapses and lung complications (Isono et al. 1982). The duration of survival is between 0% and 21%, and has not changed much over the past 15 years (Couraud and Meriot 1982; Cukingnan and Casey 1978; Maillet et al. 1982). Adjuvant radiotherapy has been suggested as a means to improve this prognosis (Rosenberg et al. 1982).

10.6.2 Radiotherapy

Epidermoid cancer of the esophagus is radiosensitive, and radiotherapy with 6000–7000 rads is sometimes curative (Yang et al. 1983). Radiation therapy is especially effective for small diameter tumors without paraesophageal involvement. Superficial and polypoid lesions appear more radiosensitive than infiltrative and ulcerative forms (Morita et al. 1985). Actually, radiotherapy usually plays a palliative purpose by reducing tumoral size, thereby possibly allowing surgery or alleviating clinical symptoms. A tracheoesophageal fistula is a contraindication for radiotherapy.

CT findings from diagnostic studies can be used to establish the radiotherapy program. Postoperative radiotherapy can reportedly reduce the frequency of local disease recurrence (Tam et al. 1987), particularly in patients with short margins of excision. Even after radiotherapy, 40% of patients die from local disease recurrence (Yang et al. 1983), and the prognosis at 5 years is only 6% (Earlam and Cunha-Melo 1980b).

10.6.3 Local Palliative Therapy

Bouginage using an endoscopic route permits dilatation of the malignant stenosis. The main risk is perforation of the normal esophagus or tumor mass (Jaffe et al. 1987).

Endoscopic laser therapy can increase the diameter of the esophageal lumen. Radiologic exploration is required beforehand to define the degree of angulation of the lumen at the level of the tumor, and to measure the distance between the tumor and the cricopharyngeus. Complications of laser therapy, including perforation and tracheoesophageal fistulae, occur in 2.1%–12.5% of patients (Cummins 1983; Wolf et al. 1986).

BICAP is a more recent technique performed after CT or sonoendoscopic measurement of wall thickness at the level of the tumor (the esophageal wall must be at least 5 mm to minimize the risk of thermal penetration). Potential complications include perforation and stricture due to scar tissue formation (Jaffe et al. 1987).

Balloon dilatation is infrequently used for neoplastic stenosis but can reduce dysphagia (Aste et al. 1985; deLange et al. 1987; Simonetti et al. 1987); it may be necessary prior to intubation (Chisholm et al. 1986). Possible complications include mucosal tears, esophageal rupture, and reflux pneumopathy.

Intubation with Livingstone or Celestin tubes is rarely indicated (0.7% of esophageal cancers for Haynes et al., 1984), being reserved for unresectable cancers and for patients with esorespiratory fistulae (Tytgat and Den Hartog Jager 1984). The frequency of complications and deaths related to intubation ranges between 6% and 58% (Chavy et al. 1986; Giradet et al. 1974; Jaffe et al. 1987). Mean survival after insertion of a stent is only 4.2 months. This technique is essentially indicated for tumors of the middle and lower thirds of the esophagus (Valbuena 1984). Complications during intubation include perforation and hemorrhage.

Post-intubation complications include airway obstruction, migration of the tube, and obstruction of the tube lumen (secondary to tumoral extension, prolapse of the edematous esophageal mucosa, iatrogenic prolapse of the stomach, impaction of food particles, new tumor growth causing blockage). Reflux esophagitis, hemorrhagic phenomena, necrosis, and perforation have also been reported.

10.7 Post-therapy Imaging Studies and Diagnosis of Complications

10.7.1 Normal Postoperative Appearance

After TTE with a left paravertebral anastomosis, the esophageal and gastric walls may appear thickened, with dilatation of the esophagus above the anastomosis. After colon interposition, the neoesophagus may be visible in the anterior mediastinum. Following THE, the high-lying anastomosis is visible on the midline or to the left of the trachea. The mediastinal fat planes are usually not altered, except in patients with postoperative inflammation; however, the density of this mediastinal fat tissue returns to normal in less than 3 months (Becker et al. 1987).

10.7.2 Early Postoperative Complications

Postoperative mortality is not rare and most often results from pulmonary complications in patients with a chronic obstructive pneumopathy (Galandiuk et al. 1986). Postoperative surveillance should include a barium swallow on the 10th postoperative day, except when an anastomotic leak is suspected, in which case water-soluble contrast is required (Agha et al. 1985). Because these patients cannot swallow a large amount of contrast medium, which results in defective visualization on standard films, the gastric tube inserted during the surgical procedure can be used. Pommeri et al. (1986) suggest opacifiation of the gastric tube in the Trendelenburg position to obtain images by reflux and to evidence any anastomotic abnormalities.

Potential early complications include anastomotic leak, cricopharyngeal incoordination (origin of a false channel), and gastric perforation. Anastomotic leaks can be treated by insertion of a balloon under fluoroscopic guidance to reduce the risk of fistula formation (de Lange et al. 1987). In practice, leakage of the proximal anastomosis and anastomotic fistulae are both common phenomena (31.8% and 34% for Larson et al. 1985). The main cause of complications is ischemia of the cervical anastomosis. Ischemic stenosis can be observed 15 days to 4 months after surgery as long, filiform narrowing, which distinguishes it from the fibrous stenosis that occurs after 3 months (short, regular narrowing) (Mouelhi et al. 1986).

Anastomotic leaks associated with clinical or biologic manifestations should be evaluated by CT to determine the impact on adjacent organs: extravasation of contrast material into the mediastinum or the pleural space, formation of a complex collection (presence of air, fluid, and contrast material), or pneumopathy.

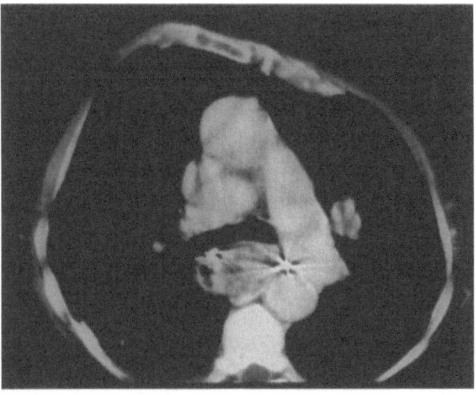

Fig. 10.28. CT study of a recurrent esophageal cancer. Solid density lesion (3-cm transverse long axis) displacing the tracheal division anteriorly. No aortic invasion

10.7.3 Late Postoperative Complications
(Figs. 10.28, 10.29)

Complications that develop more than one month after surgery generally correspond to fibrosis, and show up as short, regular anastomotic strictures on barium films or as pyloric stenosis in patients who have undergone THE. Transhiatal visceral herniation and above all tumoral recurrence are also possible. Recurrence usually develops in the 12 months following THE, often at a distance from the stomach, and the barium swallow is frequently negative (Becker et al. 1987). Postoperative fibrosis can also hinder detection of relapses (Thompson 1983). CT is thus particularly indicated for detection of mediastinal recurrence. By contrast, barium studies are better than CT for detection of small anastomotic recurrences. The frequency of anastomotic or mediastinal recurrence after TTE is 16% for Tam et al. (1987).

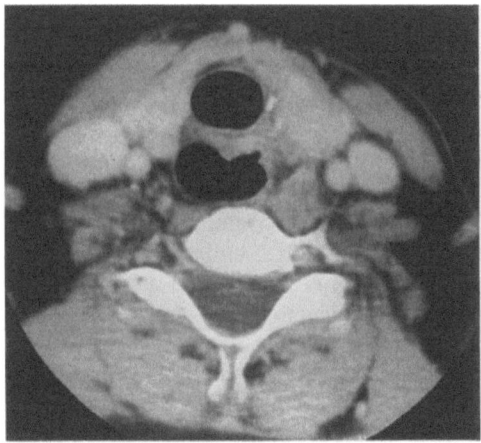

Fig. 10.29. Anastomotic recurrence of an esophageal cancer treated by surgery. This recurrence was detected endoscopically

10.7.4 Surveillance After Radiotherapy

10.7.4.1 Normal Appearance After Radiotherapy

Mediastinal radiotherapy causes pleural and pericardial thickening and perimediastinal pulmonary fibrosis, but does not obliterate the mediastinal fat planes. This fact must be kept in mind to avoid wrongly incriminating radiotherapy as the source of a solid mass within the mediastinal fat.

10.7.4.2 Complications of Radiotherapy

Postirradiation complications are rare provided an esotracheal fistula has not been overlooked. Radiation-induced perforations are readily demonstrated by CT, especially when an esotracheal fistula is detected. Hishikawa et al. (1986) reported fibrous narrowing on barium films more than 2 years after radiotherapy in 25% of the surviving patients. Because 40% of all deaths after radiotherapy are due to local disease recurrence, follow-up CT scans are indicated to detect mediastinal recurrence in the form of solid tissue-density masses within the mediastinal fat or in contact with the respiratory axis or aorta (Yang et al. 1983).

10.7.5 Surveillance After Other Types of Treatment

A barium swallow with a water-soluble contrast medium can reveal signs of perforation after bouginage, endoscopic laser therapy, BICAP, balloon dilatation, or intubation. CT can distinguish between intramural perforation and free perforation. Standard X-rays and especially CT scans are excellent means to visualize reflux pneumopathies and abscess formation. Most complications due to intubation can be detected by standard radiographs, when necessary after oral opacification with a water-soluble product.

10.8 Adenocarcinoma of the Esophagus

This malignant tumor originates either from spread of a gastric lesion into the distal esophagus or from Barrett's esophagus (a columnar epithelium-lined esophagus secondary to prolonged reflux esophagitis): 8% of all cases of reflux investigated for Sarr et al. (1985). Of all esophageal adenocarcinomas, 86% occur in patients with Barrett's esophagus (Thompson 1983). Malignant degeneration of Barrett's esophagus occurs in 2%–15% of all cases (Agha 1986; Sarr et al 1985; Sjogren and Johnson 1983). Factors known to increase the risk of cancer in patients with Barrett's esophagus include male sex, smoking, intesti-

nal-type metaplasia with severe reflux, and dysplasia (Skinner et al. 1983).

Overall, adenocarcinomas of the esophagus account for 75% of all tumors of the gastroesophageal junction. The prognosis is less favorable than for epidermoid cancers because esophageal adenocarcinoma is not radiosensitive (Mahoney and Condon 1987). Few patients can be cured surgically because of the very rapid disease course. The prognosis at 5 years is thus very low; even at 2 years, it is only between 31% and 34% (Mahoney and Condon 1987; Sanfey et al. 1985).

10.8.1 Radiographic Features
(Figs. 10.30, 10.31)

Adenocarcinoma of the esophagus generally associates radiographic evidence of malignancy with features of Barrett's esophagus (Agha 1986), a condition involving esophagitis, hiatal hernia with gastroesophageal reflux, a reticular pattern of the distal esophageal mucosa on double-contrast films (Levine et al. 1983), a high esophageal stricture, and a Barrett ulcer (a chronic peptic ulcer situated in the columnar-lined segment) (Agha 1986). A diagnosis of Barrett esophagus is very probable when high stricture, an ulcer, or a reticular mucosal appearance is seen on barium films. The risk of Barrett esophagus is less probable for low strictures and/or reflux esophagitis, and it is always nil when none of these lesions is present. Barium esophagography can detect 94% of all cancers of the gastroesophageal junction, and the false-negative errors tend to correspond to achalasia (Freeny and Marks 1982).

For Agha (1985), the radiologic features of esophageal carcinoma arising from Barrett esophagus include signs of chronic gastroesophageal reflux, chronic esophagitis, and hiatal hernia plus, in order of frequency, infiltrative stricture (60%), a varicoid pattern (40%), a mixed pattern (32%), a polypoid pattern (24%), and ulceration (20%). Esophageal carcinoma can occasionally have the same features as linitis plastica (Chejfec et al. 1983).

CT workups can accurately determine surgical resectability in 86% of cases, more thanks to precise detection of metastases than to evalua-

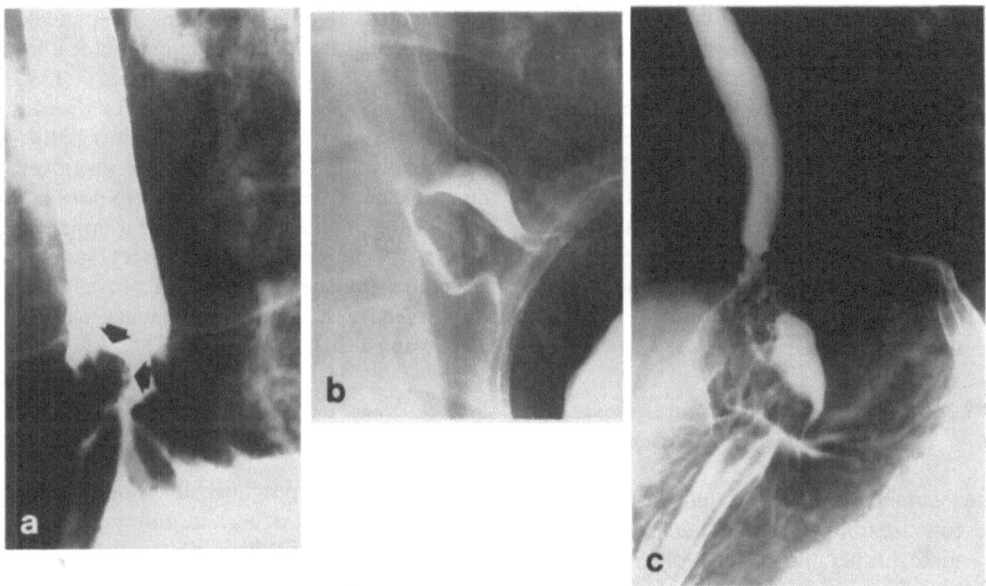

Fig. 10.30 a-c. Adenocarcinoma of the esophagus: polypoid lesion on a Barrett's esophagus (**a** and **b**), infiltrating lesion on a Barrett's esophagus (**c**)

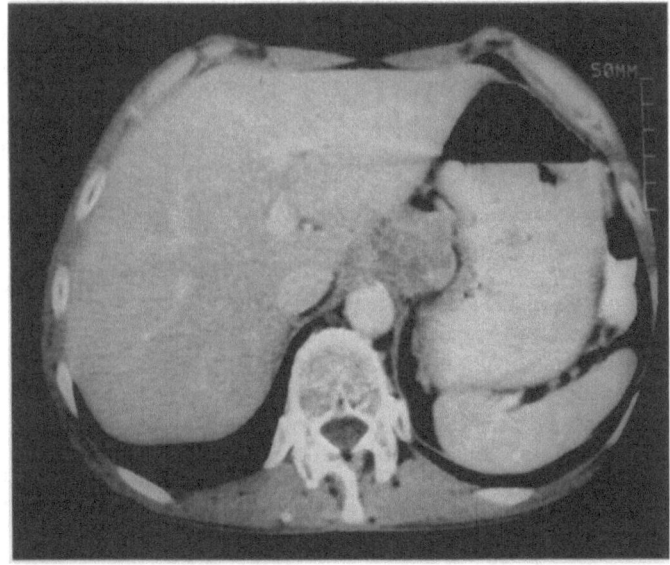

Fig. 10.31. Adenocarcinoma of the esophagus: bulky tumoral lesion (4-cm transverse diameter) (CT scan)

tion of local tumoral extension. Overall, however, CT is of limited interest. The presence or absence of fat around the lower esophagus has no diagnostic value for tumoral spread because of the high incidence of false-negative errors (30% for Freeney and Marks 1982). Pseudomasses at the normal gastroesophageal junction can usually be correctly identified by examining the patient in the left lateral decubitus position after the stomach has been sufficiently distended by gas or fluid.

10.8.2 Differences Between Adenocarcinoma and Epidermoid Cancer of the Esophagus

Adenocarcinoma of the esophagus generally presents the following characteristics that differentiate this pathology from epidermoid cancer:

- Localization in the lower third.
- Presence of a hiatal hernia and reflux esophagitis.
- Infiltrating form more common, polypoid form less common.
- Varicoid pattern more frequent (Agha 1985).
- Poorer prognosis (average survival 7 months for Fein et al. 1985).

10.8.3 Adenocarcinoma of the Esophagus and Gastric Adenocarcinoma

Both of these malignancies tend to be bulky, locally invasive tumors that metastatize early to the regional lymph nodes. Adenocarcinoma of the esophagus differs from the gastric variety in that hepatic metastases rarely occur early in the disease course, and the tumor tends to spread proximally throughout the rest of the esophagus (Mahoney and Condon 1987).

The male-to-female ratio for adenocarcinoma is higher than for gastric adenocarcinoma (6:1 versus 2:1). Chronic reflux occurs in 25% of patients with esophageal adenocarcinomas versus only 3% of patients with gastric adenocarcinoma. Likewise, hiatal hernia is present in 51% of all esophageal carcinomas but only 11% of all gastric adenocarcinomas (MacDonald and MacDonald 1987). Esophageal ade-

nocarcinoma frequently occurs in patients with a history of chronic inflammation or a hiatal hernia. Imaging techniques and CT in particular appear of limited value for disease staging (Orringer 1984), especially if a palliative operative procedure seems necessary from the outset. However, because surgery does not improve the prognosis of incurable esophageal tumors, the number of unnecessary surgical procedures may be reduced if CT proves to be truly effective in improving patient staging (Thompson 1983).

10.9 Conclusion

In conclusion, the prognosis for cancer of the esophagus remains poor, and only patients at high risk can benefit from effective screening by endoscopy and double-contrast barium esophagography. CT can define potential tumor resectability by evaluating metastatic spread and direct local invasion of the aorta and/or the tracheobronchial tree, which are contraindications for TTE and THE. However, disease extension into the paraesophageal soft tissues, the presence of adenopathies, and invasion of the pericardium and the pleura are compatible with THE for palliative purposes. Imaging techniques are also helpful for post-therapy patient follow-up to detect iatrogenic complications and disease recurrence.

10.10 References

Agha FP (1985) Barrett carcinoma of the esophagus: clinical and radiographic analysis of 34 cases. AJR 145: 41–46

Agha FP (1986) Radiologic diagnosis of Barrett's esophagus: critical analysis of 65 cases. Gastrointest Radiol 11: 123–130

Agha FP, Orringer MB, Amendola MA (1985) Gastric interposition following transhiatal esophagectomy: radiographic evaluation. Gastrointest Radiol 10: 17–24

Akiyama H (1980) Surgery for carcinoma of the esophagus. Curr Probl Surg SVII: 55–120

Akiyama H, Tsurumaru M, Kawamura T, Ono Y (1981) Principles of surgical treatment for carcinoma of the esophagus. Analysis of lymph node involvement. Ann Surg 194: 438–446

American Joint Committee Staging of Cancer of the Esophagus (1978) Manual for staging of cancer, pp 65: 70

Aste H, Munizzi F, Martines H, Pugliese V (1985) Esophageal dilation in malignant dysphagia. Cancer 56: 2713-2715

Balfe DM, Mauro MA, Koehler RE, Lee LKT, Weyman PJ, Picus D, Peterson RR (1984) Gastrohepatic ligament: normal and pathologic CT anatomy. Radiology 150: 485-490

Barajas Martinez JM, Loeches Prado N, Alcala-Santaella R (1986) Carcinoma esofagico primario; presentacion di clinica y valoracion de los metodos diagnosticos. Rev Esp Enferm Apar Dig 70: 211-213

Beatty JD, De Boer G, Rider WD (1979) Carcinoma of the oesophagus. Pretreatment assessment, correlation of radiation treatment parameters with survival, and identification and management of radiation treatment failure. Cancer 43: 2254-2267

Becker CD, Barbier P, Porcellini B (1986) CT evaluation of patients undergoing transhiatal esophagectomy for cancer. J Comput Assist Tomogr 10: 607-611

Becker CD, Barbier PA, Terrier F, Porcellini B (1987) Patterns of recurrence of esophageal esophagectomy and gastric interposition. AJR 148: 273-277

Campbell WR, Taylor SA, Pierce GE, Hermreck AS, Thomas JH (1985) Therapeutic alternatives in patients with esophageal cancer. Am J Surg 150: 665-668

Chavy AL, Rougier PM, Pieddeloup C, Kac J, Laplanche AC, Elias DM, Ducreux MP, Zummer-Rubinstein K, Zimmermann PA, Charbit MA, Crespon BM (1986) Esophageal prosthesis for neoplastic stenosis. A prognostic study of 77 cases. Cancer 57: 1426-1431

Chejfec G, Jablokow VR, Gould VE (1983) Linitis plastica carcinoma of the esophagus. Cancer 51: 2139-2143

Chisholm RJ, Stoller JL, Carpenter CM, Burhenne HJ (1986) Radiologic dilatation preceding palliative surgical tube placement for esophageal cancer. Am J Surg 151: 397-399

Collin CF, Spiro RH (1984) Carcinoma of the cervical esophagus: changing therapeutic trends. Am J Surg 148: 460-466

Correa P (1982) Precursors of gastric and esophageal cancer. Cancer 50: 2554-2565

Coulomb M, Lebas JF, Sarrazin R, Geindre M (1981) L'apport de la tomodensitométrie au bilan d'extension des cancers de l'oesophage. Incidences thérapeutiques. A propos de 40 observations. J Radiol 62: 475-487

Couraud L, Meriot S (1982) Le traitement des cancers du tiers inférieur et du tiers moyen de l'oesophage par résection et gastroplastie tubulée isopéristaltique. Chirugie 108: 703-707

Cozzi G, Bellomi M, Gariboldi M, Ostinelli O, Lo Gullo C, Ravasi G, Severini A (1987) Esophageal carcinoma. Radiologic appearance of minimal lesions. Acta Radiol [Diagn] (Stockh) 28: 177-180

Crummy AB, Wegner GP, Flaherty TT, Benfield JR, Brunette KW, Francyk WP (1968) Azygos venography. An aid in the evaluation of esophageal carcinoma. Ann Thorac Surg 6: 522-527

Cukingnan RS, Casey JJ (1978) Carcinoma of the esophagus. Ann Thorac Surg 26: 276-286

Cummins L (1983) Laser tissue interactions. In: Fleischer D, Jensen D, Bright-Asare P (eds) Therapeutic laser endoscopy in gastrointestinal disease. Nijhoff, Boston, pp 9-28

Daffner RH, Postlethwait RW, Putnam CE (1978) Retrotracheal abnormalities in esophageal carcinoma: prognostic implications. AJR 130: 719-723

Daffner RH, Halber MD, Postlethwait RW, Korobkin M, Thompson WM (1979) CT of the esophagus. II. Carcinoma. AJR 133: 1051-1055

Dancygier H, Classen M (1986) How can we diagnose the depth of cancer invasion in the esophagus? Endoscopy 18 (Suppl 3): 19-21

De Lange EE, Shaffer HA, Daniel TM, Kron IL (1987) Esophageal anastomotic leaks: preliminary results of treatment with balloon dilatation. Radiology 165: 45-47

Earlam R, Cunha-Melo JR (1980a) Oesophageal squamous cell carcinoma. I. A critical review of surgery. Br J Surg 67: 384-390

Earlam R, Cunha-Melo JR (1980b) Oesophageal squamous cell carcinoma. II. A critical review of radiotherapy. Br J Surg 67: 457-461

Endo M, Takeshita K, Yoshida M (1986) How can we diagnose the early stage of esophageal cancer? Endoscopic diagnosis. Endoscopy 18 (Suppl 3): 11-18

Fein R, Kelsen DP, Geller N, Bains M, McCormack P, Brennan MF (1985) Adenocarcinoma of the esophagus and gastroesophageal junction. Prognostic factors and results of therapy. Cancer 56: 2512-2518

Freeny PC, Marks WM (1982) Adenocarcinoma of the gastroesophageal junction: barium and CT examination. AJR 138: 1077-1084

Galandiuk S, Herman RE, Gassman JJ, Cosgrove DM (1986) Cancer of the esophagus. The Cleveland clinic experience. Ann Surg 203: 101-108

Ghadirian P (1985) Familial history of esophageal cancer. Cancer 56: 2112-2116

Giradet RE, Ransdell HT, Wheat MW (1974) Palliative intubation in the management of esophageal carcinoma. Ann Thorac Surg 18: 417-430

Glazer GM, Gross BH, Quint LE, Francis IR, Bookstein FL, Orringer MB (1985) Normal mediastinal lymph nodes: number and size according to American Thoracic Society mapping. AJR 144: 261-265

Goffman TE, McKeen EA, Curtis RE, Schein PS (1983) Esophageal carcinoma following irradiation for breast cancer. Cancer 52: 1808-1809

Graziani L, Bearzi I, Romagnoli A, Pesaresi A, Montesi A (1985) Significance of diffuse granularity and nodularity of the esophageal mucosa at double-contrast radiography. Gastrointest Radiol 10: 1-6

Gua-Qing W (1981) Endoscopic diagnosis of early esophageal carcinoma. J R Soc Med 74: 502-503

Halpert RD, Laufer I, Thompson JJ, Feczko PJ (1983) Adenocarcinoma of the esophagus in patients with scleroderma. AJR 140: 927-930

Halvorsen RA, Thompson WM (1987) Computed tomographic staging of gastrointestinal tract malignancies. Part I. Esophagus and stomach. Invest Radiol 22: 2-16

Halvorsen RA, Magruder-Habib K, Foster WL, Roberts L, Postlethwait RW, Thompson WM (1986) Esophageal cancer staging by CT: long-term follow-up study. Radiology 161: 147-151

Haynes JW, Miller PR, Steiger Z, Leichman LP, Kling GA (1984) Celestin tube use: radiographic manifestations of associated complications. Radiology 150: 41-44

Hermanek P, Sobin LH (1987) TNM. Classification of malignant tumours. Springer, Berlin, Heidelberg, New York, London, Paris, Tokyo

Hishikawa Y, Kamikonya N, Tanaka S, Miura T (1986) Esophageal stricture following high-dose-rate intracavitary irradiation for esophageal cancer. Radiology 159: 715-716

Hopkins A, Postlethwait RW (1981) Caustic burn and carcinoma of the esophagus. Ann Surg 194: 146-148

Huang GJ (1981) Early detection and surgical treatment of esophageal carcinoma. Jpn J Surg 11: 399-405

Isono K, Onada S, Ishikawa T, Sato H, Nakayama K (1982) Studies on the cause of deaths from esophageal carcinoma. Cancer 49: 2173-2179

Jaffe MH, Fleischer D, Zeman RK, Benjamin SB, Choyke PL, Clark LR (1987) Esophageal malignancy: imaging results and complications of combined endoscopic-radiologic palliation. Radiology 164: 623-630

Jones DA, Steger A, Goolden AWG (1985) Carcinoma of the oesophagus after radiotherapy for Hodgkin's disease. Br J Radiol 58: 1131

Kakegawa T, Yamana H, Ando N (1985) Analysis of surgical treatment for carcinoma situated in the cervical esophagus. Surgery 97: 150-157

Kelsen D (1982) Treatment of advanced esophageal cancer. Cancer 50: 2576-2581

Kondo M, Ando N, Kosuda S, Lian SL, Kubo A, Masaki H, Hashimoto S, Tsutsui T, Takegawa T (1982) Ga-67 scan in patients with intrathoracic esophageal carcinoma planned for surgery. Cancer 49: 1031-1034

Kron IL, Cantrell RW, Johns ME, Joob A, Minor G (1984) Computerized axial tomography of the esophagus to determine the suitability for blunt esophagectomy. Ann Surg 199: 173-174

Kuylenstierna R, Munck-Wikland E (1985) Esophagitis and cancer of the esophagus. Cancer 56: 837-839

Larson TC, Shuman LS, Libshitz HI, McMurtrey MJ (1985) Complications of colonic interposition. Cancer 56: 681-690

Lawson TL, Dodds WJ (1976) Infiltrating carcinoma simulating achalasia. Gastrointest Radiol 1: 245-248

Levine MS, Kressel HY, Caroline DF, Laufer I, Herlinger H, Thompson JJ (1983) Barrett esophagus: reticular pattern of the mucosa. Radiology 147: 663-667

Levine MS, Dillon EC, Saul SH, Laufer I (1986) Early esophageal cancer. AJR 146: 507-512

MacDonald WC, MacDonald JB (1987) Adenocarcinoma of the esophagus and/or gastric cardia. Cancer 60: 1094-1098

Maeta M, Koga S, Andachi H, Yoshioka H, Wakatsuki T (1986) Esophageal cancer developed after gastrectomy. Surgery 99: 87-91

Mahoney JL, Condon RE (1987) Adenocarcinoma of the esophagus. Ann Surg 205: 557-562

Maillet P, Baulieux J, Boulez J, Benhaim R (1982) Carcinoma of the thoracic esophagus. Results of one-stage surgery (271 cases). Am J Surg 143: 629-634

Mandard AM, Chasle J, Marnay J, Villedieu B, Bianco C, Roussel A, Elie H, Vernhes JC (1981) Autopsy findings in 111 cases of esophageal cancer. Cancer 48: 329-335

Marx MV, Balfe DM (1987) Computed tomography of the esophagus. Semin Ultrasound CT MR 8: 316-348

Moore C (1958) Visceral squamous cancer in children. Pediatrics 21: 573-581

Mori S, Kasai M, Watanabe T, Shibuya I (1979) Preoperative assessment of resectability for carcinoma of the thoracic esophagus. Part I. Esophagogram and azygogram. Ann Surg 190: 100-105

Morita K, Takagi I, Watanabe M, Niwa K, Kanazawa H (1985) Relationship between the radiologic features of esophageal cancer and the local control by radiation therapy. Cancer 55: 2668-2676

Moss AA, Schnyder P, Thoeni RF, Margulis AR (1981) Esophageal carcinoma: pretherapy staging by computed tomography. AJR 136: 1051-1056

Mouelhi MM, Gayet B, Grenier P, Biagini J, Fekete F, Nahum H (1986) Les complications des oesophagoplasties coliques. Aspects radiologiques. J Radiol 67: 605-611

Norton GA, Postlethwait RW, Thompson WM (1980) Esophageal carcinoma: a survey of populations at risk. South Med J 73: 25-27

O'Connell EW, Seaman WB, Ghahremani GG (1984) Radiation-induced esophageal carcinoma. Gastrointest Radiol 9: 287-291

Parisot P, Robin P, Huten N, Vandooren M (1985) Cancers de l'oesophage. Etude rétrospective de 225 cas. Ann Chir 39: 383-389

Picus D, Balfe DM, Koehler RE, Roper CL, Owen JW (1983) Computed tomography in the staging of esophageal carcinoma. Radiology 146: 433-438

Orringer MB (1984) Transhiatal esophagectomy without thoracotomy for carcinoma of the thoracic esophagus. Ann Surg 200: 282–288

Pomerri F, Pittarello F, Tremolada C, Ruol A, Muzzio PC (1986) Metodologie radiologiche nella valutazione delle esofagoplastiche alte. Radiol Med 72: 853–855

Postlethwait RW (1978) Carcinoma of the esophagus. Curr Probl Cancer 2: 1–44

Quint LE, Glazer GM, Orringer MB (1985a) Esophageal imaging by MR and CT: study of normal anatomy and neoplasms. Radiology 156: 727–731

Quint LE, Glazer GM, Orringer MB, Gross BH (1985b) Esophageal carcinoma: CT findings. Radiology 155: 171–175

Reboud E, Pradoura JP, Giudicelli R, Fuentes P (1983) Multicentricité du cancer de l'oesophage. Chirurgie 109: 41–46

Rosenberg JC, Schwade JG, Vaitkevicius VK (1982) Cancer of the esophagus. In: De Vita VT, Hellman S, Rosenberg SA (eds) Cancer. Principles and practice of oncology. Lippincott, Philadelphia, pp 499–533

Rousset JF, Prevost F, Roos S, Fourtanier G, Escat J (1986) Cancer de l'oesophage. Evaluation comparée de l'extension médiastinale par le scanner et la chirurgie. Ann Chir 40: 311–312

Saldana JA, Cone RO, Hopens TA, Bannayan GA (1982) Carcinoma arising in an epiphrenic esophageal diverticulum. Gastrointest Radiol 7: 15–18

Salonen O, Kivisaari L, Standertskjold-Nordenstram CG, Somer K, Virkkunen P (1987) Computed tomography in staging of oesophageal carcinoma. Scand J Gastroenterol 22: 65–68

Samuelsson L, Hambraeus GM, Mercke CE, Tylen U (1984) CT staging of oesophageal carcinoma. Acta Radiol [Diagn] 25: 7–11

Sanfey H, Hamilton SR, Smith RL, Cameron JL (1985) Carcinoma arising in Barrett's esophagus. Surg Gynecol Obstet 161: 570–574

Sarr MG, Hamilton SR, Marrone GC, Cameron JL (1985) Barrett's esophagus: its prevalence and association with adenocarcinoma in patients with symptoms of gastroesophageal reflux. Am J Surg 149: 187–193

Sato T, Sakai Y, Kajita A, Fujino Y, Taniguchi K, Kabuto T, Ishiguro S (1986) Radiographic microstructures of early esophageal carcinoma: correlation of specimen radiography with pathologic findings and clinical radiography. Gastrointest Radiol 11: 12–19

Schneekloth G, Terrier F, Fuchs WA (1983) Computed tomography in carcinoma of esophagus and cardia. Gastrointest Radiol 8: 193–206

Schottenfeld D (1984) Epidemiology of cancer of the esophagus. Semin Oncol 11: 92–100

Sherrill DJ, Grishkin BA, Galal FS, Zajtchuk R, Graeber GM (1984) Radiation associated malignancies of the esophagus. Cancer 54: 726–728

Silber W (1985) Carcinoma of the oesophagus: aspects of epidemiology and aetiology. Proc Nut Soc 44: 101–110

Simonetti G, Urigo F, Meloni BB, Canalis GC, Rovasio S, Frasson F, Di Toma F (1987) Transluminal esophagoplasty (TEP). Our experience in over fifty patients. Ann Radiol 30: 158–160

Sjogren RW, Johnson LF (1983) Barrett's esophagus: a review. Am J Med 74: 313–321

Skinner DB, Dowlatshahi KD, Demeester TR (1982) Potentially curable cancer of the esophagus. Cancer 50: 2571–2575

Skinner DB, Walther BC, Riddell RH, Schmidt H, Iascone C, Demeester TR (1983) Barrett's esophagus. Comparison of benign and malignant cases. Ann Surg 198: 554–566

Skinner DB, Ferguson MK, Soriano A, Little AG, Staszak VM (1986) Selection of operation for esophageal cancer based on staging. Ann Surg 204: 391–401

Soga J, Tanaka O, Sasaki K, Fawaguchi M, Muto T (1982) Superficial spreading carcinoma of the esophagus. Cancer 50: 1641–1645

Sugimachi K, Okudaira Y, Ueo H, Ikeda M, Inokuchi K (1982) Transtracheal mediastinal lymphography for visualization of metastatic lymph nodes in carcinoma of the esophagus. Surg Gynecol Obstet 154: 34–38

Sugimachi K, Maekawa S, Koga Y, Ueo H, Inokuchi K (1986) The quality of life is sustained after operation for carcinoma of the esophagus. Surg Gynecol Obstet 162: 544–546

Suzuki H, Kobayashi S, Endo M, Nakayama K (1972) Diagnosis of early esophageal cancer. Surgery 71: 99–103

Takemoto T, Ito T, Aibe T, Okita K (1986) Endoscopic ultrasonography in the diagnosis of esophageal carcinoma, with particular regard to staging it for operability. Endoscopy 18 (Suppl 3): 22–25

Tam PC, Cheung HC, Ma L, Siu KF, Wong J (1987) Local recurrences after subtotal esophagectomy for squamous cell carcinoma. Ann Surg 205: 189–194

Taylor CR (1986) Carcinoma of the esophagus. Current imaging options. Am J Gastroenterol 81: 1013–1020

Thompson WM (1983) Esophageal cancer. Int J Radiat Oncol Biol Phys 9: 1533–1565

Thompson WM (1985) Esophageal cancer. In: Bragg DG, Rubin P, Youker JE (eds) Oncologic imaging. Pergamon, New York, pp 207–242

Thompson WM, Oddson TA, Kelvin F, Daffner R, Postlethwait RW, Rice RP (1978) Synchronous and metachronous squamous cell carcinomas of the head, neck and esophagus. Gastrointest Radiol 3: 123–127

Thompson WM, Halvorsen RA, Foster WL, Williford ME, Postlethwait RW, Korobkin M (1983) Computed tomography for staging esophageal and gastroesophageal cancer: reevaluation. AJR 141: 951–958

Tio TL, Den Hartog Jager FCA, Tytgat GNJ (1986) The role of endoscopic ultrasonography in assessing local resectability of oesophagogastric malignancies. Accuracy, pitfalls, and predictability. Scand J Gastroenterol 21 (Suppl 123): 78–86

Tsang TK, Hidvegi D, Horth K, Ostrow JD (1987) Reliability of balloon-mesh cytology in detecting esophageal carcinoma in a population of US Veterans. Cancer 59: 556–559

Tytgat GNJ, Den Hartog Jager FCA (1984) Palliation of malignant obstruction with endoprosthesis. Acta Gastroenterol Belg 67: 188–194

Valbuena J (1984) Endoscopic palliative treatment of esophageal and cardial cancer: a new antireflux prosthesis. A study of 40 cases. Cancer 53: 993–998

Van Andel JG, Dees J, Dijkhuis CM, Fokkens W, Van Houten H, De Jong PC, Van Woerkam-ᴌykenboom WM (1979) Carcinoma of the esophagus. Results of treatment. Ann Surg 190: 684–689

Van Andel JG, Dees J, Eijkenboom WMH, Van Houten H, Jobsen JJ, Mud HJ, Obertop H, Van Putten WLJ (1986) Therapy of esophageal carcinoma. Results from the Joint Group on Esophageal Carcinoma in Rotterdam. Acta Radiol [Oncol] 25: 115–120

Wang HH, Antonioli DA, Goldman H (1986) Comparative features of esophageal and gastric adenocarcinomas: recent changes in type and frequency. Hum Pathol 17: 482–487

Weisburger JH, Wynder EL, Horn CL (1982) Nutritional factors and etiologic mechanisms in the causation of gastrointestinal cancers. Cancer 50: 2541–2549

Wolf EL, Frager J, Brandt LJ, Frager DH, Bernstein LH, Beneventano TC (1986) Radiographic appearance of the esophagus and stomach after laser treatment of obstructing carcinoma. AJR 146: 519–522

Wong J (1987) Esophageal resection for cancer: the rationale of current practice. Am J Surg 153: 18–24

Yang ZY, Gu XZ, Zhao S, Hong ZG, An HL, Hou FX, Xiang QC, Guo BZ, Dong JP, Tian GD, Liu XP, Xing BJ (1983) Long term survival of radiotherapy for esophageal cancer: analysis of 1136 patients surviving for more than 5 years. Int J Radiat Oncol Biol Phys 9: 1769–1773

Zornoza J, Lindell MM (1980) Radiologic evaluation of small esophageal carcinoma. Gastrointest Radiol 5: 107–111

11 Adenocarcinoma of the Stomach*

Although the incidence of gastric cancer has decreased considerably in most industrialized nations, these tumors remain a serious problem because they are often not diagnosed until an advanced stage. Furthermore, therapeutic progress has not yet succeeded in significantly improving patient survival. Imaging studies play a less important role for gastric adenocarcinoma than for other gastric pathologies or adenocarcinoma in other localizations because disease staging requires surgery (Halvorsen and Thompson 1987). Cancer of the cardia has benefited more from evaluation by modern imaging techniques than disease in other portions of the stomach, and is thus dealt with separately.

11.1 Epidemiology

11.1.1 Frequency

The prevalence of gastric adenocarcinoma varies widely from one region of the world to another. The highest frequencies are observed in Japan, whereas western Europe and the United States have markedly lower rates. These tumors are least common in Africa.

The frequency of gastric cancer has declined in nearly all regions of the world (Devesa 1982). Between 1951 and 1976, the mortality rate for gastric cancer in France dropped 48% in males and 58% in females (Audigier and Tuyns 1981). In the United States, the incidence of gastric cancer between 1974 and 1971 dropped 63% in males and 67% in women (Devesa 1982). Meyers et al. (1987) reported a rise in the frequency of cancer of the cardia during the past 40 years (21% to 44%) but a decrease in the frequency of antral malignancies during this same period (60% to 33%). The decrease in the incidence of gastric cancer appears essentially related to dietary modifications (Decarli et al. 1986). Variations in frequency have been linked to several parameters: histologic type, sex, age, socioeconomic factors, and genetic factors.

Gastric adenocarcinomas are not a homogeneous entity, but have been subdivided into intestinal and diffuse types (Lauren 1965). The intestinal type is commonly associated with chronic gastritis and intestinal metaplasia, which are less frequent in diffuse disease. Cancers of the cardia and the body of the stomach tend to be diffuse, whereas the intestinal type predominates in the antrum. The reduction in the incidence of gastric cancer is especially marked for the intestinal type, the most frequent variant in high-risk areas.

The incidence of gastric cancer is higher in males than in females in all regions of the world; overall, the sex ratio is between 1.5 and 2.5. For Grabiec and Owen (1985), the incidence of gastric carcinoma is 32.4 for individuals over 40 years of age and 0.4 for individuals younger than 40. Young patients tend to present with advanced, diffuse disease with a poor prognosis. In children, adenocarcinoma is less frequent than lymphoma and leiomyosarcoma, and is encountered in three circumstances: as a complication of gastrointestinal polyposis, after treatment of lymphoma, and, rarely, de novo (Goldthorn and Canizaro 1986).

The frequency of gastric cancer is higher in poor social classes. In migratory populations, the risk of gastric cancer often drops notably during the second generation; this has been demonstrated in particular for Japanese emigrants to the United States (Locke and King 1980). This situation, which corresponds to a

---

* Written in collaboration with A. Rogopoulos.

drop in the incidence of intestinal-type disease, suggests that environmental factors intervening early in an individual's lifetime can modify development of such gastric cancers.

A genetic factor has been evoked in the onset of diffuse-type cancers: relatives of patients with diffuse-type cancer are at higher risk for developing cancer than relatives of patients with intestinal-type disease.

11.2 Pathogenesis

11.2.1 Endogenous Factors

Chronic atrophic gastritis is a common pathology in patients at high risk for gastric cancer. For Meyers et al. (1987), 2% of all patients with gastric adenocarcinomas also have atrophic gastritis. However, surveillance of all individuals with atrophic gastritis is impractical because of the high frequency of this pathology in the elderly. Intestinal metaplasia of the stomach has been postulated as a premalignant condition for gastric carcinoma.

While most *gastric polyps* are hyperplastic lesions without any malignant predisposition (see Chap. 2), some are sentinel lesions of stomach cancer. For example, adenomatous polyps, which frequently develop on atrophic gastritis, have a high malignant potential. This is particularly true for villous adenomas (Faivre et al. 1976).

Cancers arising on a *gastrectomy stump* represent 0.4%-8.7% of findings in gastric cancer studies (Orringer 1950; Stalberg and Takidal 1971), with an average of 2.5% (Richelme et al. 1984). The risk is higher in males than in females (sex ratio of 4.3 for Stanta et al. 1986). The role of the type of surgical procedure is controversial. Certain authors claim the risk is the same regardless of the procedure; others consider vagotomy and Billroth II operations to be associated with a higher risk (Caygill et al. 1986; Dlin et al. 1985; Viste et al. 1986). The potential role of the Billroth II procedure suggests that bile reflux may be implicated in gastric carcinogenesis. The risk of adenocarcinoma is similar to that in the general population during the first few years after gastric surgery, but rises sharply after more than 20 years. The resectability of these adenocarci-

nomas is often limited because they are advanced lesions. Severe epithelial dysplasia appears to constitute a premalignant condition; this should prompt regular follow-up, in particular for gastrectomized individuals with this abnormality.

Malignant transformation of *gastric ulcers* has been the subject of numerous controversies. Two criteria are essential for diagnosis of ulcer cancer: history of a pre-existent ulcer and presence of carcinoma on one or more margins of the ulcer.

The risk of gastric cancer is three to four times higher in patients with *Bierner's anemia* than in the general population. The risk of stomach cancer in patients with *Menetrier's disease* has been estimated at 10% (Martin et al. 1962).

11.2.2 Environmental Factors

The main environmental factors responsible for the decline in the incidence of gastric cancers are related to dietary changes. Food preservation by refrigeration, in particular, has an important role. Intragastric nitrate derivatives are considered a main factor in the development of cancer: nitrosamines are stable compounds which require biologic activation to become carcinogenic, whereas nitrosamides are carcinogenic without such activation (Reed et al. 1981). Large amounts of nitrate derivatives are formed when meat is conserved by salting, whereas refrigeration prevents the formation of these compounds. Consumption of highly salted food, smoked food or fish, and canned foods increases the risk of gastric cancer whereas vitamin C (which blocks transformation of nitrites into nitrosamides), cold-preserved meats and fish, leafy green vegetables and fresh fruits correspond to the least carcinogenic diet possible, provided that it is started at an early age. Other less important etiologic factors include smoking, alcohol consumption, and vitamin deficiencies (Weisburger et al. 1982).

11.3 Pathologic Findings

Dysplasia is a premalignant condition. Intestinal metaplasia is frequent, but is not induced by dysplasia (Hattori 1986). Dysplasia associates the following abnormalities: augmentation of cell proliferation, abnormal morphology and cellular pleomorphism, architectural disorganization of the glands, and stromal changes (Ming et al. 1984).

11.3.1 Gross Anatomy

The macroscopic forms of gastric adenocarcinoma correspond to the endoscopic appearances: polypoid lesion, infiltration, and ulceration. Borrman's classification identifies the following appearances: B1 polypoid, B2 ulceratisn, B3 ulceration and infiltration, B4 diffuse infiltration (Morson and Dawson 1979).

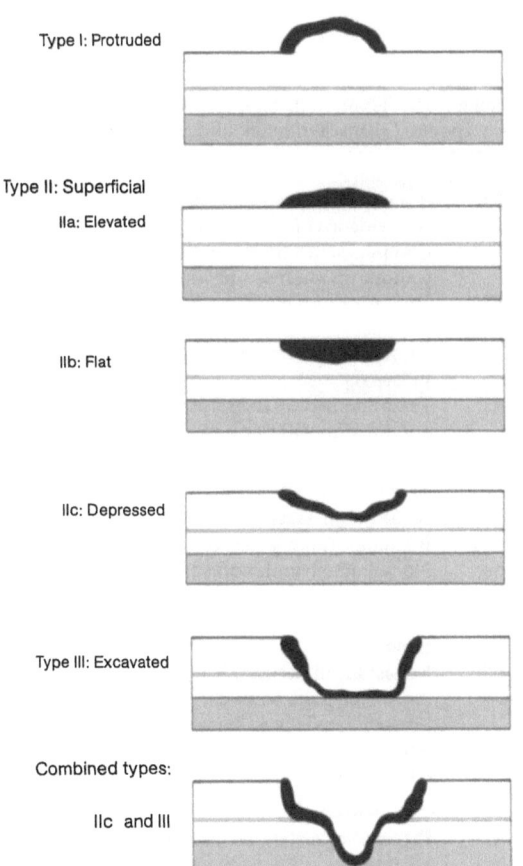

Fig. 11.1. Different patterns of early gastric carcinoma

The distribution of lesions within the stomach is as follows: upper third of the stomach, including the cardia 31%–37%; body of the stomach 10%–11%; antrum 37%–42%; diffuse disease 15% (Berger et al. 1986; Meyers et al. 1987). For Esaki et al. (1987), 17% of multiple lesions occur in elderly patients.

Early gastric cancer (EGC) has been defined as carcinoma invading the mucosa and/or mucosa and the submucosa, regardless of the presence of lymph node metastases (Japanese Research Society for Gastric Cancer 1981). The five stages of EGC are summarized in Figure 11.1 (Fernando and Nakamura 1986; Gold et al. 1984; Japanese Research Society for Gastric Cancer 1981; Ohta et al. 1987; Shirakabe 1972). EGC represents fewer than 10% of all gastric cancers in Europe and the United States (Miller et al. 1975; White et al. 1985). It is three times more common in Japan, where it represents 30%–39% of recent series (Ohta et al. 1987). The depressed type is more common than the elevated type. The depressed type is encountered in subjects aged 40-60 years; it is localized to the body or the fundus, and associated gastric lesions are present in 26.4% of cases (essentially ulceration). The elevated type occurs essentially in the antrum. Most associated lesions (present in 46.1% of cases for Ohta et al. 1987) are polyps.

11.3.2 Microscopic Features

11.3.2.1 Histologic Classification

Aside from the classification of Lauren (1965), which distinguishes intestinal and diffuse types of gastric adenocarcinoma, another staging system, based on cytologic findings, identifies papillary, tubular, and mucinous and signet-ring variants, and adenocarcinoma with independent cells (linitis plastica). Adenosquamous carcinoma is very rare, and its prognosis is not as good as that of adenocarcinoma because the lesion is more extensive and tends to invade the lymphatics (Mori et al. 1986).

11.3.2.2 Degree of Differentiation

The degree of differentiation must be specified for each anatomic form. The undifferentiated form affects young women in particular; these depressed and/or infiltrating lesions develop from the normal mucosa. Hepatic metastases are rare, but peritoneal carcinosis is frequent. By contrast, the differentiated form often affects elderly males; these elevated or depressed lesions are expansive and occur on intestinal metaplasia; hepatic metastases are frequent but peritoneal carcinosis is rare (Fernando and Nakamura 1986).

11.3.2.3 Particular Forms

Gastric linitis is an infiltrating cancer that thickens the stomach wall; the folds are obliterated or thickened by the carcinomatous infiltration; histologic diagnosis can be difficult in the absence of mucosal destruction. *Carcinoma with lymphoid stroma* (or medullary carcinoma with lymphoid infiltration) appears to represent a separate group; gross examination reveals ulcerations and well-limited lesions; histologically, the carcinomatous structures consisting of lymphocytes and plasmocytes are separated by massive lymphoid infiltration.

11.3.3 Mode of Spread

Gastric cancer can extend by contiguous spread, along lymphatic pathways, through the bloodstream, or by intraperitoneal seeding. Contiguous spread along the gastrointestinal tract wall explains the frequency of esophageal involvement (26.8%) and duodenal involvement (21.6%) regardless of the gastric localization in the literature review conducted by Yan and Brooks (1985). Spread along lymphatic pathways exists in 70.5% of cases for Yan and Brooks (1985); the lymph nodes are first invaded in the drainage area of the tumor. Extension occurs secondarily at the levels of the parapancreatic, lomboaortic, hepatic, and periesophageal chains. Hematogenous dissemination is responsible for hepatic, pulmonary, adrenal gland, ovarian, bone, and thyroid metastases. Peritoneal implants are responsible for carcinosis; this mechanism, rather than hematogenous dissemination, probably explains the appearance of Krukenberg's ovarian tumor.

11.3.4 Classifications of Gastric Adenocarcinoma

Table 11.1 summarizes the TNM classification (Hermanek and Sobin 1987). The classification systems of Gutmann et al. (1939) and Dukes are also used. The Dukes classification distinguishes four stages (Morson and Dawson 1979):

Stage A Tumor confined to the serosa, no nodal involvement
Stage B Involvement of the serosa
Stage C Intact serosa but adenopathies
Stage D Metastases, regardless of the local status

Table 11.1. TNM clinical classification of gastric carcinoma. (From Hermanek and Sobin 1987)

T – Primary tumor	
TX	Primary tumor cannot be assessed
T0	No evidence of primary tumor
Tis	Carcinoma in situ: intraepithelial tumor without invasion of the lamina propria
T1	Tumor invades lamina propria or submucosa
T2	Tumor invades muscularis propria or subserosa
T3	Tumor penetrates the serosa (visceral peritoneum) without invasion of adjacent structures
T4	Tumor invades adjacent structures
N – Regional lymph nodes	
NX	Regional lymph nodes cannot be assessed
N0	No regional lymph node metastasis
N1	Metastasis in perigastric lymph node(s) within 3 cm of the edge of the primary tumor
N2	Metastasis in perigastric lymph node(s) more than 3 cm from the edge of the primary tumor or in lymph nodes along the left gastric, common hepatic, splenic, or coeliac arteries
M – Distant metastasis	
MX	Presence of distant metastasis cannot be assessed
M0	No distant metastasis
M1	Distant metastasis

While combined use of biopsies and cytologic studies increases the chance of diagnosing cancer, in particular during follow-up of premalignant lesions, examination of the surgical specimen is indispensable for accurate classification of gastric adenocarcinoma. The entire surgical specimen must be examined because 15%-16% of all early gastric cancers are multicentric (Ohta et al. 1987).

11.4 Diagnostic Data Other than Imaging

11.4.1 Circumstances of Discovery and Screening

Screening programs have not been set up for gastric cancer in the United States or Europe because of the low incidence of this pathology and the fact that such screening is prohibitively expensive (Gold et al. 1984). So long as double-contrast gastric examinations and endoscopy are reserved for symptomatic patients, no increase should be expected in the percentage of EGC compared to all gastric cancers. To increase this percentage, the indications for gastric investigation techniques would have to be widened to all cases of unexplained dyspepsia in patients beginning at 50 years of age (Goldstein et al. 1983). Along with individual screening by fiberoptic endoscopy or double-contrast studies, mass screening is impractical in Western nations; even in Japan, cost effectiveness remains controversial.

11.4.2 Clinical Symptoms

Patients with EGC may be asymptomatic or have only minor clinical symptoms (pain, weight loss); hemorrhage is rare. The clinical manifestations of invasive cancers, the type usually encountered in western countries, include weight loss (72%-90%), abdominal pain (51%-62%), nausea and vomiting (40%-84%), bleeding (27%), dysphagia (22%), abdominal mass (17%-32%) (Meyers et al. 1987; Naraynsingh 1985). Dysphagia is a fairly frequent sign encountered with gastric cancer. Barium studies must not be limited to the esophagus because achalasia can occur secondary to a gastric cancer (Halpert et al. 1985).

11.4.3 Endoscopy

The gross features of invasive cancer include:

- *Polypoid lesion* protruding into the gastric lumen, often with a shallow, central ulceration. When this ulceration increases in size and the nodular form spreads out, an ulcerated infiltrating polypoid lesion (the most frequent form) can be seen: the elevated ulceration of variable form and depth bleeds easily and is surrounded by a hard irregular rim. This rim consists of the extremities of the folds that converge towards the ulcer.
- *A large mass* can occupy a great portion of the stomach; diagnosis of these lesions with their irregular, friable surface is no problem.
- *Infiltrating forms* localized to a small part of the body of the stomach may be difficult to identify; the mucosa is thickened. Modifications of the global morphology of the stomach may become visible after air is insufflated into the gastric cavity; gastric wall pliability must also be evaluated. Linitis plastica is the typical form of these infiltrating lesions.

Overall, nodular lesions represent 44% of all gastric cancers; ulcerated lesions account for 40%; the remainder are polypoid and infiltrating lesions (Morson and Dawson 1979).

Compared to barium radiology studies, endoscopy is of particular interest: in addition to use for biopsies, it can detect minute gastric cancers less than 5 mm in diameter (Iishi et al. 1985; Oohara et al. 1984). For the diagnosis of this type of cancer, the value of endoscopy compared to anatomic data after gastric surgery is between 22.5% and 44.3% (solitary cancers and cancers associated with another, larger gastric cancers considered together).

Overall, endoscopy successfully diagnoses 83%-100% of all gastric cancers; for EGC, it can reach 100% when 8-12 biopsies are performed, but drops to only 50% if only one or two biopsies are used (Chevrel et al. 1985). Detection of EGC can be improved by the endoscopic Congo red test combined with methylene blue staining (Tatsuta et al. 1982). In addition to the difficulties inherent to the small size of these lesions and their submucosal nature, the cardia is a difficult sector to visualize endoscopically (Milnes et al. 1982).

Laparoscopy has also been used for the work-up of gastric cancers (Possik et al. 1986). This technique has a value of 88.5% for serosal infiltration, 81.2% for tumor fixation, 58.2% for metastatic lymph nodes, 89.4% for peritoneal involvement, and 96.5% for hepatic metastases.

11.5 Imaging Studies

11.5.1 Contrast Studies

11.5.1.1 Techniques

Several techniques can be used to examine the stomach, with either water-soluble iodinated products (indicated essentially for postoperative studies) or barium. Examination can be completed by a compression study, evaluation of mucosal relief, and full-column views. An association of these different techniques increases the accuracy of barium studies from 9% to 18% (Gelfand et al. 1987). Fluoroscopy can be used to guide percutaneous gastrostomy, an alternative to surgical gastrectomy for patients with very advanced local or general disease (Wills 1986).

11.5.1.2 Value of Barium Studies

Barium studies have a kappa index of 0.91 for diagnosis of cancer, which is very satisfactory (Shaw et al. 1987). Although there are no diagnostic problems for invasive cancers, particular mention is warranted for the value of radiology studies for EGC. Single-contrast studies have a false-negative rate of 25%, and 4%–14% of all benign-appearing ulcers are actually malignant (Barentsz et al. 1986; Cotton 1973; Schulman and Simpkins 1975). Double-contrast barium meal examinations can usually diagnose ulcerations smaller than 1 cm (Levine et al. 1988; Shirakabe 1972), and appear more effective for detecting elevated EGC (5 mm) than depressed lesions (10 mm) (Fernando and Nakamura 1986). However, for Montesi et al. (1982), double-contrast barium studies have a false-negative error rate of 33% for diagnosis of EGC. For minute gastric cancers (under 5 mm), double-contrast studies

have a sensitivity of 15.5% for both solitary lesions and lesions associated with a larger gastric adenocarcinoma (Gold et al. 1984). Overall, regardless of the type of cancer, barium studies are less effective than endoscopy.

11.5.1.3 Radiographic Features of EGC (Figs. 11.2–11.5)

The macroscopic features of EGC visualized radiographically (Table 111.1) are as follows:

Type I   Protruded type, causing elevation of the mucosa, with a smooth or nodular surface

Type II   Superficial cancer (referred to as mucoerosive cancer by Gutmann et al. (1939). Four times more frequent than type I, type II may be elevated, flat, or depressed. The mucosa loses its shiny appearance and becomes granular; it can be associated with a flat-edged ulceration whose limits are formed by raised up mucosa or radiating folds. The gastric wall contour is irregular and rounded. Extension is often multifocal, with islands of healthy mucosa. This lesion can vary from 3–40 mm. Radiographic healing is present in 71% of EGC with ulceration (Sakita et al. 1971).

Type III Excavated cancer: association of a chronic ulcerous structure and a cancer

Ulcerations can be defined as benign or malignant with an excellent sensitivity. The radiologic features of neoplastic ulcers are as follows (Thompson et al. 1983):

- En face views: radiating mucosal folds with nodularity, clubbing, fusion, penciling or amputation; presence of an ulcer crater with sharply angled margins and an irregular surrounding mass.
- profile view: ulcer lying inside the stomach wall; absence of a "Hampton" line; no ulcer collar, irregular ulcer mound.

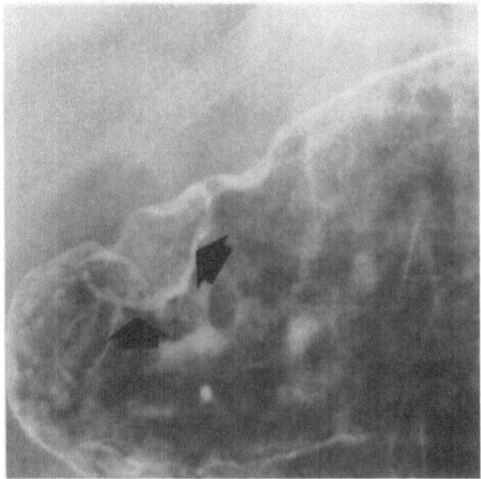

Fig. 11.2. Early carcinoma, type I

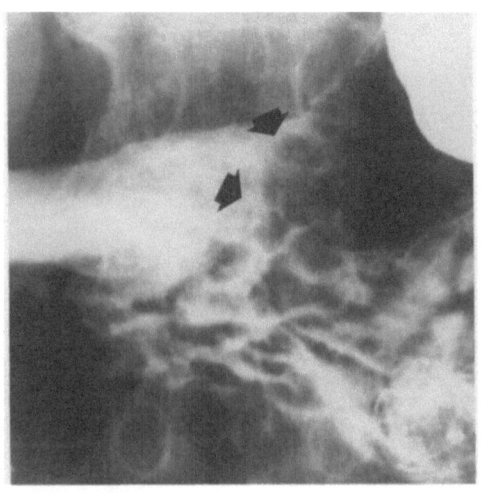

Fig. 11.4. Early carcinoma, combined type (IIA and IIC) *(arrows)*

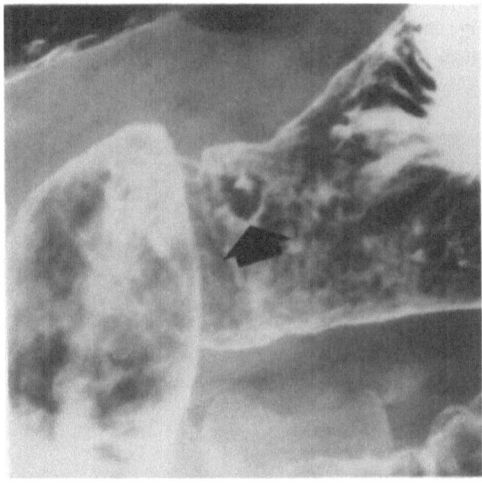

Fig. 11.3. Early carcinoma, type II

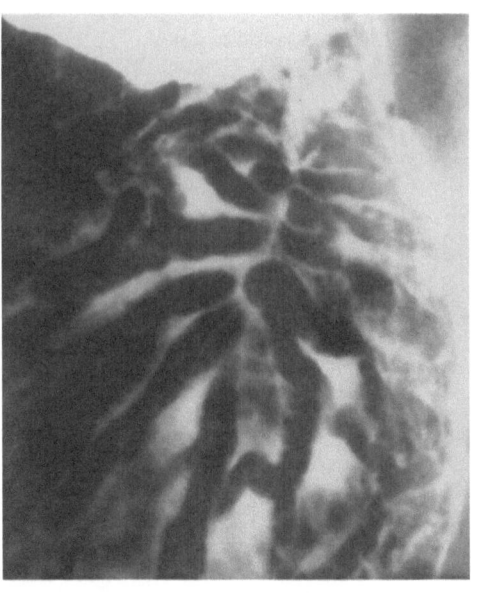

Fig. 11.5. Early carcinoma, combined type (IIA and IIC)

11.5.1.4 Advanced Cancer (Figs. 11.6–11.10)

The three main forms are more or less associated:

– Polypoid lesions often occur in the cardia and the upper third of the stomach; these ulcerated lesions have an irregular surface.

– Ulcerated lesions are composed of an ulceration and a peripheral rim; they protrude at the periphery and infiltrate in depth. The depth and width of the ulceration varies, and the concave inferior surface may be smooth or irregular. The height and thickness of the rim delimiting the ulceration are also variable.

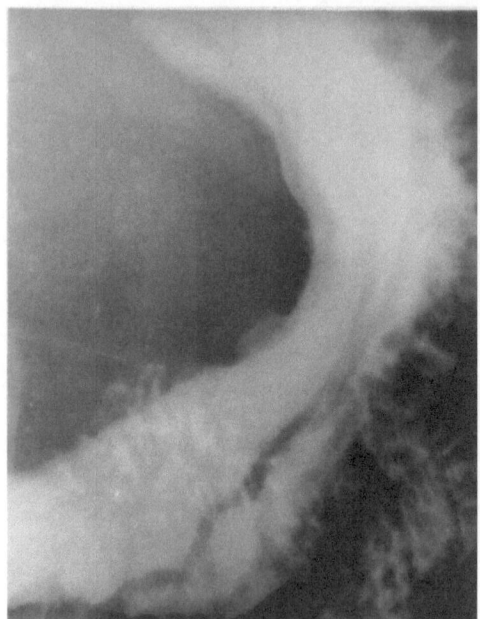

Fig. 11.6. Ulcerated gastric cancer

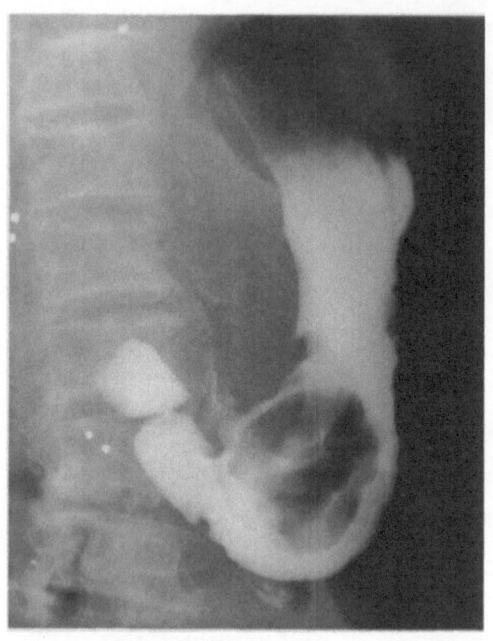

Fig. 11.8. Polypoid cancer in the body of the stomach

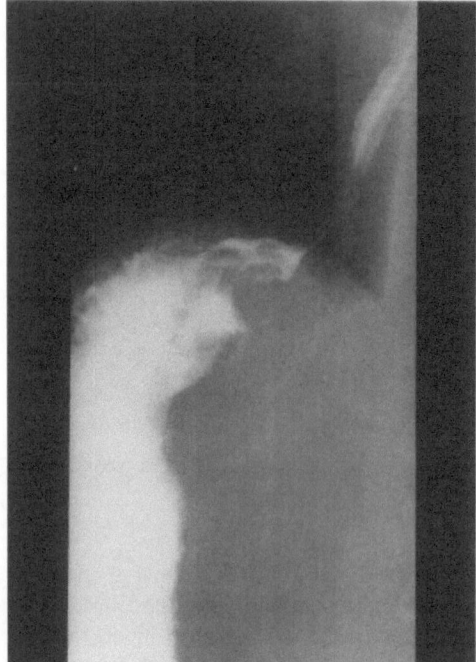

Fig. 11.7. Ulcerated cancer of the upper third of the
stomach

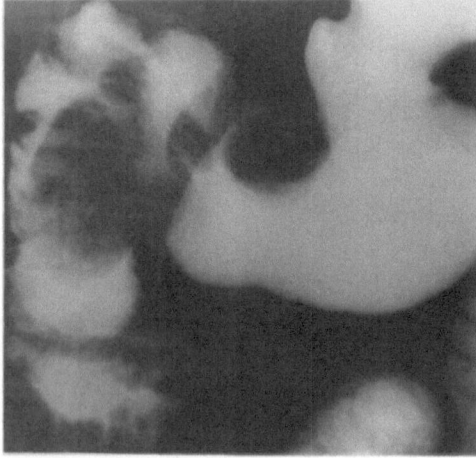

Fig. 11.9. Antral cancer that has prolapsed into the
duodenum

– The ulcero-infiltrating type is rarer; the
poorly delimited ulceration is only partially
surrounded by a raised rim, which is more
or less continuous with the healthy mucosa.

Other forms of advanced gastric cancer also
exist. Linitis plastica, the most classic form,

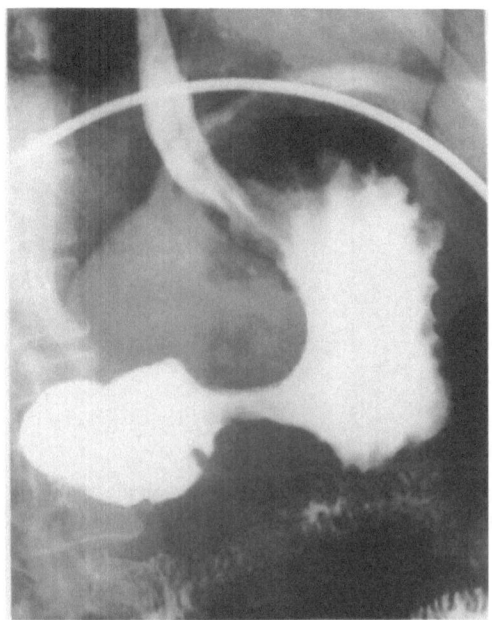

Fig. 11.10. Linitis plastica of the stomach

represents fewer than 15% of all gastric carcinomas. It often affects the antrum and the fundus, but may extend to the entire stomach and other segments of the gastrointestinal tract. The gastric wall is considerably thickened and is hard and rigid. Circumferential involvement of the stomach leads to circular retraction and transforms the stomach into a narrow rigid tube. The mucosa may be normal, atrophic, or associated with longitudinal folds; associated ulcerations may be visible. Malignant gastric tumors may cause duodenal intussusception, but this phenomenon is more common with benign tumors (Joffe et al. 1977; Kleinhaus et al. 1986). It is important to search for signs of duodenal and esophageal extension on radiographic studies.

11.5.1.5 Cancer on a Gastric Stump
(Figs. 11.11, 11.12)

The radiologic appearance (polypoid, infiltrating, or ulcerating) varies with the site of the cancer: involvement of the gastroesophageal

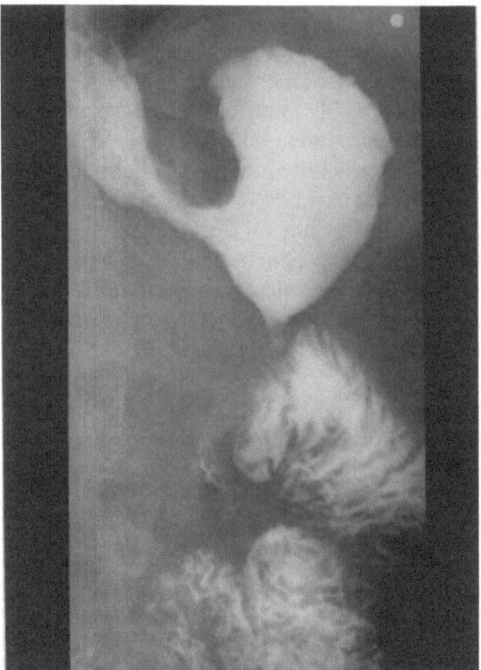

Fig. 11.11. Cancer of the stomach on the gastric stump

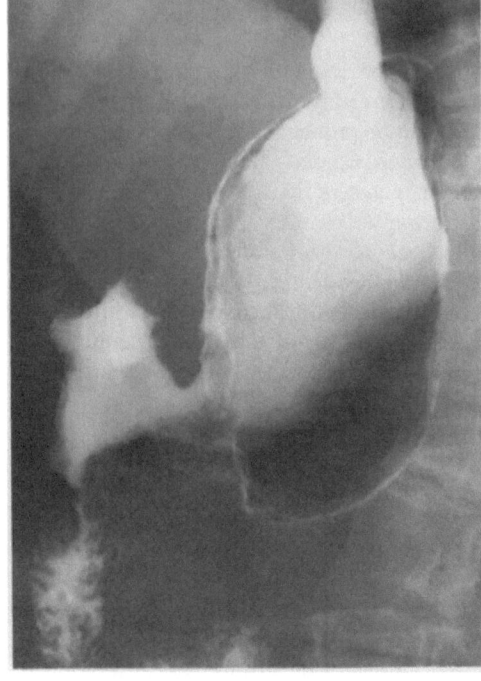

Fig. 11.12. Cancer of the stomach on the gastric stump

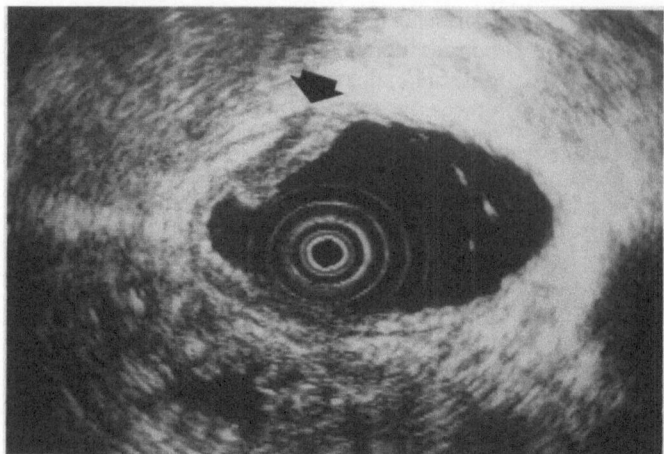

Fig. 11.13. Gastric endosonography: this superficial gastric cancer *(arrow)* invaded the mucosa to a depth of 3 mm, corresponding to initial involvement of the muscularis propria. (Courtesy of Dr. Valette, Lyons, France)

junction, cancer of the anastomotic region (filling defect, infiltrating lesion, exceptionally ulceration on a filling defect), diffuse form with a total filling defect of the stump.

11.5.1.6 Differential Diagnosis

Whereas the malignant nature of advanced cancers is readily demonstrated, detection of EGC can be problematic; this underscores the importance of good quality radiologic examinations. Cancers that develop on an anterior gastrectomy are rarely diagnosed radiologically because the lesions are often very advanced and evident. In other cases, the differential diagnosis of cancer requires differentiation from gastritis of the stump, peptic ulcer, jejunogastric intussusception, or parietoepiploic prolapse.

11.5.2 Ultrasonography

11.5.2.1 Endosonography (Figs. 11.13–11.15)

Although still in the developmental stage, this technique will be increasingly used for workups of gastric wall lesions and evaluation of peritumoral adenopathies (Heyder and Lux 1986; Lambert et al. 1988). Examinations are currently unsatisfactory in a third of cases, especially because of the size of available transducers. The tumor manifests as a hypoechoic lesion whose depth of penetration can be determined fairly accurately. Compared to lymphoma, adenocarcinomas are more echogenic, and extend less longitudinally but more in depth (Bolondi et al. 1987). Ultrasonography can demonstrate other localizations and determine the possibly multifocal character of even small cancers. Enlarged nodes at least 10 mm in size are generally assumed to be metastatic (Lambert et al. 1988). Endosonography is more sensitive than CT for evaluation of the depth of tumoral penetration through the gastric wall. In favorable cases, it can even reveal involvement of contiguous viscera (body of the pancreas for example).

11.5.2.2 Abdominal Ultrasonography
(Figs. 11.16, 11.17)

Abdominal sonograms are useful for preoperative patient workups. Advanced tumors are almost always visualized (Derchi et al. 1983). The tumor may image as a mass, as gastric wall thickening, or a combination of both features (Yeh and Rabinowitz 1981). For Derchi et al. (1983), ultrasonography had a sensitivity of 85.7% for detection of lymph node metas-

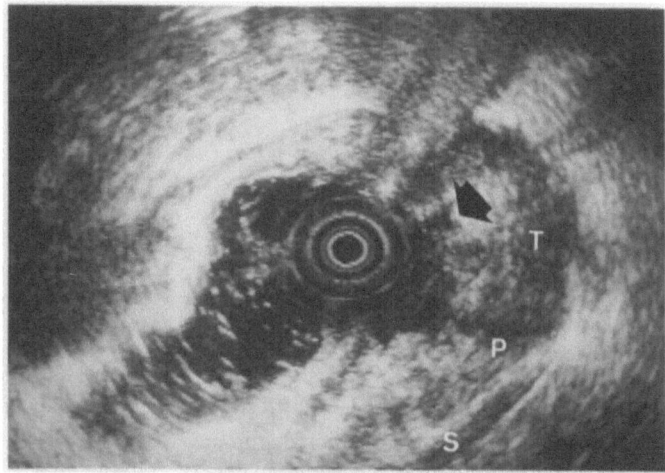

Fig. 11.14. Endosonography of the stomach: bulky gastric tumor *(T)* with an ulceration *(arrow)*. This tumor invaded the pancreas *(P)*. S, splenic vein. (Courtesy of Dr. Valette, Lyons, France)

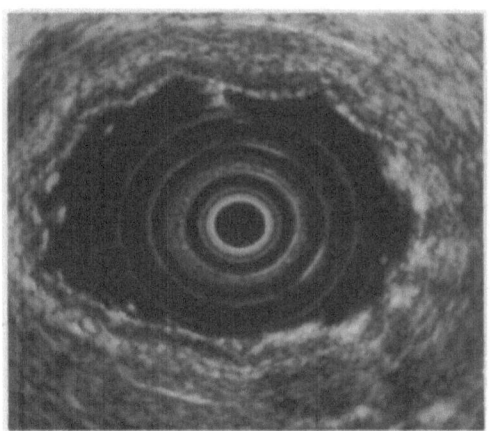

Fig. 11.15. Endosonography of the stomach: linitis plastica presenting as gastric wall thickening and loss of differentiation of the normal sonographically defined layers. (Courtesy of Dr. Valette, Lyons, France)

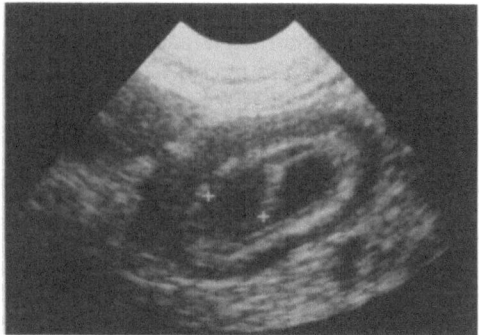

Fig. 11.16. Small cancer of the gastric antrum visualized by ultrasound (10 mm between the *two crosses*)

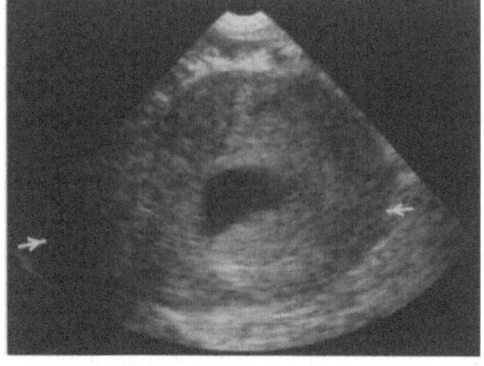

Fig. 11.17. Bulky cancer of the gastric antrum (23 cm between the *two arrows*)

tases and a specificity of 85.7% provided any nodal mass 5 mm or more was considered metastatic. For patients without interfering intestinal gas, ultrasound can correctly evaluate tumoral invasion of the pancreatic region and transverse colon. Multidirectional ultrasound scans render ultrasonography better than CT for evaluation of this type of extension. Ultrasound can also demonstrate ascites and hepatic metastases, but early peritoneal carcinosis usually cannot be diagnosed (Derchi et al. 1983).

11.5.2.3 Intraoperative Ultrasonography

Machi et al. (1986) have stressed the value of intraoperative ultrasonography for detection of small gastric wall lesions. Real-time examination with a 7.5-MHz linear array transducer can assess both the depth of tumoral penetration and degree of lateral wall extension after the stomach is distended with saline solution. The normal stomach wall measures 3–5.5 mm, and has been imaged as five distinct anatomic layers. Layer 1 (innermost layer) is hyperechoic, and corresponds to the mucosal surface; layer 2 is hypoechoic and corresponds to the mucosa; layer 3 is hyperechoic and corresponds to the submucosa; layer 4 is hypoechoic and corresponds to the muscularis propria; layer 5 is hyperechoic and corresponds to the subserosa-serosa interface (Machi et al. 1986). Diagnosis of EGC can be confirmed if the first three layers show distortions but layer 4 is intact.

11.5.3 Computed Tomography

11.5.3.1 Technique

CT examination requires adequate distention of the stomach with fluid or air; otherwise, the number of false-negative and false-positive errors is very high except for obvious bulky tumors. The thickness of the normal stomach wall does not exceed 1 cm (Balfe et al. 1981). The antrum is the most difficult region to examine because of the transverse plane of section at this level. CT evaluation of the antral region is thus best complemented by ultrasonography, which can define tumoral relationships with contiguous structures that are sometimes poorly demonstrated by transverse scans.

Exploration of a gastric cancer by CT requires scans from the diaphragm down to the pelvic brim. Digestive tract and intravenous contrast medium injection facilitates identification of metastatic lymph nodes, particularly in the gastrohepatic ligament.

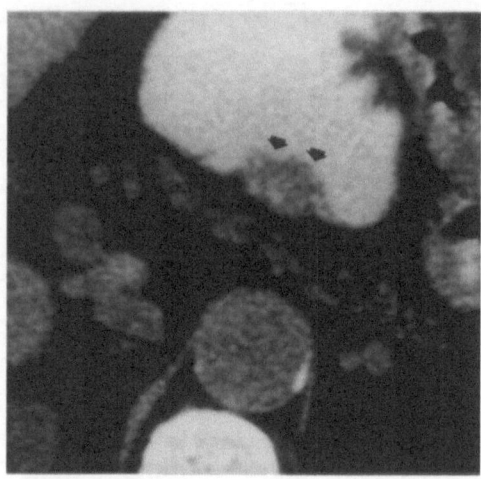

Fig. 11.18. Small cancer of the posterior edge of the stomach *(arrows)*

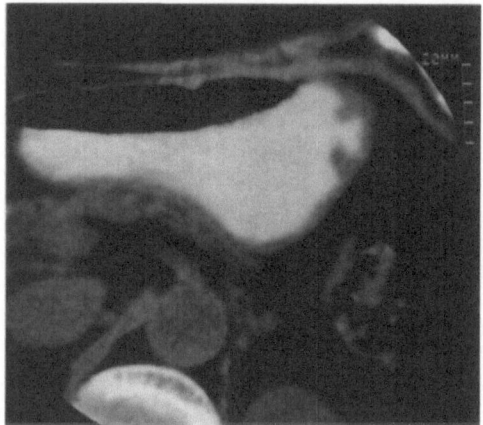

Fig. 11.19. Ulcerated gastric cancer

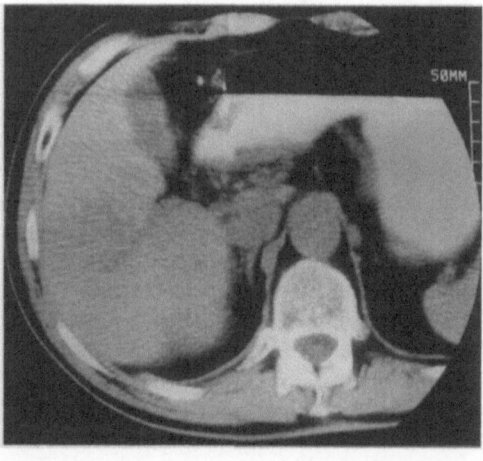

11.5.3.2 Radiologic Features
(Figs. 11.18–11.23)

Gastric cancer is not always visualized by CT; this is especially true for EGC and minute cancers. Lesions may present as an exophytic intraluminal mass or focal wall thickening, with or without ulceration (Scatarige et al. 1988). Calcifications are rare, but suggest the diagnosis of mucin-secreting adenocarcinoma (Nishimura et al. 1984). The primary role of CT is detection of regional and retroperitoneal adenopathies, peritoneal metastases, and omental invasion, hepatic metastases and ovarian metastases.

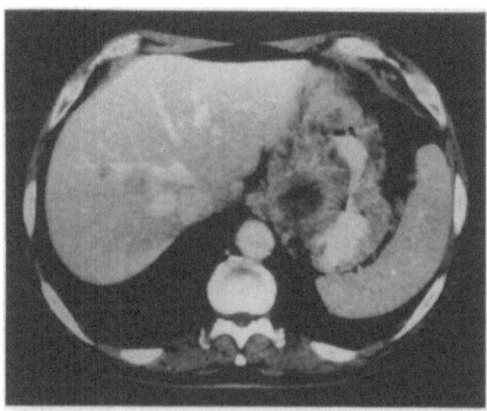

Fig. 11.21. Bulky cancer of the body of the stomach associated with nodal infiltration and hepatic metastases

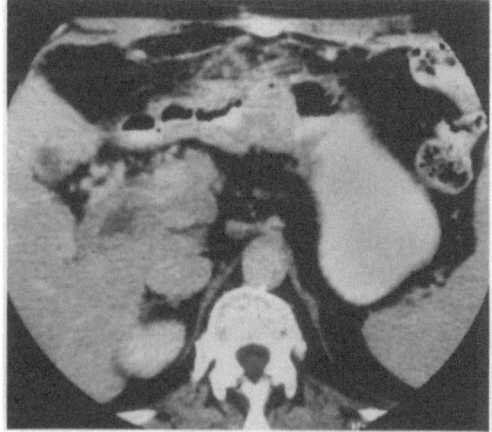

Fig. 11.22. Bulky cancer of the gastric antrum, with anterior infiltration of the peritoneum and hepatic metastases

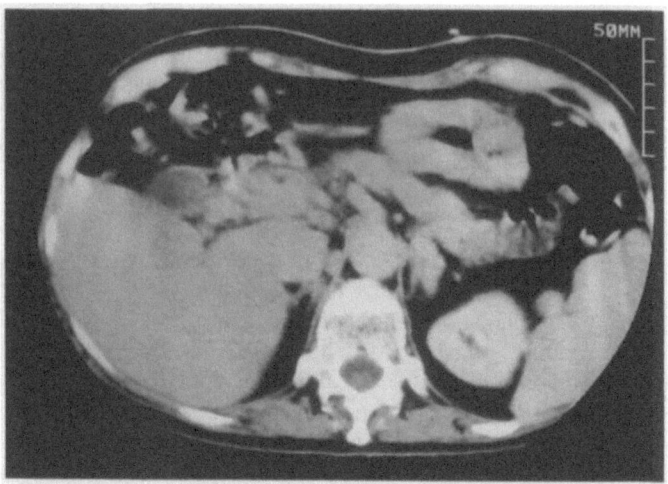

◀ **Fig. 11.20.** Infiltrating cancer of the gastric antrum, with small nodal masses posterior to the tumor

Fig. 11.23. Linitis plastica of the stomach, with severe gastric wall thickening. This lesion remained separate from the adjacent gastrointestinal viscera

11.5.3.3 Value of CT for Pretherapy Workup of Gastric Adenocarcinoma

The overall accuracy of CT for tumor staging and treatment planning is between 53% and 72.5% (Kleinhaus and Militianu 1988; Sussman et al. 1988; Triller et al. 1986). For Sussman et al. (1988), 16% of all gastric cancers are overstaged and 31% are understaged. Tumor resectability is correctly assessed in 80%–82% of cases (Kleinhaus and Militianu 1988; Triller et al. 1986). As for other gastrointestinal cancers, CT is least sensitive for the detection of adenopathy; for gastric cancers, it ranges from 52.5% to 64% (Sussman et al. 1988; Triller et al. 1986). Any node with a diameter of τ mm or greater is considered metastatic by Triller et al. (1986). False-negative errors can thus result from metastatic nodes that are normal in diameter (peritumoral adenopathies, gastrohepatic ligament, or greater curvature chain nodes). False-positive errors correspond to postinflammatory hypertrophy or reactive hyperplasia. Pancreatic involvement by extensive gastric cancers is sometimes difficult to evaluate, and CT accurately depicts pancreatic invasion in only 82% of cases (Sussman et al. 1988). CT thus appears of limited utility for preoperative staging of gastric adenocarcinomas (Cook et al. 1986), but can spare patients with extensive disease (N2 tumors for example) from undergoing unnecessary laparotomy.

11.5.3.4 Indications

Preoperative workup is based on physical examination and complementary techniques such as hepatic function tests, possibly carcinoembryonic antigen assays, chest X-rays and hepatic ultrasonography (in France). When there are symptoms suggestive of advanced lesions, CT examination can be offered. Owing to the routine availability of endoscopy and the fact that this technique is required for positive diagnosis of gastric adenocarcinoma, this examination, completed by sonoendoscopy in the same session, generally replaces barium studies. If endoscopy and sonoendoscopy determine the focal nature of the lesion, abdominal ultrasonography may be sufficient for preoperative workup. If, on the contrary, extensive lesions are visualized, CT is indicated to assess the extent of disease spread and, in particular, peritoneal carcinosis, retroperitoneal involvement, and pelvic extension.

11.6 Treatment and Prognosis

The only currently effective treatment for gastric cancer is surgical resection. Adjuvant therapies (radiotherapy or chemotherapy) have not yet proved effective in improving survival.

11.6.1 Surgical Management of Gastric Adenocarcinoma

When lesions extend to adjacent organs, resection may be extended towards the spleen, the tail of the pancreas, the transverse colon, or the left liver. Subtotal procedures for unresectable lesions and palliative operations aimed at improving the quality of patient survival are associated with a high operative mortality rate. Gastrojejunostomy-type procedures are generally performed for unresectable antral lesions. Percutaneous gastrostomy, which allows enteral nutrition, is sometimes an alternative to surgical gastrostomy for patients with cancer of the cardia. Regardless of the technique, the initial surgical procedure depends on extemporaneous histologic examination, and actually corresponds to disease staging. Intraoperative sonography may be justified for examination of the gastric wall, with particular attention to exploration of the liver for possible metastases. Lymph nodes are sampled for extemporaneous examination.

11.6.2 Radiotherapy

The role of irradiation for the treatment of gastric cancers is currently debated, and primarily concerns external beam radiotherapy. Radiotherapy is reserved for unresectable tumors or after insufficient surgical resection. Preoperative radiotherapy does not improve survival; exclusive radiotherapy has a very mediocre effect for inoperable, non-resectable, and metastatic tumors; adjuvant postoperative radiotherapy has not been found effective. Intraoperative radiotherapy is currently the subject of ongoing evaluations. Radiochemotherapy combinations appear more promising.

11.6.3 Chemotherapy

The benefits of chemotherapy remain debatable. For Inokuchi et al. (1984), there is no improvement in survival for patients with advanced cancers; by contrast, for Friedman et al. (1983), mean survival is 2 years for patients with disseminated gastric cancers.

11.6.4 Indications

The indications for surgery depend on the location and extent of the lesion, on the results of extemporaneous histologic examination of the pedicular nodes, and the presence or absence of metastases.

Adenocarcinomas of the gastric antrum are best treated by distal gastrectomy, provided that the sections pass at a sufficient distance from the lesion and that the surgical margins are free of tumoral involvement. Adenocarcinomas of the body and upper portion of the stomach are managed by total gastrectomy. In the series of Nagata et al. (1983), 78.6% of patients were treated by partial gastrectomy and 21.1% by total gastrectomy. For Chevrel et al. (1985), EGC requires total gastrectomy with omentectomy and dissection of the first nodal level of the three lymphatic chains draining the stomach. Resectability rates vary considerably between Japanese series (84.6% resectability for Nagata et al. 1983) and other authors (62%–64% resectability: Berger et al. 1986; Diehl et al. 1983; Naraynsingh 1985).

11.6.5 Prognostic Factors

The most important prognostic factor is the extent of lesions at surgery, hence the major role played by surgery for staging (Stark and Sauter 1985). The TNM classification is the main system used to evaluate prognostic factors. Local invasion, presence of adenopathies, and metastases are the most important factors

(Meyers et al. 1987), but sex and patient age are also important. For Bozzetti et al. (1986), female sex and age over 60 years are favorable prognostic factors.

11.6.6 Survival

Outside of Japan, global survival varies by country from 6% to 10.7% (Bizer 1983; Hollender et al. 1983; Meyers et al. 1987) and this rate does not appear to have changed for the last 30 years (Meyers et al. 1987). Overall survival of gastric cancer patients is 64% at 5 years, but rises to 74.6% after curative resection (Nagata et al. 1983). All non-Japanese authors have confirmed the better prognosis for resectable tumors: the prognosis at 5 years is between 15% and 32% (Berger et al. 1986; Bizer 1983; Scott et al. 1985).

Cancers of the gastric stump have a particularly unfavorable prognosis at 5 years (6.9% for Dlin et al. 1985), whereas EGC has a satisfactory prognosis if postoperative deaths are excluded. For Japanese authors, the 5-year survival rate is 90-95% (Kidodura 1971; Ohta et al. 1987). In the United States, the prognosis is nearly as favorable (68%-93% for Gold et al. 1984). The prognosis appears better for depressed forms than for elevated lesions (Kodama et al. 1983).

11.7 Patient Follow-up

11.7.1 Clinical Pictures and Frequency of Complications

Postoperative complications (generally respiratory pathologies or local problems) develop in 15%–34% of patients (Hollender et al. 1983; Yan and Brooks 1985). Fistulization and necrosis of the gastric stump are the main complications after gastroduodenostomy; leaking of the duodenal stump and acute pancreatitis are the main complications after gastrojejunostomy; anastomotic fistulae are the major problem after total gastrectomy. Anastomotic leaks constitute the greatest risk (Berger et al. 1986).

Postoperative mortality after total gastrectomy ranged from 12.5% to 41% between 1950 and

1974 in the review of Hollender et al. (1983). It is currently between 4.6% and 13.7% (Bizer 1983; Saario et al. 1986; Yan and Brooks 1985). In addition to complications due to the total gastrectomy or not, patients who have undergone metastasectomy or partial hepatectomy may develop complications related to the liver resection (Okuyama et al. 1985). Overall, like Meyers et al. (1987), we can consider that complications or postoperative death occur in only 25% of patients after gastric surgery for adenocarcinoma.

11.7.2 Disease Recurrence

Along with detecting immediate complications, follow-up examinations are aimed at discovery of recurrent adenocarcinomas (local recurrence or hepatic metastases) and such non-carcinologic complications as esophagitis, a dumping syndrome, weight loss, and anastomotic stenosis due to scar tissue formation. Recurrent disease is focal in 20% of cases and generalized in 80% (with 50% local recurrences) for Iwanaga et al. (1978). For these same authors, the frequency of recurrences within 2 years is 56%.

11.7.3 Follow-up Algorithm

For patient surveillance, hepatic function tests can be performed every 3 or 4 months along with carcinoembryonic antigen assays and a chest X-ray. This combined follow-up technique (clinical, biologic and imaging) can become annual after the 2nd year. If local recurrence is suspected, fibroscopy is indicated.

11.7.4 Imaging Studies for Follow-up of Patients with Gastric Adenocarcinoma

In addition to ultrasonography, which can visualize essentially hepatic metastases, two other techniques may be proposed: one before endoscopy (barium studies), and the other as a second intention technique in case of extensive disease recurrence (CT).

11.7.4.1 Barium Studies (Figs. 11.24–11.26)

Outside of the immediate postoperative period, potential non-neoplastic complications after partial gastrectomy include a chronic blind fistula, gastrojejunal evagination, intussusception of a jejunal loop into the gastric stump, stomitis or an inflammatory granuloma, parietoepiploic prolapse, or a postoperative peptic ulcer. Neoplastic recurrences on the gastrectomy stump, generally associated with the reappearance of clinical symptoms, may be imaged (especially infiltrating lesions); polypoid masses and ulcerated lesions are less common.

After upper pole gastrectomy, the usual finding is gastroesophageal reflux complicated by peptic esophagitis. Regardless of the type of surgical procedure, non-tumoral complications after total gastrectomy may include: often clinically asymptomatic blind fistula, granuloma, rarely jejunoesophageal intussusception, esophageal reflux with esophagitis. Recurrence after total gastrectomy for cancer generally occurs at the esojejunal junction, with filling defects in the anastomotic region

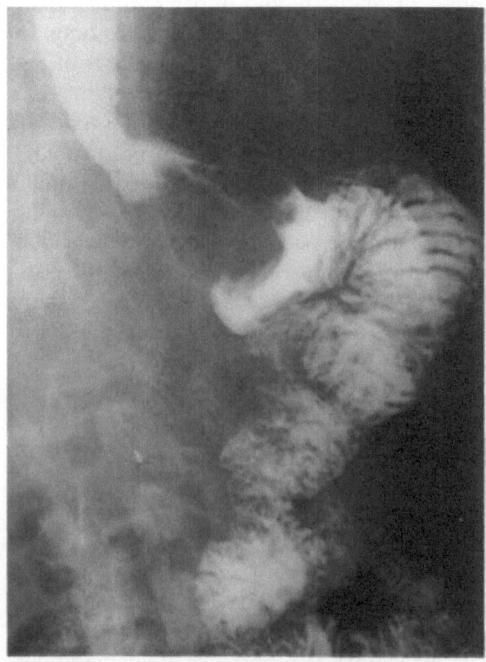

Fig. 11.24. Recurrence after partial gastrectomy

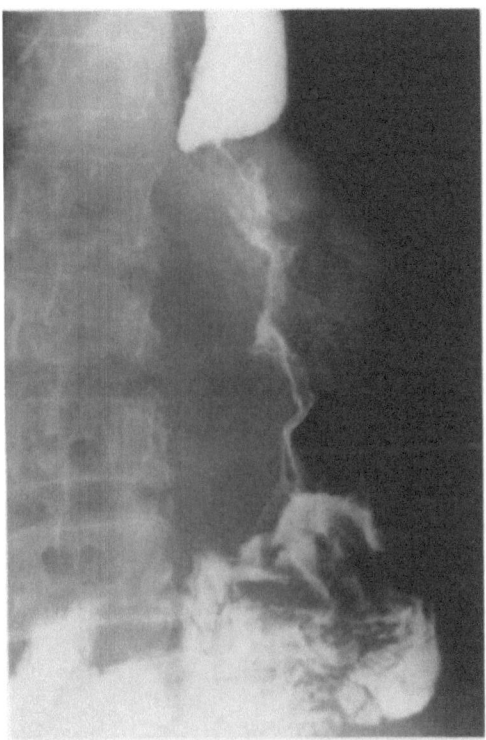

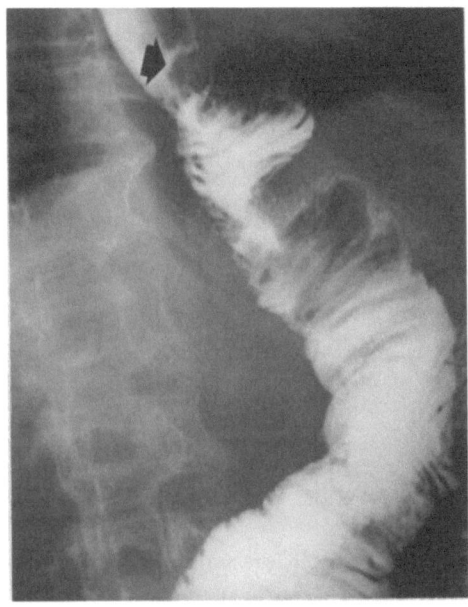

Fig. 11.25. Recurrence after total gastrectomy

Fig. 11.26. Small anastomotic nodule *(arrow)* corresponding to a granuloma. No radiologic or endoscopic signs of recurrence

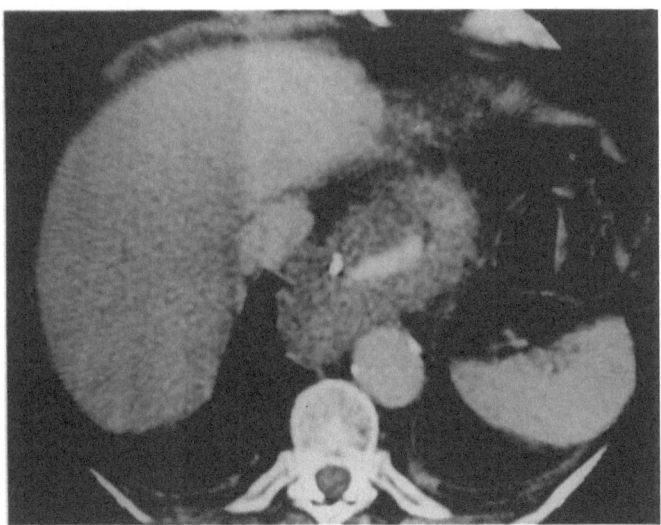

Fig. 11.27. Recurrence of a cancer of the cardia

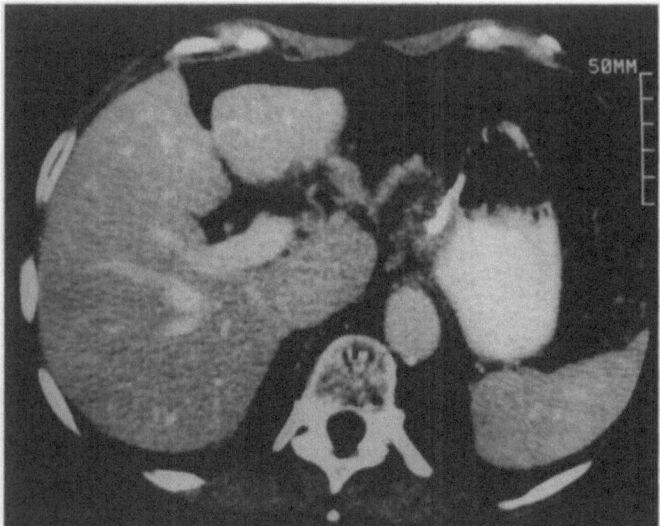

Fig. 11.28. Anastomotic recurrence of a gastric cancer

or the terminal esophagus, and stasis above this point.

11.7.4.2 Computed Tomography
(Figs. 11.27–11.29)

After gastrectomy, CT may demonstrate local recurrence as a soft tissue mass (average size 3 cm); obliteration of the fat plane between the area of anastomosis and the pancreatic bed confirms the diagnosis. CT may thus be useful for monitoring response to treatment, especially for patients who develop clinical symptoms. Although the sensitivity of CT is not very satisfactory (as in pretherapy work-ups), CT is helpful for diagnosis of recurrent disease and for guiding percutaneous biopsies.

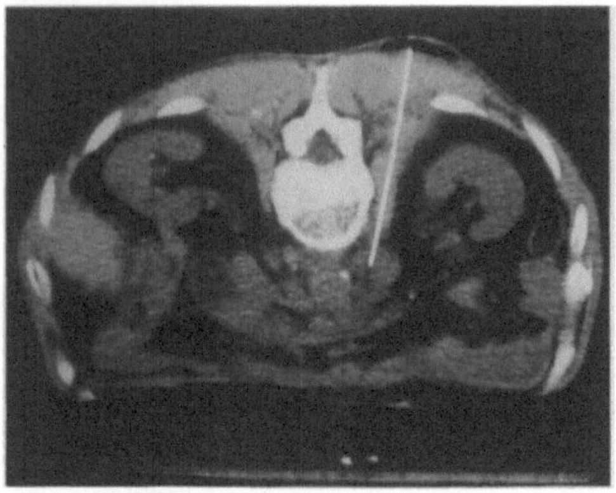

Fig. 11.29. Retroperitoneal adenopathies in a patient treated for gastric cancer with no local signs of recurrent disease. Aspiration biopsy under CT guidance diagnosed nodal metastases of the treated gastric cancer

11.8 Cancer of the Cardia

Only the characteristics specific to this region are dealt with here; the diagnostic imaging features are comparable to those for the lower esophagus (see Chap. 10).

11.8.1 General Features

Cancer of the cardia is on the rise, and 96% of these lesions are adenocarcinomas (Sons and Borchard 1986). Extension to the esophagus occurs in 60% of cases (Fierst 1972; Okamura et al. 1987). The patient is generally elderly; individuals under 35 years account for only 3% of all cases (Bloss et al. 1980). Dysphagia

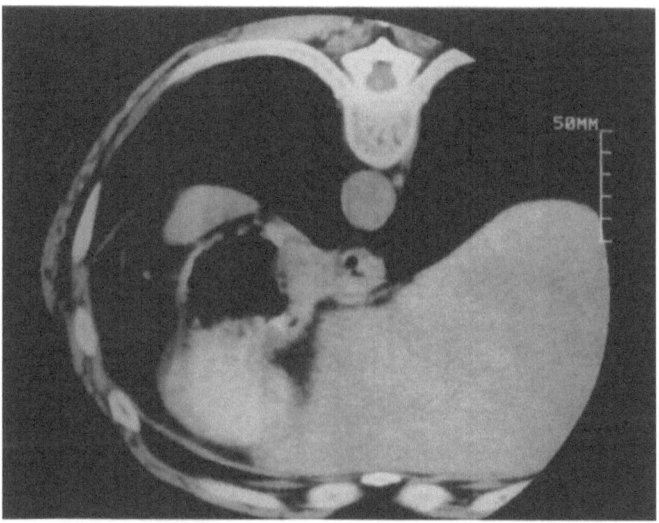

Fig. 11.30. CT study of cancer of the cardia: examination with the patient lying on the side facilitates imaging of the tumor and disease extension towards the stomach

is the most common clinical symptom, being mentioned in 65%–80% of cases (Levine et al. 1983).

Adverse prognostic factors include a Bormann type IV lesion, tumor size greater than 5 cm, serosal infiltration, and the presence of adenopathies (Okamura et al. 1987). Surgical management consists in resection of the esophagus and proximal stomach, or total resection of the esophagus and stomach. Wilson et al. (1985) have suggested use of preoperative radiotherapy to attempt to improve survival. The prognosis varies widely depending on the authors: it was 7%–10% in series prior to 1981 (Block and Lancaster 1964; MacDonald 1972). For Paolini et al. (1986), the average prognosis was 26.5% at 5 years. Okamura et al. (1987) emphasized the prognostic role of esophageal involvement; for these authors, the 5-year prognosis after curative surgery is 70% in the absence of esophageal involvement versus only 26.9% in case of esophageal involvement.

11.8.2 Imaging (Figs. 11.30–11.32)

Barium studies can evidence a tumor regardless of its type (polypoid, infiltrating, or ulcerated); searches should be made for extension

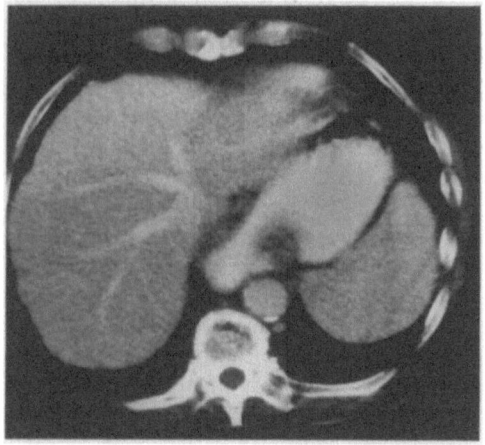

Fig. 11.31. Pseudotumoral syndrome of the cardia: this image actually corresponds to a normal variant, as revealed by the control examination performed with the patient lying on the side

to the esophagus. Barium studies can be very useful, especially when severe stenosis hampers passage of the endoscope. *CT* of the gastroesophageal junction can involve diagnostic problems if the examination is not performed correctly. In particular, a hiatal hernia or redundant mucosa prolapsing into the cardia when the hernia is partially or completely re-

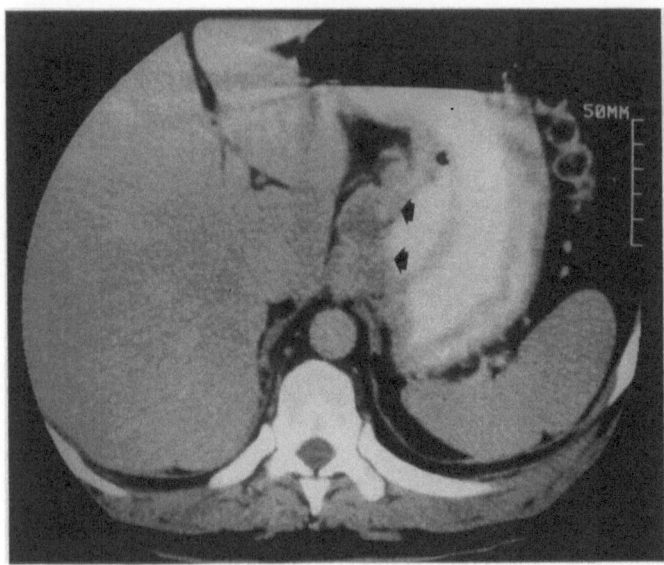

Fig. 11.32. Gastric extension of cancer of the cardia *(arrows)*

duced may be confused with a cancer of the cardia (Pupols and Ruzicka 1984). CT may be useful if resection appears possible, because its specificity for detection of metastases, adenopathies, and invasion of contiguous structures is excellent (its sensitivity is not as good).

11.9 Conclusion

Gastric adenocarcinoma remains a considerable health problem because of its frequency and poor prognosis. Improvement of therapeutic results rests on two factors:

- Early diagnosis, which justifies regular follow-up of high-risk individuals and screening programs. Endoscopy, which allows morphologic analysis of the stomach, may be replaced by double-contrast barium studies which are often better accepted by the patient.
- New, more effective therapeutic strategies as complements to surgery, which remains indispensable for both staging and radical treatment of gastric adenocarcinoma.

11.10 References

Audigier JC, Tuyns A (1981) Evolution de la mortalité par cancer de l'oesophage et de l'estomac en France entre 1951 et 1976. Gastroenterol Clin Biol 5: 243–250

Balfe DM, Koehler RE, Karstaedt N, Stanley RJ, Sagel SS (1981) Computed tomography of gastric neoplasms. Radiology 140: 431–436

Barentsz JO, Rosenbusch GR, Strijk SP, Yap SH (1986) Radiologic examination in gastric cancer. A retrospective study in 188 patients. Acta Radiol [Diagn] (Stockh) 27: 547–552

Berger F, Huten N, Robin P, Benatre A, Vandooren M (1986) Etude rétrospective de 225 cancers gastriques observés en chirurgie de CHU de 1968 à 1980. Ann Chir 40: 14–20

Bizer LS (1983) Adenocarcinoma of the stomach: current results of treatment. Cancer 51: 743–745

Block GE, Lancaster JR (1964) Adenocarcinoma of the cardioesophageal junction. Arch Surg 88: 852–858

Bloss RS, Miller TA, Copeland EM (1980) Carcinoma of the stomach in the young adult. Surg Gynecol Obstet 150: 883–886

Bolondi L, Casanova P, Caletti GC, Grigioni W, Zani L, Barbara L (1987) Primary gastric lymphoma versus gastric carcinoma: endoscopic US evaluation. Radiology 165: 821–826

Bozzetti F, Bonfanti G, Morabito A, Bufalino R, Menotti V, Andreola S, Doci R, Gennari L (1986) A multifactorial approach for the prognosis of patients with carcinoma of the stomach after curative resection. Surg Gynecol Obstet 162: 229–234

Caygill CPJ, Hill MJ, Kirkham JS, Northfield TC (1986) Mortality from gastric cancer following gastric surgery for peptic ulcer. Lancet ii: 929-931

Chevrel JP, Sarfati E, Dachez R, Costil P (1985) Les cancers superficiels de l'estomac. J Chir (Paris) 122: 171-174

Cook AO, Levine BA, Sirinek KR, Gaskill HV (1986) Evaluation of gastric adenocarcinoma: abdominal computed tomography does not replace celiotomy. Arch Surg 121: 603-606

Cotton PB (1973) Fibreoptic endoscopy and the barium meal. Results and implications. Br Med J 2: 161-165

Decarli A, La Vecchia C, Cislaghi C, Mezzanotte G, Marubini E (1986) Descriptive epidemiology of gastric cancer in Italy. Cancer 58: 2560-2569

Derchi LE, Biggi E, Rollandi GA, Cicio GR, Neumaier CE (1983) Sonographic staging of gastric cancer. AJR 140: 273-276

Devesa SS (1982) Time trends in stomach cancer incidence in the United States by age and region. In: Magnus K (ed) Trends in cancer incidence. Hemisphere, Washington, pp 155-164

Diehl JT, Hermann RE, Cooperman AM, Hoerr SO (1983) Gastric carcinoma. A ten-year review. Ann Surg 198: 9-12

Dlin C, Sarfati E, Chevrel JP (1985) Les cancers dits "du moignon gastrique". Revue de la littérature à propos de quatre observations. J Chir (Paris) 122: 193-200

Esaki Y, Hirokawa K, Yamashiro M (1987) Multiple gastric cancers in the aged with special reference to intramucosal cancers. Cancer 59: 560-565

Faivre J, Respaud G, Bruhiere J, Moulinier B (1976) Les tumeurs villeuses de l'estomac. Lyon Med 235: 19-24

Fernando SSE, Nakamura K (1986) Japanese technique of early gastric cancer diagnosis. Am J Gastroenterol 81: 757-768

Fierst SM (1972) Carcinoma of the cardia and fundus of the stomach. Am J Gastroenterol 57: 403-409

Friedman MA, Ogawa M, Carter SK, Sakurai Y, Kimura K, Hannigan J (1983) Chemotherapy of disseminated gastric cancer. A joint effort of the Northern California Oncology group and the Japanese Gastric Cancer Chemotherapy group. Cancer 52: 1771-1777

Gelfand DW, Chen YM, Ott DJ (1987) Multiphasic examinations of the stomach: efficacy of individual techniques and combinations of techniques in detecting 153 lesions. Radiology 162: 829-834

Gold RP, Green PHR, O'Toole KM, Seaman WB (1984) Early gastric cancer: radiographic experience. Radiology 152: 283-290

Goldstein F, Kline TS, Kline IK, Thornton JJ, Abramson J, Bell L (1983) Early gastric cancer in a United States hospital. Am J Gastroenterol 78: 715-719

Goldthorn JF, Canizaro PC (1986) Gastrointestinal malignancies in infancy, childhood, and adolescence. Surg Clin North Am 66: 845-861

Grabiec J, Owen DA (1985) Carcinoma of the stomach in young patients. Cancer 56: 388-396

Gutmann RA, Bertrand I, Peristiant TJ (1939) Le cancer de l'estomac au début. Doin, Paris

Halpert RD, Spickler E, Feczko PJ (1985) Dysphagia in patients with gastric cancer and a normal esophagram. Radiology 154: 589-591

Halvorsen RA Jr, Thompson WM (1987) Computed tomographic staging of gastrointestinal malignancies. Part I. Esophagus and stomach. Invest Radiol 22: 2-16

Hattori T (1986) Development of adenocarcinomas in the stomach. Cancer 57: 1528-1534

Hermanek P, Sobin LH (1987) TNM. Classification of malignant tumours. Springer, Berlin Heidelberg New York London Paris Tokyo

Heyder N, Lux G (1986) Malignant lesions of the upper gastrointestinal tract. Scand J Gastroenterol 21 (Suppl 123): 47-51

Hollender LF, Kauffmann JP, Bur F, Meyer C, Bahnini J, Keller D, Cordeiro F, Pigache P (1983) Etude rétrospective de 384 exérèses pour cancers gastriques. Chirurgie 109: 731-741

Iishi H, Tatsuta M, Okuda S (1985) Endoscopic diagnosis of minute gastric cancer of less than 5 mm in diameter. Cancer 56: 655-659

Inokuchi K, Hattori T, Taguchi T, Abe O, Ogawa N (1984) Postoperative adjuvant chemotherapy for gastric carcinoma. Analysis of data in 1805 patients followed 5 years. Cancer 53: 2393-2397

Iwanaga I, Koyama H, Furukawa H, Taniguchi H, Wada A, Tateishi R (1978) Mechanism of late recurrence after radical surgery for gastric carcinoma. Am J Surg 135: 637-640

Japanese Research Society for Gastric Cancer (1981) The general rules for the gastric cancer study in surgery and pathology. Jpn J Surg 11: 127-139

Joffe N, Goldman H, Antonioli DA (1977) Transpyloric prolapse of polypoid gastric carcinoma. Gastroenterology 72: 1326-1330

Kidodura T (1971) Frequency of resection, metastases and five-year survival rate of early-gastric cancer in a surgical clinic. Jpn J Cancer Res 11: 45-49

Kleinhaus U, Militianu D (1988) Computed tomography in the preoperative evaluation of gastric carcinoma. Gastrointest Radiol 13: 97-101

Kleinhaus U, Weich YL, Maoz S (1986) Gastroduodenal intussusception secondary to prolapsing gastric tumors. Gastrointest Radiol 11: 229-232

Kodama Y, Inokuchi K, Soejima K, Matsusaka T, Okamura T (1983) Growth patterns and prognosis in early gastric carcinoma. Superficially spreading and penetrating growth types. Cancer 51: 320-326

Lambert R, Souquet JC, Valette PJ (1988) L'endosonographie digestive en 1988. Principes et perspectives. Gastroenterol Clin Biol 12: 376-386

Lauren P (1965) The two histological main types of gastric carcinoma: diffuse and so-called intestinal type carcinoma. An attempt at a histoclincial classification. Acta Pathol Microbiol Scand 64: 31–49

Levine MS, Laufer I, Thompson JJ (1983) Carcinoma of the gastric cardia in young people. AJR 140: 69–72

Levine MS, Rubesin SE, Herlinger H, Laufer I (1988) Double-contrast upper gastrointestinal examination: technique and interpretation. Radiology 168: 593–602

Locke FB, King H (1980) Cancer mortality risk among Japanese in the United States. J Natl Cancer Inst 65: 1149–1156

MacDonald WC (1972) Clinical and pathologic features of adenocarcinoma of the gastric cardia. Cancer 29: 724–731

Machi J, Takeda J, Sigel B, Karegawa T (1986) Normal stomach wall and gastric cancer: evaluation with high-resolution operative US. Radiology 159: 85–87

Martin E, Potet F, Debray C, Lambling A (1962) Etude anatomopathologique de la gastrite hypertrophique géante. Acta Gastroenterol Belg 25: 514–551

Meyers WC, Damiano RJ, Postlethwait RW, Rotolo FS (1987) Adenocarcinoma of the stomach. Changing patterns over the last 4 decades. Ann Surg 205: 1–8

Miller G, Kaufmann M (1975) Das Magenfrühkarzinom in Europa. Dstch Med Wochenschr 100: 1946–1949

Milnes JP, Hine KR, Holmes GKT, Cohen MEL (1982) Limitations of endoscopy in the diagnosis of carcinoma of the cardia of the stomach. Br J Radiol 55: 593–595

Ming SC, Bajtai A, Correa P, Elster K, Jarvi O, Munoz N, Nagayo T, Stemmerman GN (1984) Gastric dysplasia. Significance and pathologic criteria. Cancer 54: 1794–1801

Montesi A, Graziani L, Pesari A, De Nigris E, Bearzi I, Ranaldi R (1982) Radiologic diagnosis of early gastric cancer by routine double-contrast examination. Gastrointest Radiol 7: 205–215

Mori M, Iwashita A, Enjoji M (1986) Adenosquamous carcinoma of the stomach. A clinicopathologic analysis of 28 cases. Cancer 57: 333–339

Morson BC, Dawson IMP (1979) Gastrointestinal pathology. Blackwell Scientific, Oxford

Nagata T, Ikeda M, Nakayama F (1983) Changing state of gastric cancer of Japan. Am J Surg 145: 226–233

Naraynsingh V (1985) Gastric carcinoma in the West Indies: a Trinidad study. Cancer 56: 2117–2119

Nishimura K, Togashi K, Tondo G, Dodo Y, Tanada S, Nakano Y, Torizuka K (1984) Computed tomography of calcified gastric carcinoma. J Comput Assist Tomogr 8: 1010–1011

Ohta H, Noguchi Y, Takagi K, Nishi M, Kajitani T, Kato Y (1987) Early gastric carcinoma with special reference to macroscopic classification. Cancer 60: 1009–1106

Okamura T, Tsujitani S, Marin P, Haraguchi M, Korenaga D, Baba H, Sugimachi K (1987) Adenocarcinoma in the upper third part of the stomach. Surg Gynecol Obstet 165: 247–250

Okuyama K, Isono K, Juan IK, Onoda S, Ochiai T, Yamamoto Y, Koide Y, Satoh H (1985) Evaluation of treatment for gastric cancer with liver metastasis. Cancer 55: 2498–2505

Oohara T, Aono G, Ukawa S, Takezoe K, Johjima Y, Kurosawa H, Asakura R, Tohma H (1984) Clinical diagnosis of minute gastric cancer less than 5 mm in diameter. Cancer 53: 162–165

Orringer D (1950) Carcinoma of the stomach after gastric operation. Am J Surg 141: 487–491

Paolini AP, Tosato F, Cassese M, De Marchi C, Grande M, Paoletti P, Gherardini P, Fegiz G (1986) Total gastrectomy in the treatment of adenocarcinoma of the cardia. Review of the results in 73 resected patients. Am J Surg 151: 238–243

Possik RA, Franco EL, Pires DR, Wohnrath DR, Ferreira EB (1986) Sensitivity, specificity, and predictive value of laparoscopy for the staging of gastric cancer and for the detection of liver metastases. Cancer 58: 1–6

Pupols A, Ruzicka FF (1984) Hiatal hernia causing a cardia pseudomass on computed tomography. J Comput Assist Tomogr 8: 699–700

Reed PL, Smith PLR, Haines K, House FR, Walters C (1981) Gastric juice N-nitrosamines in health and gastroduodenal disease. Lancet ii: 550–552

Richelme H, Ceccanti JP, Bourgeon A (1984) Les cancers du moignon gastrique. A propos de 14 observations récentes. Ann Gastroenterol Hepatol (Paris) 20: 23–26

Saario I, Schroder T, Tolppanen EM, Lempinen M (1986) Total gastrectomy with esophagojejunostomy. Analysis of 100 consecutive patients. Am J Surg 151: 244–246

Sakita T, Ogura Y, Takasu S, Fukutomi H, Miwa T, Yoshimori M (1971) Observations on the healing of ulcerations in early gastric cancer. Gastroenterology 60: 835–844

Scatarige JC, Fishman EK, Jones B (1988) CT of the stomach. In: Fishman EK, Jones B (eds) Computed tomography of the gastrointestinal tract. Churchill Livingstone, New York, pp 55–84

Schulman A, Simpkins KC (1975) The accuracy of radiological diagnosis of benign, primarily and secondarily malignant gastric ulcers and their correlation with 3 simplified radiological types. Clin Radiol 26: 317–325

Scott HW, Adkins RB, Sawyers JL (1985) Results of an aggressive surgical approach to gastric carcinoma during a twenty-three-year period. Surgery 97: 55–59

Shaw PC, Van Romunde LKJ, Griffioen G, Janssens AR, Kreuning J, Eilers GAM (1987) Peptic ulcer and gastric carcinoma: diagnosis with biphasic radiography compared with fiberoptic endoscopy. Radiology 163: 39–42

Shirakabe H (1972) Double contrast studies of the stomach. Thieme, Stuttgart

Sons HU, Borchard F (1986) Cancer of the distal esophagus and cardia. Incidence, tumorous infiltration and metastatic spread. Ann Surg 203: 188–195

Stalberg H, Takidal S (1971) Stomach cancer following gastric surgery for benign conditions. Lancet ii: 1175–1177

Stanta G, Sasco AJ, Riboli E, Cocchi A, Rossitti P (1986) Prevalence of gastric cancer in a large necropsy series. Lancet ii: 624

Stark RH, Sauter KE (1985) Surgical treatment of adenocarcinoma of the stomach in a community hospital. Surg Gynecol Obstet 160: 153–156

Sussman SK, Halvorsen RA, Illescas FF, Cohan ʀ, Saeed M, Silverman PM, Thompson WM, Meyers WC (1988) Gastric adenocarcinoma: CT versus surgical staging. Radiology 167: 335–340

Tatsuda M, Okuda S, Tamura H, Taniguchi H (1982) Endoscopic diagnosis of early gastric cancer by the endoscopic Congo red-methylene blue test. Cancer 50: 2956–2960

Thompson G, Somers S, Stevenson GW (1983) Benign gastric ulcer: a reliable radiologic diagnosis? AJR 141: 331–333

Triller J, Roder R, Stafford A, Schroder R (1986) CT in advanced gastric carcinoma: is exploratory laparotomy avoidable? Eur J Radiol 6: 181–186

Viste A, Bjornestad E, Opheim P, Skarstein A, Thunold J, Hartveit F, Eide GE, Eide TJ, Soreide O (1986) Risk of carcinoma following gastric operations for benign disease. A historical cohort study of 3470 patients. Lancet ii: 502–504

Weisburger JH, Wynder EL, Horn CL (1982) Nutritional factors and etiologic mechanisms in the causation of gastrointestinal cancers. Cancer 50: 2541–2549

White RM, Levine MS, Enterline HT, Laufer I (1985) Early gastric cancer. Recent experience. Radiology 155: 25–27

Wills JS (1986) Percutaneous gastrostomy: applications in gastric carcinoma and gastroplasty stoma dilatation. AJR 147: 826–827

Wilson SE, Hiatt JR, Stabile BE, Williams RA (1985) Cancer of the distal esophagus and cardia: preoperative irradiation prolongs survival. Am J Surg 150: 114–121

Yan CJ, Brooks JR (1985) Surgical management of gastric adenocarcinoma. Am J Surg 149: 771–774

Yeh HC, Rabinowitz JG (1981) Ultrasonography and Computed tomography of gastric wall lesions. Radiology 141: 147–155

12 Adenocarcinoma of the Small Intestine*

The infrequency of intestinal adenocarcinoma is reflected by the fact that only 2400 cases had been reported in the literature up until 1973 (Morgan and Busutill 1977). Other intestinal neoplasms have been the subject of publications describing modifications in the diagnostic or therapeutic attitude following use of new radiologic techniques: CT for lymphomas and connective tissue tumors; angiography for hepatic embolization, which at least temporarily alleviates flushing in patients with metastatic carcinoid liver tumor. By contrast, there are few recent studies on adenocarcinoma of the small intestine. Diagnosis of this type of tumor has thus not benefitted from the technologic advances in radiology, and its prognosis has not been improved by the introduction of new therapeutic options.

12.1 General Features

These rare tumors have an annual incidence of 0.3 per 100 000 population (Smith et al. 1980). In autopsy series, the duodenum is involved in 0.04% of cases (Burgeman et al.1956; Hoffman and Pack 1937). Compared to other gastrointestinal tract cancers, intestinal adenocarcinomas represent approximately 0.3% (Lillimoe and Imbembo 1980; Spelberg and Schmidtler 1980); they are 40-60 times less frequent than colonic adenocarcinoma (Swift 1980). Compared to other malignant tumors of the small intestine, adenocarcinoma accounts for an average of 47.1% (Darling and Welch 1959; Gerard et al. 1962; McPeak 1967; Ostermiller et al. 1966; Pagtalunan et al. 1964; Rochlin and Longmire 1961), with values

ranging from 23% to 69% (Cohen et al. 1971; Ebert and Zuidema 1965).

The three gross types of intestinal adenocarcinomas may exist alone or in combination: infiltrating lesions, the most common (Brenner and Brown 1955); ulcerating lesions, a frequent cause of hemorrhage (Pringot and Bodart 1970); and polypoid lesions, which are rarer (Mittal and Bodzin 1980). Histologically, Lieberkühnian forms predominate; Brunnerian and mucus-secreting forms are exceptional; undifferentiated and anaplastic epitheliomas are very rare.

Tumoral spread occurs through the nodal pathways, then along a hepatic route; the frequency of disease extension is directly correlated with the histologic grade (Ostermiller et al. 1966). At surgery, usually performed soon after diagnosis, 38.6% of patients already have nodal involvement and 25.1% have hepatic metastases. In a review of 657 cases (Bruneton et al. 1983), 27.4% of patients had duodenal involvement, 35.4% had jejunal involvement, and 26.8% had ileal involvement. Duodenal adenocarcinomas can be divided into three groups: suprapapillary, peripapillary, and subpapillary (Crawford Barclay and Kent 1962). Peripapillary forms (51.6%) and subpapillary forms predominate (40.2%); suprapapillary tumors are very rare (Bruneton et al. 1983). These figures correspond to literature reviews beginning in the 1950s (Resnik and Cooper 1958; Spira et al. 1977). Before this period, statistics indicated a marked predominance of peripapillary lesions because authors included vaterian ampullomas in their studies and histology techniques were unable to clearly distinguish adenocarcinomas of duodenal origin from biliary and pancreatic lesions (Berger and Koppelman 1942; Kleinerman et al. 1950; Stewart and Lieber 1937). Half of all adenocarcinomas in the jejunum

---

* Written in collaboration with C. Balu-Maestro.

occur within 5 cm of the ligament of Treitz; in the ileum, 62% of these lesions lie within 5 cm of Bauhin's valve (Chanoine 1955).

In a review of 126 cases (Bruneton et al. 1983), 51.6% of lesions were less than 5 cm in diameter, 37.3% were between 5 and 10 cm, and 11.1% were larger than 10 cm. Most lesions smaller than 5 cm are found in the duodenum, because examination of this region often allows diagnosis before they reach a larger size.

Numerous etiologic hypotheses have attempted to explain the rarity of intestinal adenocarcinoma: impaired immunity and rapid cell turnover have both been postulated. However, several predisposing factors have been identified: adenoma, and especially villous adenoma, which degenerates in 30% of cases for Spira et al. (1971); Lieberkühnian adenomas degenerate in only 7% of cases (Perzin and Bridge 1981). Brunner's adenomas have no malignant propensity. Peutz-Jeghers syndrome undergoes malignant transformation on rare occasions (Dozois et al. 1969). Ulcerous degeneration was controversial for a long time (Jefferson 1916-1917) but is now a well-recognized factor. Other implicated conditions include Crohn's disease (essentially multifocal ileal lesions) (Kerber and Frank 1984; Meiselman et al. 1987; Smith et al. 1980), gluten intolerance (Javier and Lukie 1980), Gardner's syndrome (Schnur et al. 1973), familial colonic polyposis, and Torre syndrome (Lillemoe and Imbembo 1980).

Intestinal adenocarcinoma is associated with discrete male predominance; mean age is 55 years. In 620 cases reviewed (Bruneton et al. 1983), clinical signs cited alone or in combination included: pain (62.5%), weight loss (53.7%), vomiting (51.7%), hemorrhage (40.8%), intestinal obstruction (37.2%), anorexia (26.9%), jaundice (24.6%), mass (17.9%), constipation (16.7%), diarrhea (13.2%). The non-specificity of these manifestations explains the delay before diagnosis and the relative frequency of obstruction and a palpable abdominal mass. The average interval between the onset of clinical symptoms and diagnosis is 5 months. At diagnosis, besides lesions with a malignant potential, the following pathologic associations have been reported: an associated cancer (20.3% of cases for Barclay and Schapira 1983), celiac disease (Javier and Lukie 1980), and cystic pancreatic heterotopia.

Endoscopy almost always leads to diagnosis of duodenal adenocarcinomas by permitting biopsy; however, in a few cases, lesion size can preclude satisfactory exploration, and results are not always positive (Maillet et al. 1975).

Neither radiotherapy nor chemotherapy have succeeded in improving patient survival compared to surgery alone (Morgan and Busutil 1977). Analysis of surgical series reveals increased use of total resection during the past years: from 43% in 1966 (Serrano and McPeak 1966) to 70% in 1980 (Lillemoe and Imbembo 1980). However, regardless of the technique used, in those studies providing details on mortality, the prognosis is only 12.8% survival at 2 years and 7.8% at 5 years. These results are hardly better than those of Berger and Koppelman back in 1942; only operative mortality has really decreased. The prognosis for intestinal adenocarcinoma is thus markedly worse than for other intestinal malignancies.

12.2 Imaging

Owing to the rarity of intestinal adenocarcinomas, there are few recent reports on imaging with CT and ultrasound. In a review of 379 cases (Bruneton et al. 1983), the frequency of false-negative results for barium examinations was 13.5%. After radiologic examination, a diagnosis of cancer is made in nearly 70% of cases; in fewer than 10% of cases the presumptive diagnosis is a benign tumor (Spira et al. 1977).

The imaging patterns of intestinal adenocarcinoma are well known (Koehler 1983). In a review of 95 cases (Bruneton et al. 1983), three patterns were seen alone or in combination: stenosis (60%), filling defect (41%), ulceration (27.4%). Differential diagnosis can be difficult. Annular stenosis localized in the duodenum, with or without ulceration, suggests adenocarcinoma, but other lesions (metastases, lymphoma, carcinoids) occasionally have the same appearance (Gallego et al. 1986; Levine et al. 1987; Papadopoulos and Nolan 1985) (Figs. 12.1-12.5).

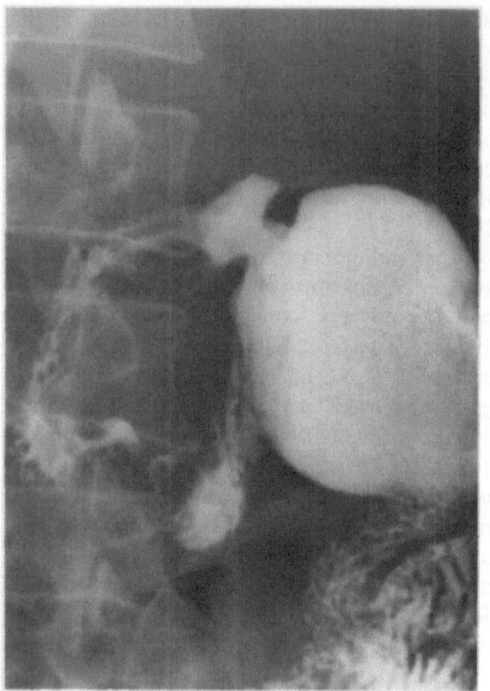

Fig. 12.1. Ulcerated duodenal adenocarcinoma

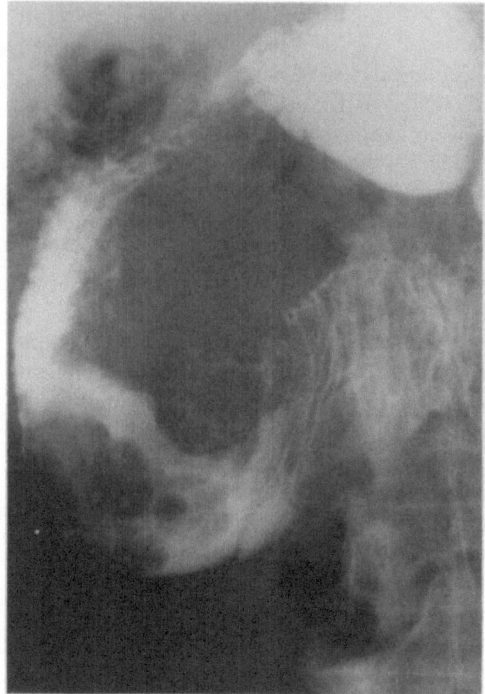

Fig. 12.2. Bulky ulcerated adenocarcinoma of the duodenum

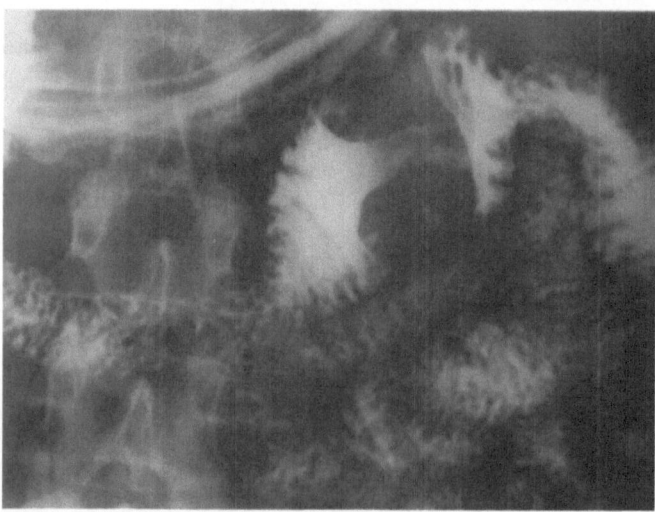

Fig. 12.3. Adenocarcinoma of the duodenojejunal flexure causing stenosis

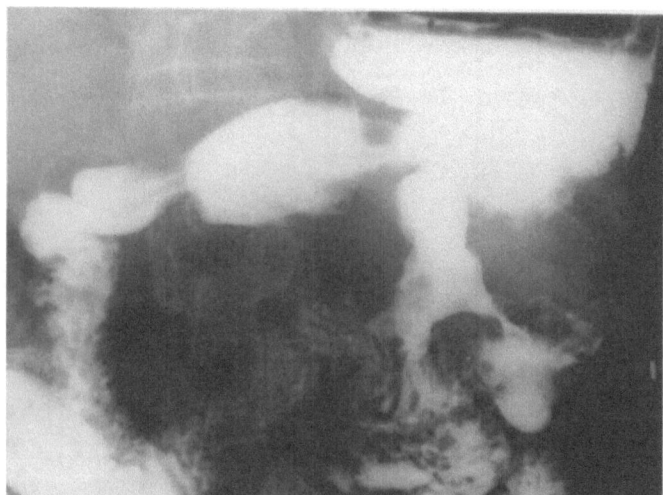

Fig. 12.4. Bulky adenocarcinoma of the duodenojejunal flexure (infiltrating and ulcerated lesion)

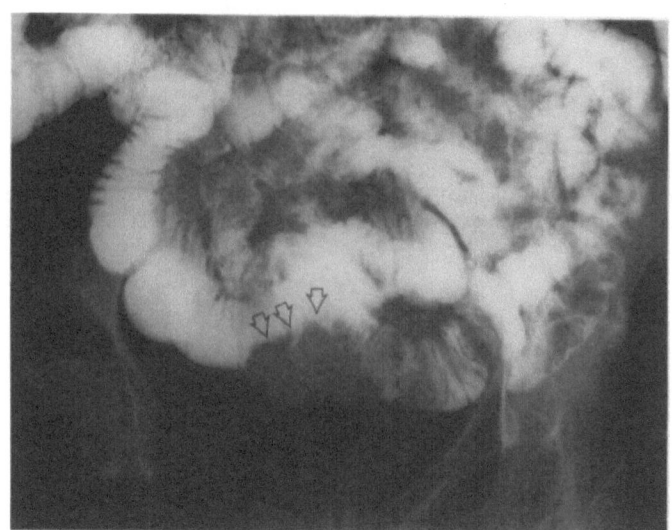

Fig. 12.5. Ileal adenocarcinoma *(arrows)*

Angiography demonstrates arteriolar irregularities with tumoral hypovascularity; the presence of neovessels is less common. Arterial wall infiltration may suggest the extent of local spread (Ekberg and Ekholm 1980) although less accurately than ultrasonography and especially CT (Figs. 12.6, 12.7).

Ultrasonography can visualize duodenal lesions, but the remainder of the small intestine is often poorly explored because of overlying intestinal gas. A duodenal adenocarcinoma may present as a solid, heterogeneous image or target lesion; the parietal thickening has no specific echostructure. The duodenal origin of the lesion is identified by its vascular relations (vena cava and aorta posteriorly, superior mesenteric vessels anteriorly) and especially by continuity with the normal duodenum or duodenum dilated above the lesion site. However, differential diagnosis from focal adenopathies is not always possible (Derchi et al. 1986).

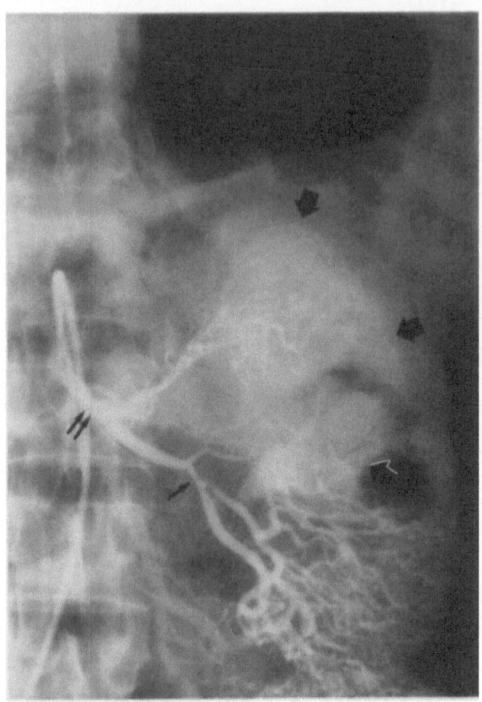

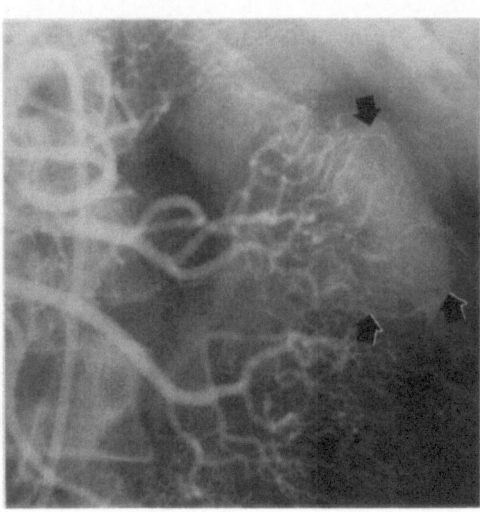

Fig. 12.6. Angiographic study of an adenocarcinoma at the duodenojejunal flexure: arterial stenoses *(small arrows)* and very discrete tumor hypervascularity *(large arrow)*

Fig. 12.7. Arteriographic study of a jejunal adenocarcinoma: discrete arteriolar irregularities *(arrows)* without any other angiographically visible abnormality

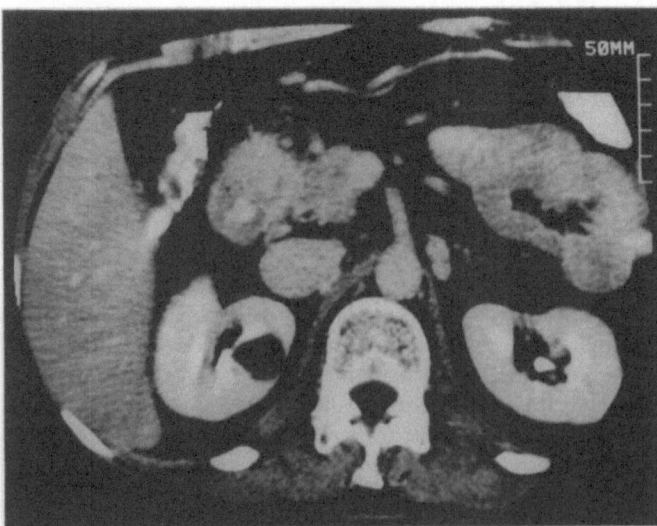

Fig. 12.8. Duodenal adenocarcinoma: CT revealed anterior infiltration of the lesion. No extension towards the pancreas; the bile duct is normal

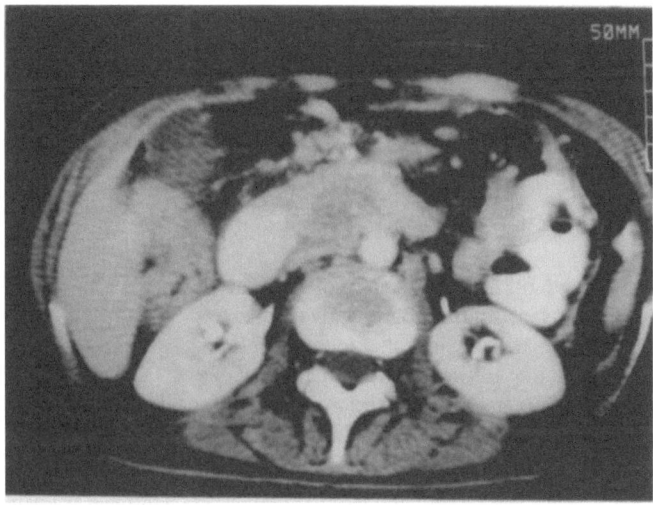

Fig. 12.9. Duodenal adenocarcinoma: CT could not accurately differentiate components of a pancreatic cancer from duodenal adenocarcinoma

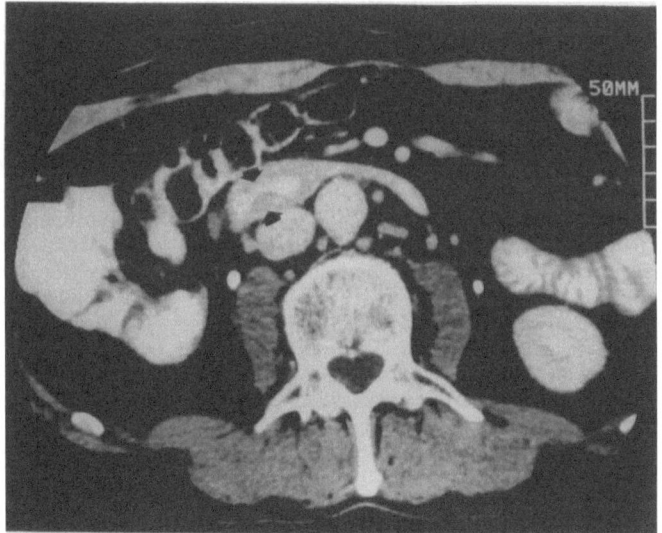

Fig. 12.10. Small duodenal adenocarcinoma causing early stenosis *(arrows)*

Few publications concern CT (Farah et al. 1987; Scatarige et al. 1987), but incorporation of this technique in pretherapy workups (Figs. 12.8–12.10) offers the following advantages:

- Exact lesion localization (for example, by demonstrating the normal aspect of the pancreas and the kidneys in case of a duodenal adenocarcinoma).

- Demonstration of vascular extension, infiltration of the mesenteric and/or retroperitoneal fat.

Morphologically, the tumor may present as a mass with intestinal wall thickening or as a polypoid filling defect; ulcerations are often too small to be seen by CT. These images have no specificity, however, and are also encountered with lymphomas and metastases. In fact, barium studies can actually reveal smaller lesions that are often more suggestive of the diagnosis of adenocarcinoma. After surgery, CT is indicated for detection of disease recurrence (Thompson and Halvorsen 1987).

12.3 Conclusion

Intestinal adenocarcinoma has not benefitted from diagnostic and therapeutic advances over the past 20 years, outside of duodenal endoscopy; this is due to the insidious nature of the pathology. Surgery appears the only effective treatment at present; neither radiotherapy nor chemotherapy have yet proven to be of significant therapeutic benefit.

12.4 References

Barclay THC, Chapira DV (1983) Malignant tumors of the small intestine. Cancer 51: 878-881

Berger L, Koppelman H (1942) Primary carcinoma of the duodenum. Ann Surg 116: 738-750

Brenner RL, Brown CH (1955) Primary carcinoma of duodenum: report of 15 cases. Gastroenterology 29: 189-198

Bruneton JN, Drouillard J, Bourry J, Roux P, Lecomte P (1983) L'adénocarcinome de l'intestin grêle. Etat actuel du diagnostic et du traitement. Etude de 27 cas et revue de la littérature. J Radiol 64: 117-123

Burgeman A, Baygenstoss AH, Cain JC (1956) Primary malignant neoplasms of the duodenum including the papilla of Vater. A clinico-pathologic study of 31 cases. Gastroenterology 30: 421-431

Chanoine F (1955) Contribution à l'étude des tumeurs malignes primitives du jéjuno-iléon. Acta Gastroenterol Belg 18: 163-199

Cohen A, McNeill D, Terz JJ, Lawrence W (1971) Neoplasms of the small intestine. Am J Dig Dis 16: 815-824

Coscina WF, Arger PH, Levine MS, Herlinger H, Cohen S, Coleman BG, Mintz MC (1986) Gastrointestinal tract focal mass lesions: role of CT and barium evaluations. Radiology 158: 581-587

Crawford Barclay TH, Kent HP (1962) The diagnosis of primary tumors of the duodenum. Gut 3: 49-59

Darling RC, Welch CE (1959) Tumors of the small intestine. N Engl J Med 260: 397-408

Derchi LE, Ierace T, De Pra L, Solbiati L, Rizzatto G, Musante F (1986) The sonographic appearance of duodenal lesions. J Ultrasound Med 5: 269-273

Dozois RR, Judd E, Dahlin DC, Bartholomen LG (1969) The Peutz-Jeghers syndrome. Is there a predisposition to the development of intestinal malignancy? Arch Surg 98: 509-517

Ebert PA, Zuidema GD (1965) Primary tumors of the small intestine. Arch Surg 91: 452-455

Ekberg O, Ekholm S (1980) Radiology in primary small bowel adenocarcinoma. Gastrointest Radiol 5: 49-53

Farah MC, Jafri SZH, Schwab RE, Mezwa DG, Francis IR, Noujaim S, Kim C (1987) Duodenal neoplasms: role of CT. Radiology 162: 839-843

Gallego MS, Pulpeiro JR, Arenas A, Colina F (1986) Primary adenocarcinoma of the terminal ileum simulating Crohn's disease. Gastrointest Radiol 11: 355-356

Gerard A, Bremer A, Jacobs E, Deloyers L (1962) A propos de 17 cas de tumeurs primitives de l'intestin grêle. Acta Gastroenterol Belg 25: 846-857

Hoffman WJ, Pack GT (1937) Cancer of the duodenum, clinical and roentgenographic study of 18 cases. Arch Surg 35: 11-63

Javier J, Lukie B (1980) Duodenal adenocarcinoma complicating celiac sprue. Dig Dis Sci 25: 150-153

Jefferson G (1916-17) Carcinoma of the suprapapillary duodenum casually associated with preexisting simple ulcer. Br J Surg 4: 209-226

Kerber GW, Frank PH (1984) Carcinoma of the small intestine and colon as a complication of Crohn disease: radiologic manifestations. Radiology 150: 639-645

Kleinerman J, Yardumian K, Tamaki HT (1950) Primary carcinoma of duodenum. Ann Intern Med 32: 451-465

Koehler RE (1983) Small bowel neoplasms. In: Margulis AR, Burhenne HJ (eds) Alimentary tract radiology, 3rd edn. Mosby, St Louis, pp 962-980

Levine MS, Drooz AT, Herlinger H (1987) Annular malignancies of the small bowel. Gastrointest Radiol 12: 53-58

Lillemoe K, Imbembo AL (1980) Malignant neoplasm of the duodenum. Surg Gynecol Obstet 150: 822-826

McPeak CJ (1967) Malignant tumors of the small intestine. Am J Surg 114: 402-411

Maillet P, Baulieux J, Barbier B, Boulez J, Otto JP (1975) Les tumeurs malignes primitives du duodenum. Lyon Chir 71: 388-394

Meiselman MS, Ghahremani GG, Kaufman MW (1987) Crohn's disease of the duodenum complicated by adenocarcinoma. Gastrointest Radiol 12: 333-336

Mittal VK, Bodzin JH (1980) Primary malignant tumors of the small bowel. Am J Surg 140: 396-399

Morgan DF, Busutill RW (1977) Primary adenocarcinoma of the small intestine. Am J Surg 134: 331-333

Ostermiller W, Joerfenson EJ, Weibel L (1966) A clinical review of tumors of the small bowel. Am J Surg 111: 403-409

Pagtalunan RJG, Majo CW, Dockerty MB (1964) Primary malignant tumors of the small intestine. Am J Surg 108: 13-18

Papadopoulos VD, Nolan DJ (1985) Carcinoma of the small intestine. Clin Radiol 36: 409-413

Perzin KH, Bridge MF (1981) Adenomas of the small intestine; a clinicopathological review of 51 cases and a study of their relationship to carcinoma. Cancer 48: 799-819

Pringot J, Bodart P (1970) Le diagnostic des tumeurs bénignes et malignes du duodénum. Revue de la littérature et des cas diagnostiqués dans le service de 1960 à 1968. Acta Gastroenterol Belg 33: 137-172

Resnik HLP, Cooper DR (1958) Carcinoma of the duodenum. Review of the literature from 1948 to 1956. Am J Surg 95: 946-952

Rochlin DB, Longmire WP (1961) Primary tumors ot the small intestine. Surgery 50: 586-592

Scatarige JC, Allen HA, Fishman EK (1987) Computed tomography of the small bowel. Semin Ultrasound CT MR 8: 403-423

Schnur PL, David E, Brown PW, Beahrs OH, Remine H, Harrisch EG (1973) Adenocarcinoma of the duodenum and the Gardner syndrome. JAMA 223: 1229-1232

Serrano JF, Mc Peak CJ (1966) Primary neoplasms of the duodenum. Surgery 59: 199-202

Smith TR, Conradi H, Bernstein R, Greweldinger J (1980) Adenocarcinoma arising in Crohn's disease; report of 2 cases. Dis Colon Rectum 23: 498-503

Spelberg F, Schmidtler F (1980) Primary malignant tumors in the small bowel. A report about 43 of our own cases and 1134 cases from literature. Acta Chir Jugosl 27: 39-46

Spira IA, Ghazi A, Wolff WI (1977) Primary adenocarcinoma of the duodenum. Cancer 39: 1721-1726

Stewart HL, Lieber MM (1937) Carcinoma of the suprapapillary portion of the duodenum. Arch Surg 35: 99-129

Swift AC (1980) Dual primary adenocarcinoma of the duodenum and jejunum in a patient with a previous colonic cancer. Postgrad Med J 56: 871-874

Thompson WM, Halvorsen RA (1987) Computed tomographic staging of gastrointestinal malignancies. Part II. The small bowel, colon, and rectum. Invest Radiol 22: 96-105

13 Adenocarcinoma of the Colon and Rectum*

13.1 General Features

Colorectal cancers are the most prevalent gastrointestinal tract tumors and the second most common malignancy in the United States after lung cancer. In 1980, 114 000 new cases of colorectal cancer and 117 000 new cases of lung cancer were recorded in the United States. The survival rate has changed very little in recent decades, and is currently around 42% at 5 years (Leffall 1981).

13.1.1 Epidemiology

13.1.1.1 Frequency

Colorectal cancers occur with an irregular distribution. The frequency is greatest in most western countries with a high standard of living. Japan was formerly a low-incidence area, and the marked increase noted in recent years is probably related to dietary modifications. Changes in frequency have also been noted with time. Between 1967 and 1980, Vobecky et al. (1984) found a decrease in the incidence of sigmoid cancers in both men and women, and an increase in cecal cancer in women. Overall, the frequency of right colon cancer has risen; in their study covering 1945-1978, Slater et al. (1986) reported a rise in the frequency of right colon cancer from 18.7% to 27.5%.

13.1.1.2 Risk Factors

Sex. Male predominance has been noted for rectal cancer (sex ratio between 1.5:1 and 2:1); colon cancer affects both sexes equally. There is discrete female predominance for cancers of the right colon and transverse colon (Halvorsen 1986). Although the risk of cancer actually exists beginning at age 40, it does not become appreciable until 45 years, and then doubles each decade thereafter.

Age. Average patient age at diagnosis is around 70 years; only 0.6%-3.7% of colorectal cancer patients are under 30 years of age (Rao et al. 1985). These tumors are usually not diagnosed until an advanced stage (two-thirds of cases are already stage D), and poorly differentiated histologic types are common (Behbehani et al. 1985; Odone et al. 1982).

Race. For Johnson and Carstens (1986), sigmoid cancer is more common in whites than in blacks (50.9% versus 36.6%) whereas whites are less affected by right colon cancer (24.5% versus 35.3%).

Predisposing Conditions. Nearly all premalignant colorectal lesions are adenomas. This factor is discussed in more detail further on in this chapter. The frequency of the adenoma-adenocarcinoma sequence is discussed in the chapter on adenomas (see Chap. 1). Development of epithelial dysplasia during ulcerative colitis increases the risk of cancer. This risk is very high when colitis affects the entire colon; it is lower when only the left colon is involved. The risk at 30 years is 25.3% for diffuse colonic disease versus 3.7% for left colitis only (Mir-Madjlessi et al. 1986). Multiple colorectal tumors are common (8%-43% of cases in the review by Greenstein et al. 1986); one-third of

---

* Written in collaboration with G. Schmutz and M.Y. Mourou.

cases are poorly differentiated histologic types (Mir-Madjlessi et al. 1986; Stevenson et al. 1984). The risk of colorectal cancer in patients with Crohn's disease is lower, and in fact certain authors feel that there is not even any increased risk (Johnson et al. 1983). Those Crohn's disease patients who do go on to develop cancer have usually had long-standing disease (Kerber and Frank 1984). Individuals with a prior history of cancer are at increased risk for colorectal cancer; this is particularly true for women. In subjects with a history of breast cancer, for example, the relative risk is multiplied by 2 or 3 (Agarwal et al. 1986; Rozen et al. 1986). By contrast, no correlation has been found between biliary lithiasis and colorectal cancer (Linos et al. 1982).

Hereditary Factors. Familial polyposis, characterized by the presence of numerous adenomatous polyps throughout the colon and rectum, is inevitably complicated by cancer of the colon or rectum (see Chap. 2). Lynch and Krush (1967) described the features of the familial colon cancer syndrome, an autosomal dominant pathology transmitted in a direct vertical manner affecting both sexes. The cumulative risk of colonic cancer is approximately 50%. This syndrome is characterized by the young age of patients, the preferential localization in the right colon, the absence of colorectal polyposis, the frequency of recurrent disease after resection, and the high frequency of associated cancers (in particular breast and uterine malignancies).

Environmental Factors. Study of environmental factors is complex, but dietary factors are known to play a preponderant role. Epidemiologic studies have not yet succeeded in identifying the exact carcinogens involved; they merely suggest that western-type diets increase the risk of colorectal cancer. The most common hypotheses implicate excessive intake of animal fats (fat theory) and a deficit in fibers and raw fruits and vegetables (fiber theory) (Rose et al. 1986). Other personal factors may or not intervene; bowel habits apparently have no role in the frequency of colorectal cancers (Nakamura et al. 1984), whereas tobacco use has an adverse effect. In smokers, colorectal tumors are usually diagnosed at a later stage, with a high frequency of stage C and D lesions, perhaps the result of alterations in the host's immune anti-tumor defenses (Daniell 1986).

13.1.2 Pathologic Anatomy

13.1.2.1 Gross Appearance

Morphology. The most common macroscopic appearance is an ulcerative-infiltrating lesion. Ulcerative carcinomas manifest as a central ulceration surrounded by a roughly circular shoulder with raised borders. The lateral borders of cancers that develop in a narrow segment may join together and become attached; a secondary ulceration forms a rim, producing annular narrowing of the colon. The possibilities for tumoral growth condition the presentation of these cancers: small-caliber segments like the transverse colon and descending colon are the sites of annular stenosing lesions; right colon cancers are large polypoid masses which can become very bulky, especially in the cecum. Pure polypoid lesions are rare; these exophytic masses often have a wide base on the colon wall. Infiltrating lesions (such as linitis plastica) are infrequent, and cause circular infiltration without ulceration.

Size and Associated Lesions. Colorectal tumors are generally solitary; average size is 5 cm. *De novo* colorectal cancers are rare (Lev and Grover 1981); these small, non-infiltrating lesions are found in the rectum (Parturier-Albot and Albot 1985) where they develop on the flat, non-polypoid mucosa (Shamsuddin et al. 1985). Synchronous colorectal cancer is encountered overall in 2%–6% of patients (Chawla et al. 1986; Kaibara et al. 1984; Langevin and Nivatvonge 1984; Lee et al. 1982), although the frequency is markedly higher in individuals with polyposis (21%–44%) or ulcerative colitis (8%–43% in the study by Greenstein et al. 1986). For Langevin and Nivatvonge (1984), 28% of patients with colorectal cancer also have one or more polyps.

Location and Frequency. The frequency of involvement of the various segments of the colon and rectum varies, depending on the series: right colon 24.6%–29%; left colon 37.9%–46%; rectum 25%–39.6% (Newland et al. 1981; Wolmark et al. 1983). Right colon carcinomas tend to occur in young individuals and in women (Rao et al. 1985). The distribution of colorectal cancers in patients with ulcerative colitis is the same as for colorectal adenocarcinomas (Slater et al. 1985).

13.1.2.2 Histology

Colorectal adenocarcinomas can be divided into well-differentiated tubular or tubulovil-lous types and moderately or poorly differentiated cancers. These two types of cancers account for around 80% of all colorectal cancers. Tubular adenocarcinoma accounts for 87% of these lesions (Toman et al. 1982). Mucoid adenocarcinoma, which accounts for slightly under 20% of cases, tends to affect young subjects: it represents over 80% of cases in persons under age 30 (Rao et al. 1985) and 28% in patients between 30 and 40 years (Beckman et al. 1984). The other histologic types (anaplastic carcinoma and squamous cell carcinoma) are very rare (Berardi et al. 1986).

13.1.2.3 Tumoral Spread

Colorectal cancers generally spread perpendicular to the wall rather than longitudinally. Lymphatic and hematogeneous metastases rarely appear before the tumor has penetrated the muscularis propria and infiltrated the extraparietal tissues. Lymphatic involvement is thus often predictable, and the frequency of adenopathies is correlated with the depth of tumoral penetration. By contrast, there is no correlation between tumor size and the frequency of metastatic lymph nodes (Wolmark et al. 1984b). In addition to nodal involvement, the veins often contain neoplastic emboli. Sites of metastases, in order of frequency, include the lymph nodes, liver, bones, lungs, peritoneum, and brain. Associated cancers, present in 4.5% of cases for Lee et al. (1982), may occur in the bladder, prostate, breast, cervix uteri, and lungs.

Table 13.1. TNM clinical classification. (From Hermanek and Sobin 1987)

T – Primary tumor	
TX	Primary tumor cannot be assessed
T0	No evidence of primary tumor
Tis	Carcinoma in situ
T1	Tumor invades submucosa
T2	Tumor invades muscularis propria
T3	Tumor invades through muscularis propria into subserosa or into non-peritonealized pericolic or perirectal tissues
T4	Tumor perforates the visceral peritoneum or directly invades other organs or structures
N – Regional lymph nodes	
NX	Regional lymph nodes cannot be assessed
N0	No regional lymph node metastasis
N1	Metastasis in one to three pericolic or perirectal lymph nodes
N2	Metastasis in four or more pericolic or perirectal lymph nodes
N3	Metastasis in any lymph node along the course of a named vascular trunk
M – Distant metastasis	
MX	Presence of distant metastasis cannot be assessed
M0	No distant metastasis
M1	Distant metastasis

13.1.2.4 Classifications

The multiplicity of staging classifications for colorectal cancers complicates comparison of the diagnostic and therapeutic indications and results published in the literature. Figure 13.1 lists the different classifications, after Zinkin (1983). Two of these eight classifications are identical (Astler and Coller 1954; Dukes 1929, 1932; Dukes and Bussey 1958; Gabriel et al. 1935; Kirklin et al. 1949; Lockhart-Mummery 1927-1928; Simpson and Mayo 1939). The 1987 TNM classification (Hermanek and Sobin 1987) (Table 13.1) now takes the number of nodes into account. This factor was not previously taken into consideration in earlier TNM classifications, which limited their efficacy for prognosis (Wolmark et al. 1986).

13.1.2.5 Histoprognosis

For Newland et al. (1981), 45.5% of all low-grade lesions are stage A while 58.1% of high-grade lesions are stage D.

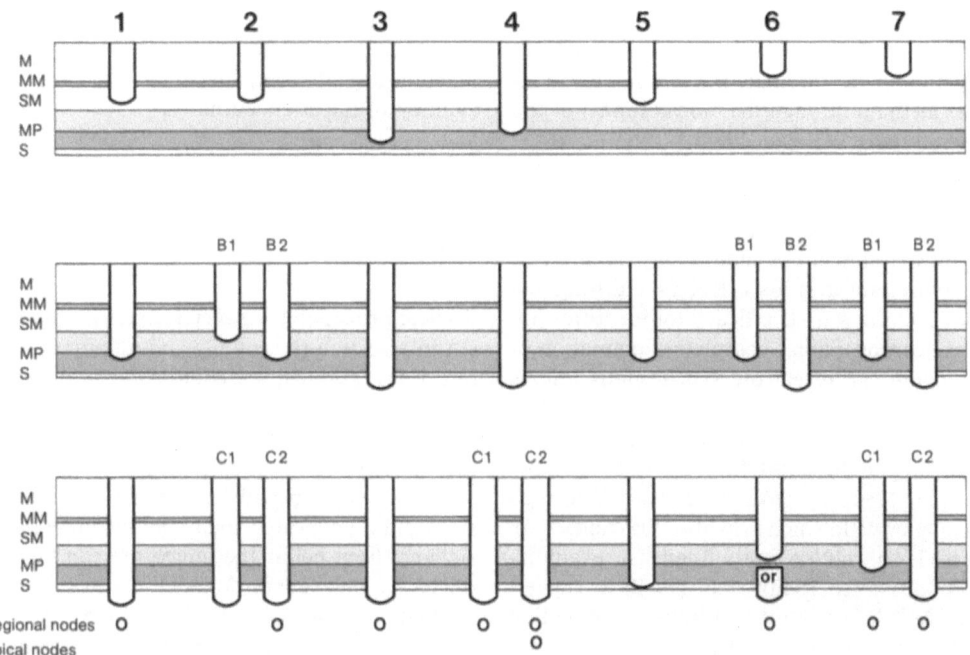

Fig. 13.1. Different classifications and stages A,B,C according to Zinkin (1983). *1,* Lockhart-Mummcry (1927-1928); *2,* Duke's (1929); *3,* Duke's (1932); *4,* Duke's and Bussey (1958); *5,* Simpson and Mayo (1938); *6,* Lirklin et al. (1949); *7,* Astler and Coller (1954); *M,* mucosa; *MM,* muscularis mucosa; *MP,* muscularis propria; *S,* serosa; *SM,* submucosa

13.1.3 Clinical Study

Clinical manifestations include diarrhea, rectal bleeding, pain, deterioration of general condition and, on rare occasions, obstruction. A constellation of these signs should prompt endoscopic and radiologic exploration of the colon and rectum.

Right colon cancer generally manifests as systemic deterioration, anemia, or fever; a palpable cecal mass (possibly due to intussusception) is present with over a third of right colon cancers. Left colon cancers usually grow in an annular manner, causing alterations in bowel habits such as constipation, partial obstruction, and sometimes acute large bowel obstruction. Clinical latency is a common feature of rectal tumors, which may be a fortuitous discovery at routine physical examination. Rectal bleeding is the most common and most suggestive symptom of rectal cancer.

Complications occur in fewer than 10% of cases (Labrosse et al. 1983); they include, in decreasing order of frequency, acute obstruction, intraperitoneal perforation, fistula between the rectum and another organ, or subperitoneal abscess. These clinical pictures usually occur in elderly subjects and individuals with advanced disease (stages C and D); the resultant resectability rate is under 50% and the prognosis is only 10% at 5 years. Paraneoplastic syndromes are rare; dermatomyositis is the most frequent (Triboulet et al. 1981).

13.1.4 Diagnosis by Non-imaging Techniques

13.1.4.1 Endoscopy

Endoscopy can be performed with a rigid proctosigmoidoscope or a flexible fiberoptic sigmoidoscope, or by total colonoscopy. Colonoscopy is the most effective technique because the entire left colon and rectum can be observed; by contrast, the ascending colon and the cecum are explored in only 80% of cases. When examination of the right colon is difficult, radiologic films can be obtained after injection of an iodinated water-soluble contrast medium through the biopsy tunnel of the colonoscope (Wu et al. 1982).

Endoscopy has an excellent sensitivity (95.5% for Beggs and Thomas 1983) and plays an important role in screening, staging, and post-therapy follow-up. Colonoscopy is increasingly used for diagnosis (Kelvin and Maglinte 1987). Along with its efficacy for identification of cancerous lesions, complete examination of the colon can reveal the synchronous lesions present in 49% of cases for Weber et al. (1986). The frequency of synchronous cancers varies, according to the series, from 2% to 6% (Chawla et al. 1986; Thorson et al. 1986). The high frequency with which synchronous cancers are missed on routine barium enema examinations prompted Reilly et al. (1982) to suggest routine colonoscopy as an initial examination technique. Increasing use of this approach has markedly reduced the role of radiologic examinations for the detection of colon cancer.

13.1.4.2 Biological Tests

Serum carcinoembryonic antigen (CEA) assays are of little value for the diagnosis of intestinal cancers because the CEA level is often normal for small tumors and can even remain within normal limits for metastatic tumors. Elevations in CEA may also occur with non-cancerous gastrointestinal pathologies (intestinal inflammation, pancreatitis, cirrhosis) and high levels may reflect non-intestinal or non-digestive cancers. However, CEA has a better sensitivity than other markers; for Putzki et al. (1987) the specificity of CEA is 85% using a threshold of 2.6 ng/ml and 95% for a threshold of 4.7 ng/ml. While CEA assays are not very sensitive for resectable tumors (Moertel et al. 1986), elevated levels found during pretherapy workup often correspond to the following picture: large stenosing tumor, advanced disease stage, differentiated histologic type (Midiri et al. 1985; Wolmark et al. 1984a). Other biochemical tumor markers such as carbohydrate antigen 19-9 (CA 19-9) and tissue polypeptide (TPA) appear of limited utility. The hemogram often reveals

hypochromic anemia and the erythrocyte sedimentation rate is frequently elevated. Liver function test abnormalities may assist in recognition of hepatic metastases.

13.1.5 Therapeutic Options

13.1.5.1 Surgery

Radical procedures for rectal carcinomas consist in resection (essentially abdominoperineal resection); perineal resection and Hartmann's operation are used less often. Conservative management includes anterior resection and, increasingly, abdominotransanal resection. Anterior resection with a coloanal anastomosis is often advocated today because the classic 5-cm limit below the tumor site can be reduced to only 2 cm. Automatic suture clips facilitate this type of operation, which is much less mutilating than abdominoperineal resection, but is reserved for cancers of the middle and upper rectum. Palliative repeat resection for recurrence of a resected rectal tumor can provide symptomatic relief that improves patient comfort (Adloff and Arnaud 1985). Palliative rectal interventions consist in external bypasses (left colostomy) which prevent obstruction but do not eliminate the functional problems created by the rectal tumor.

The only radical treatment for colon cancer is segmental colectomy. Presence of a synchronous adenoma may prompt complete colectomy (Dowling et al. 1985). Extended colectomy may be used when there are tumoral adhesions to adjacent viscera because such adhesions are not necessarily neoplastic, and the prognosis at 5 years is the same as for a normal colectomy for Le Treut et al. (1986). Palliative interventions in the colon include partial resection and bypass operations (external or internal). Hepatic metastases are increasingly treated by surgery because improvements in surgical and reanimation techniques have reduced postoperative mortality (Fortner et al. 1984a). Ligation of the hepatic artery gives a mean survival of only 9.5 months for Petreli et al. (1981), and use of this procedure is on the decline.

13.1.5.2 Radiotherapy

External beam radiotherapy may be administered preoperatively, postoperatively, both preoperatively and postoperatively, as an intraoperative procedure, or using interstitial implants. Preoperative external beam irradiation increases the resectability rate, permitting over 30% of initially inoperable candidates to later undergo surgery (Salmon et al. 1983; Tepper 1983); it reduces the frequency of hepatic metastases but not the incidence of local recurrence (Mohiuddin et al. 1985). Postoperative external beam radiotherapy improves local control (Sischy 1982); in the rectum, Baillet (1007) reported a reduction in local recurrences from 34% to 12% thanks to postoperative radiotherapy. For Mohiuddin et al. (1985), a combination of pre- and postoperative radiotherapy gives a survival rate of 78% at 5 years versus 34% without irradiation. Intraoperative radiotherapy is currently limited by technical difficulties. Interstitial implants are useful for very focal rectal cancers with a low propensity for lymphatic spread (only 10%–15% of all rectal cancers). Contact radiation therapy with or without iridium-192 provides a prognosis of 74% at 5 years (Papillon et al. 1983).

For relatively small rectal cancers, radiotherapy combined with surgery permits preservation of anal sphincter function while ensuring a relatively low recurrence rate (Gingold et al. 1983; Ramming et al. 1986; Rich et al. 1985).

13.1.5.3 Laser

Laser destruction of cancerous tissue is currently used in two extreme clinical situations: eradication of small polypoid colorectal cancers and partial destruction of the surface of large inoperable cancers.

13.1.5.4 Chemotherapy

Chemotherapy may be administered to patients with advanced colorectal cancers or, on the contrary, used as an adjuvant modality for patients who have undergone curative surgery. 5-Fluorodeoxyuridine (FUDR) is used alone or in combination with other chemotherapeutic agents, but results of systemic administration currently do not appear very satisfactory. Boulis Wassif et al. (1984) reported that a combined radiochemotherapeutic regimen discretely improved survival, although it also increased non-tumoral complications in the intestines and urinary tract. Likewise, for inoperable tumors, combined radiochemotherapy might increase the survival from 15% to 20% at 5 years, at the cost of urinary and gastrointestinal complications (Boulis Wassif 1983).

Intra-arterial chemotherapy of colorectal tumors can be given by drug injection into the two hypogastric arteries (Patt et al. 1985). The one-third of patients who subsequently develop cutaneous perianal erythema can be treated by concomitant corticotherapy. While intra-arterial chemotherapy can alleviate pain, it has no other benefits. Surgically implanted pumps (Infusaid pump) have recently been introduced for the treatment of hepatic metastases, usually by FUDR. For Johnson and Rivkin (1985) and Niederhuber et al. (1984), half of patients achieve a response, with a survival longer than 1 year.

13.1.6 Results and Prognosis

13.1.6.1 Prognostic Factors

The best prognostic factors are histologic differentiation, the depth of penetration into the colonic wall, the absence of a mucinous component, and the presence of lymphoplasmocytic infiltration within or around the tumor (De Mascarel et al. 1981). Histologic differentiation plays an important role because 37%–44% of undifferentiated cancers recur versus only 21%–25% of differentiated cancers (Doutre et al. 1982; Phillips et al. 1984).

Colonic wall penetration can be staged in several manners:

- Dukes' stage: recurrence occurs in fewer than 10% of cases for stage A and B1 lesions, 30%–45% for stage B2 and C1 lesions, and over 50% in stage C2 tumors (Olson et al. 1980; Rich et al. 1983; Russel et al. 1984).
- Number of adenopathies (Wolmark et al. 1986).

Other less important prognostic factors include:

- Better prognosis of exophytic tumors (Steinberg et al. 1986b).
- Lesion diameter: 17% recurrence rate for lesions under 4 cm versus 33% for lesions over 4 cm (Doutre et al. 1982).
- Location of the cancer (Olson et al. 1980): recurrence in the transverse colon is very rare, as opposed to rectosigmoid localizations (Malcolm et al. 1981). The rectum includes two highly vulnerable zones located less than 8-10 cm from the sphincter: first, the prerectal space between the rectum and the pelvic tissue (absence of fascia); second, the subperitoneal pelvic space (owing to anatomic continuity of the levator ani muscle with the rectal wall). The distance between the rectum and the lower and middle hemorrhoidal lymphatics precludes anatomically complete nodal resection (Guernelli and Briccoli 1985).
- CEA level: an elevated initial CEA value corresponds to a shorter survival for a given degree of tumoral spread (Wanebo et al. 1978). Elevation in the CEA level during stage C disease is an adverse factor (Moertel et al. 1986).
- Female sex (the prognosis is less good in women owing to the difficulties for radical treatment; the lymphatic drainage is more complex than in men, and there are numerous anastomoses).
- Age under 60 years: whereas late diagnosis (especially stage D) is responsible for a poor prognosis for individuals younger than 30 yr (Rao et al. 1985; Safford et al. 1981), not all authors agree that individuals under 60 years have a less favorable prognosis (Araujo Teixeira et al. 1985).
- Presence of clinical symptoms: symptomatic right colon lesions are an adverse factor: these lesions tend to be larger than those in asymptomatic patients (Wright and Higgins 1982). Regardless of the stage, obstruction and perforation are adverse prognostic factors (Steinberg et al. 1986a; Wolmark et al. 1983).

13.1.6.2 Results

Overall, colorectal cancers have a prognosis of 54% at 5 years and 40% at 10 years (Araujo Texeira et al. 1985). Results for colorectal cancers classified using Dukes' system are as follows (Eisenberg et al. 1982): 5 year survival rate of 79.6% for stage A lesions, 74.4% for stage B, 37.3% for stage C, and 4.1% for stage D. At 10 years, the prognosis is 76.3% for stage A, 65.2% for stage B, 28.8% for stage C, and 3.7% for stage D. These values are approximately the same for both the colon and the rectum (Rich et al. 1983).

Patients who present with recurrent disease after surgery are not always candidates for additional surgery or abdominoperineal resection (impossible in 27%-60.5% of cases) (Deveney and Way 1984; Martin et al. 1980). Average survival after repeat surgery is 1 year (Polk and Spratt 1971). At 5 years, the prognosis is 0%-15% (Mosnier and Guivarc'h 1987).

The overall survival for patients with hepatic metastases after curative resection is 25%-34% at 5 years (Butler et al. 1986; Coppa et al. 1985; Wagner et al. 1984). Intra-arterial chemotherapy gives a prognosis at 2 years of 37% when metastases involve less than 50% of the liver (Fortner et al. 1984b).

13.2 Pretherapy Staging of Colorectal Adenocarcinomas

13.2.1 Barium Enema Examination
(Figs. 13.2-13.9)

The role of radiologic examinations for the detection of colorectal tumors has declined considerably the past few years as increasing use has been made of colonoscopy. However, barium enema examinations are still often requested by the attendant physician and barium studies are indicated when technical factors prevent total colonoscopy. Furthermore, barium enema examination is usually better tolerated and more easily accepted by patients than colonoscopy.

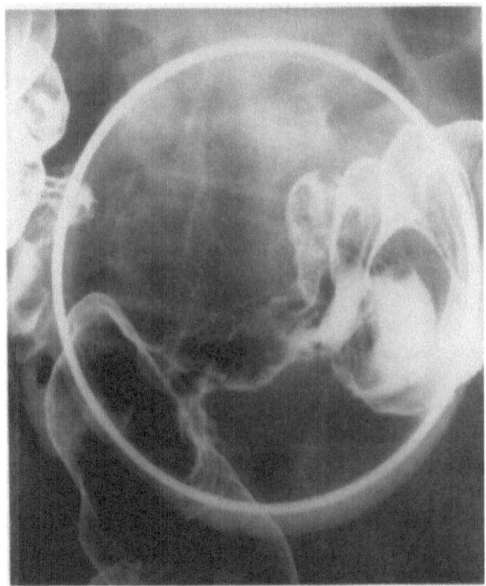

Fig. 13.2. Adenocarcinoma of the sigmoid

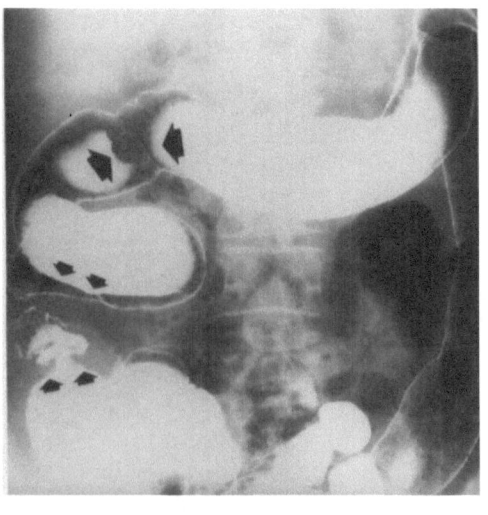

Fig. 13.4. Adenocarcinoma of the right colon *(small arrows)* associated with a degenerated polyp of the hepatic flexure *(large arrows)*

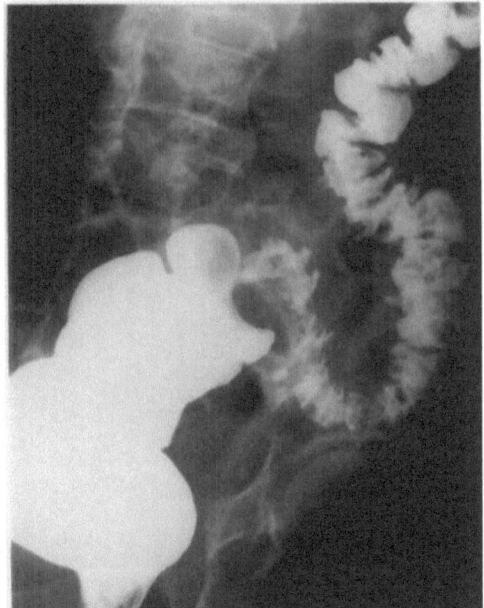

Fig. 13.3. Adenocarcinoma of the sigmoid with severe stenosis

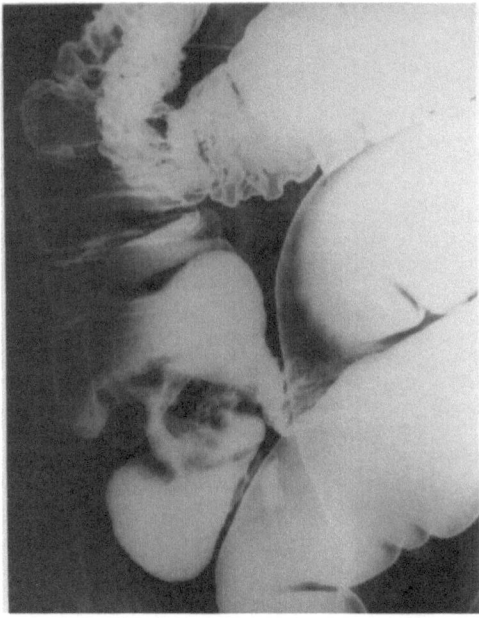

Fig. 13.5. Stenosing adenocarcinoma of the cecum

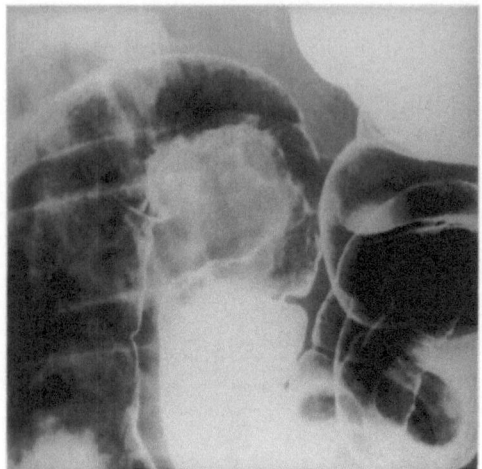

Fig. 13.6. Degenerated polyp of the left colon

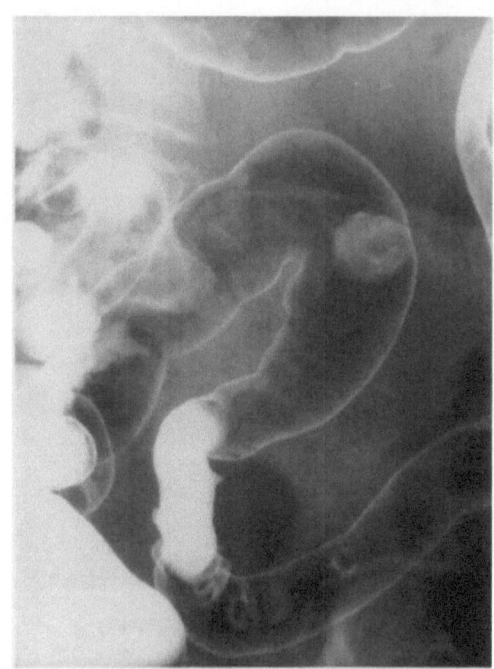

Fig. 13.8. Degenerated polyp of the left colon   ▶

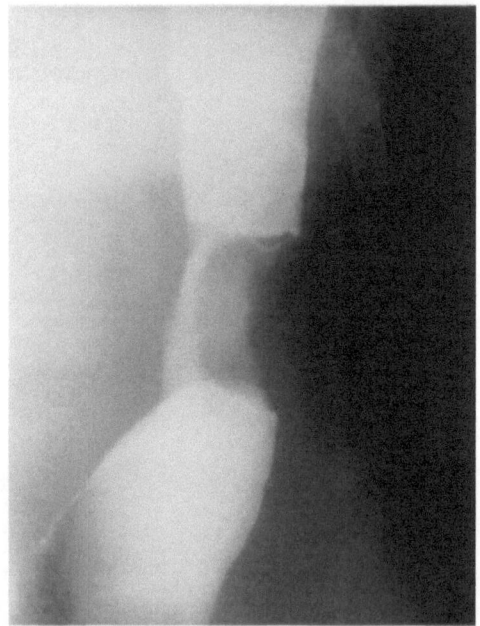

Fig. 13.7. Polypoid adenocarcinoma of the left colon

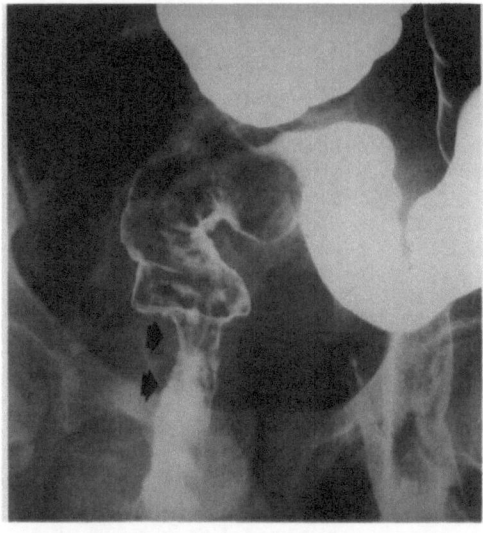

Fig. 13.9. Infrequent, extensive stenosing rectal cancer *(arrows)*

13.2.1.1 Technique and Value

Two techniques are available: double-contrast barium enema (DCBE) and single-contrast barium enema (SCBE). At present, DCBE is used more often than SCBE. In the survey conducted by Margulis and Thoeni (1988), 63.5% of the barium enema examinations performed in hospitals were double-contrast studies. Development of high-quality fluoroscopic equipment has improved analysis of the colon and reduced the rate of false-negative errors (Kewenter et al. 1987).

Regardless of the technique, the overall value of barium enema examinations is 84.9% for Brekkan et al. (1983). SCBE has a sensitivity of 78%-95.2%, depending on whether radiologic or gastroenterologic series are considered (Johnson et al. 1983; Thorson et al. 1986); the sensitivity of DCBE in similar series is 73%-95.3% (Fork et al. 1983; Johnson et al. 1983; Thorson et al. 1986). For Fork et al. (1983), DCBE correctly diagnoses 98% of all neoplastic lesions over 15 mm. Kewenter et al. (1987) emphasized the fact that half of all tumors under 1 cm are not detected by barium enema, regardless of the technique. While very few of these lesions are cancerous, barium enema examinations also often fail to diagnose synchronous cancers (Reilly et al. 1982). Although more sensitive than SCBE for small lesions, DCBE false-negative results have been reported even for bulky colorectal cancers. This can be explained by the fact that bulky masses may not deform the edges of the colon, and face-on examination of the colonic mucosa is essential for detection of mucosal changes. DCBE is currently considered the examination of choice for searches for colorectal cancer; SCBE is generally reserved for elderly patients and individuals in poor general condition.

13.2.1.2 Radiologic Appearances

Early Carcinoma. In addition to those rare cases of de novo colorectal cancer occurring as often small, non-infiltrating lesions on the flat non-polypoid rectal mucosa, nearly all other early lesions are polyps. The malignant features of such polyps are not always evident, especially when they measure less than 2 cm (Skucas et al. 1982). This underlines the importance of removing any polyp detected. Signs of malignancy detectable by DCBE include: irregular outline, broad base, size over 1 or 2 cm, retraction at the base of the polyp, significant growth between two radiologic examinations for lesions under 1 cm. In the series of Skucas et al. (1982), 43% of malignant polyps were over 2 cm while 50% of benign polyps measured less than 1 cm, and only 5% were larger than 2 cm.

Advanced Carcinoma. Many colorectal carcinomas are already fairly advanced at diagnosis, when average lesion size is at least 4 cm. The radiologic appearances reflect tumor morphology (annular, polypoid, or flat). Polypoid carcinomas vary in size; the surface of bulky lesions may be ulcerated. For this type of tumor, SCBE is often more suggestive of the diagnosis than DCBE, because luminal distention by air during DCBE may render deformation of the contour less visible. Annular carcinoma usually shows abrupt transition between the tumor and the healthy adjacent colon tissue; the mucosa of the narrowed segment is destroyed and may demonstrate ulceration. The limits of the tumoral zone are rigid, often with a ragged or nodular appearance. Annular carcinomas rarely measure over 5 cm, and have a characteristic overhanging edge (tumor shoulder or shelf). Flat lesions are unusual; the corresponding filling defect is often associated with ulceration; this type of cancer is often not detected by SCBE. The rare reports of calcifications all concern mucoid adenocarcinoma.

Specific Forms. Linitis plastica is rare; the diverticular zones are intact and the involved segment is always rather long (over 5 cm); the concentrically narrowed lumen shows progressive transition between the lesion and the healthy tissue (Sibilly et al. 1980). An intraluminal lenticular ulcer surrounded by a meniscoid lucency of tumor is another rare form (Siskind and Burrell 1986).

Barium enema examinations performed less than 15 days after interventional endoscopy may be the source of diagnostic difficulties: spasms after electrocoagulation of multiple lesions; persistent ulceration after a deep biopsy; small, elevated sequellar zone with irregular borders and a smooth center after electrocoagulation of a small sessile polyp; small residual lesion of uncertain diagnosis (Bartram and Hall-Craggs 1987).

Associated Lesions. In addition to synchronous cancers, one or more polyps may be present; the frequency varies depending on the literature series (Faivre et al. 1979). These lesions are often small, and over half of cases are not detected by barium enema examination (Thorson et al. 1986). Coexistence of sigmoid diverticula increases the diagnostic difficulties; 6.6% of sigmoid diverticula are associated with a cancer (Boulos et al. 1985). Diffuse lymphoid follicles, probably corresponding to an immune response, are rare, especially in elderly subjects; these infrequent images are especially visible in the right colon (Bronen et al. 1984). Lesions of ulcerative colitis can also complicate recognition of an adenocarcinoma. Epithelial dysplasia, often not visible radiologically, may have a slightly nodular appearance and must be kept under surveillance because of the risk of carcinoma (Stevenson et al. 1984). Adenocarcinomas in patients with Crohn's disease generally show intraluminal growth; infiltrating lesions are less common; these lesions are not necessarily found at sites of regional enteritis (Miller et al. 1987).

Complications. The usual appearance of colorectal carcinoma may be modified by obstruction or perforation (Kelvin and Gardiner 1987). Three-quarters of all cases of colonic obstruction in the adult are caused by primary carcinomas. The site of predilection is the sigmoid colon. Adenocarcinoma causing right colon obstruction may lead to small bowel obstruction; colonic urticaria, generally due to submucosal edema, may be visualized in such cases. Barium enema examination is difficult if not impossible in patients with complete obstruction. Intussusception is rare; polypoid masses in the cecum, the major cause, often have a coiled-spring appearance on SCBE. One-third of all cases of tumoral perforation are associated with extravasation of contrast medium and half of cases show signs of inflammation. Fistulization may occur towards

the stomach and the jejunum (Hulnick et al. 1987). Necrotic lesions may be difficult to recognize on DCBE; the irregular limits of these tumors, which project outside the normal mucosal line of the colon, correspond to extramural extension. Necrotic lesions are often poorly differentiated histologic types producing abundant mucus (Hunter et al. 1983).

13.2.1.3 Sources of Error and Differential Diagnosis

Causes of Error. Kelvin et al. (1981) analyzed the causes of error for lesions averaging 3 cm: 52% of cases were purely perceptive errors (essentially filling defects, mucosal surface not seen en face), 32% were technical factors (excessive barium, insufficient distention during DCBE), 6% were errors of interpretation (false-positive errors of adenocarcinoma for hemorrhoids or benign narrowing caused by ulcerative colitis); by contrast, 10% of lesions were not visible even retrospectively. Diverticula increase the diagnostic problems; sigmoid diverticula in particular are responsible for an increased rate of error. For Baker and Alterman (1985), the median error rate in individuals with diverticula is 7.2%, and this figure increases with the number of diverticula. Poor patient preparation prior to DCBE should lead to this technique being abandoned in favor of SCBE, performed using vigorous compression.

Differential Diagnosis. Few diagnostic problems occur if the patient is prepared correctly prior to barium enema examination. Intraluminal masses suggestive of malignancy, such as neoplastic stricture, involve no diagnostic problem and prompt confirmatory endoscopy. When a solitary filling defect does not present all of the features suggestive of a carcinoma, other diagnoses may be entertained: adenoma, internal hemorrhoid, stool, endometriosis, lipoma, other neoplasm (lymphoma, metastasis). Likewise, focal narrowing of the colon may have a nonmalignant etiology: spasm, diverticulitis, inflammatory process (ulcerative colitis, Crohn's disease, ischemic or postradiation changes), amebiasis, tuberculosis, or an adjacent cancer (Kelvin and Gardiner 1987).

The possibility of cancer must not be over-looked in individuals with pre-existent lesions (ulcerative colitis or Crohn's disease, for example) and comparison of serial radiologic films may reveal signs of neoplastic transformation.

13.2.2 Ultrasonography

13.2.2.1 Sonoendoscopy

Technique. The rectum may be examined with an endorectal ultrasound probe (endoscopic transrectal ultrasonography) or by blind transrectal ultrasonography. Endoscopic ultrasound appears more sensitive because it clearly visualizes the lesions. Blind transrectal ultrasound is currently more common than the endoscopic technique but is limited by the penetration depth of only 15 cm (Tio and Tytgat 1986). Several types of transducers are available (axial, longitudinal, or a combination of both). The efficacy of examination is the same regardless of the patient's position (lithotomy position, knee-chest position, etc.) (Rifkin 1987; Silverstein et al. 1986).

Normal Appearance. The number of sonographically-visible rectal wall layers reported in the literature depends on the transducer frequency utilized (Konishi et al. 1985; Rifkin and Marks 1985). The normal thickness of the rectal wall is currently agreed to be 2–3 mm; five layers are visible when examination is performed with a 7.5-MHz transducer (Rifkin 1987):

- First (innermost) layer: hyperechoic, corresponding to the interface between the transducer and the mucosa.
- Second layer: hypoechoic, corresponding to the mucosa and the submucosa.
- Third layer: hyperechoic, corresponding to an interface between the submucosa and the muscularis propria.
- Fourth layer: hypoechoic, corresponding to the muscularis propria.
- Fifth (outermost) layer: hyperechoic, corresponding to the interface between the muscularis propria and the perirectal fat.

A certain degree of controversy exists concerning the third hyperechoic layer. Wang et al. (1987), for example, consider the third hyperechoic layer to represent the submucosa. For these authors, the normal mucosa is 0.6 mm thick, the submucosa 0.9 mm, and the muscularis externa (propria) 1.8 mm. Precise anatomic definition of this third hyperechoic layer is important because it allows differentiation of stages T1 and T2 in the TNM classification system and stages A and B1-C1 in the classification of Astler and Coller (1954).

Normal lymph nodes measure less than 1.5 cm and usually cannot be distinguished from the perirectal fat.

Difficulties. In addition to the need for precise anatomic definition of the third hyperechoic layer, several other technical difficulties merit attention. The rigidity and diameter of currently available transducers hamper and sometimes prevent sonoendoscopic examination of stenosing lesions. Adhesions can create problems with ulcerated tumors (Tio and Tytgat 1986). Mosnier et al. (1987) have underscored the technical problems created by air in the balloon, perforation due to overinflation of the balloon during examination, and hyperechoic artifacts due to the presence of fecal matter in the rectum. With a minimum of experience, intestinal loops can easily be identified in the pouch of Douglas and an extrarectal pathology can be differentiated from the normal rectal wall. The main drawback of sonoendoscopy is the impossibility of satisfactory examination of bulky tumors and stenosing lesions. CT is particularly indicated in such cases.

Ultrasonographic Appearance of Colorectal Cancers (Figs. 13.10, 13.11). Colorectal carcinomas are generally hypoechoic masses which suddenly interrupt the regular sequence of the various layers of the rectal wall. Particular attention must be paid to determining the relationships of the lesion with the muscularis propria (fourth hypoechoic layer). Fecal matter and air trapped between the tumor and the transducer occasionally image as a hyperechoic mass (Rifkin 1987). Small submucosal tumors that invade the muscularis propria at an early stage can be difficult to visualize sono-

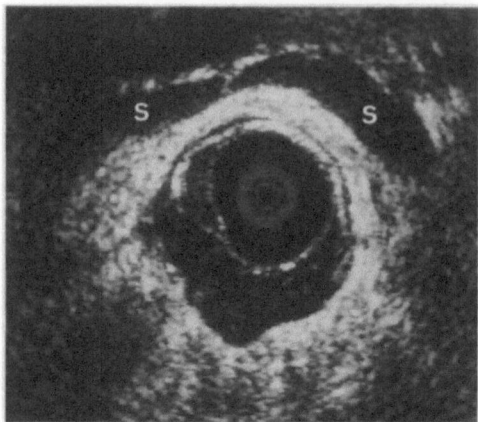

Fig. 13.10. Rectal sonoendoscopy: this bulky rectal ___er ruptured through the submucosa and infiltrated the perirectal fat. *S,* seminal vesicles. (Courtesy of Dr. Valette, Lyons, France)

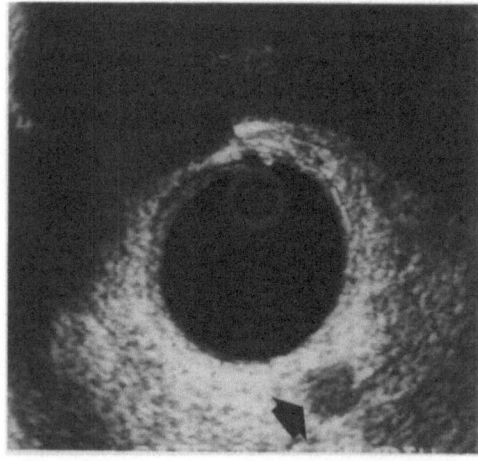

Fig. 13.11. Rectal sonoendoscopy: examination demonstrated a metastatic perirectal lymph node *(arrow)* above the rectal lesion (not visible on this film). (Courtesy of Dr. Valette, Lyons, France)

graphically. There are no morphologic differences between metastatic lymph nodes and inflammatory nodes (Di Candio et al. 1987), but endorectal ultrasound accurately analyzes the structures adjacent to the rectum (levator ani, vagina, bladder, etc.).

Value of Sonoendoscopy. Whereas sonoendoscopy has greater than 90% accuracy for tumor

identification and staging (Beynon et al. 1986; Pahlman et al. 1984; Rifkin and Wechsler 1986; Saitoh et al. 1986), its accuracy for nodal involvement is markedly lower owing to the non-specificity of nodal hypertrophy and the possibility of metastatic nodes without any detectable enlargement. The overall sensitivity of sonoendoscopy is thus between 50% and 73.2% (Di Candio et al. 1987; Rifkin et al. 1986; Rifkin 1987; Saitoh et al. 1986). Inflammatory nodes are a source of false-positive errors and for Rifkin (1987), the specificity of endorectal ultrasound is 91%.

Sonoendoscopy is superior to CT for tumor analysis (Beynon et al. 1986; Kramann and Hildebrandt 1986) and definition of perirectal fat infiltration. For Rifkin (1987), the sensitivity of endorectal ultrasound is 83% versus only 55% for CT. The value of intrarectal ultrasound was particularly emphasized by Hildebrandt and Feifel (1985), who proposed replacing the T in the TNM classification by a uT when sonoendoscopy is technically possible.

13.2.2.2 Abdominal Ultrasonography

Study of the Colorectal Tumor. For Price and Metreweli (1988), the predictive value of ultrasonography for diagnosing an abdominal mass as colonic cancer is 79%. Sonographically, these rounded or lobulated masses are echo-poor, but may have a highly echoic central zone (target sign) or clusters of eccentrically located echoes (cockade sign). Short irregular thickening may be demonstrated. In the cecum, edema of the terminal ileum may be imaged as low-echo wall thickening. Ultrasonography cannot differentiate inflammatory and tumoral masses.

Hepatic Ultrasonography. In France, ultrasonography is a first line technique for hepatic examination; it has a sensitivity between 57% and 92% for diagnosis of hepatic metastases and a specificity of 81%-96% (Bruneton et al. 1988). Sonographic evaluation of lesions over 1.5 cm is usually satisfactory. Liver metastases of colorectal cancers are generally hyperechoic, without posterior reinforcement, and usually exhibit discrete posterior attenuation.

A hypoechoic halo may be present. These features correspond to lesions that do not exceed 3–4 cm. Larger lesions acquire a complex appearance, and may undergo necrosis or calcification. Hypoechoic metastases of colorectal cancers are less frequent. Ultrasound-guided fine-needle (20–22 gauge) aspiration biopsy has a value of 85% (Bell et al. 1986). The initial surgical procedure for colorectal cancers is an exploratory procedure, with particular attention being paid to evaluation of the liver. Intraoperative ultrasound has become an indispensable technique for detection of small lesions, which can be managed by metastasectomy (Bismuth and Castaing 1987; Deixonne and Lopez 1987).

13.2.3 Computed Tomography

13.2.3.1 Technique

The quality of CT examination depends closely on the quality of preparation of the colon and the rectum. Oral and rectal administration of iodinated contrast agents and rectal air insufflation improve detection of colorectal lesions. Intravenous contrast medium injection is particularly useful for liver studies. CT scans are obtained from the diaphragm to the level of the pubic symphysis. Evaluation of relationships with the bladder is improved by iodinated opacification; likewise, a vaginal tam-

pon can aid in localization of the cervix uteri. Gothlin et al. (1987) used contiguous 5-mm scans for study of the rectum; patients were examined in the prone position after insufflation of air or intrarectal injection of contrast medium. Van Waes et al. (1983) used sagittal scans with a CT Philips Tomoscan 300.

13.2.3.2 CT Features of Colorectal Cancer (Figs. 13.12–13.15)

The possibilities of CT led Thoeni et al. (1981) to devise a classification which resembles the Dukes staging system (Table 13.2). The normal colon wall is 3 to 4 mm thick; after air insufflation or iodinated opacification of the cleansed colon and rectum, any wall thickening greater than 5 mm can be considered pathologic.

Primary colorectal cancers manifest as focal, soft-tissue density masses adjacent to the lumen of the colon or rectum. Carcinoma that has infiltrated the entire wall is visualized as concentric thickening on CT scans perpendicular to the large axis of the colon. Obstructive tumors may be demonstrated as concentric wall thickening, in particular if the CT scans are perpendicular to the longitudinal axis of the colon (Kelvin and Gardiner 1987). Mucus-secreting adenocarcinomas may contain punctate calcifications. The transverse colon and the splenic and hepatic flexures are the two

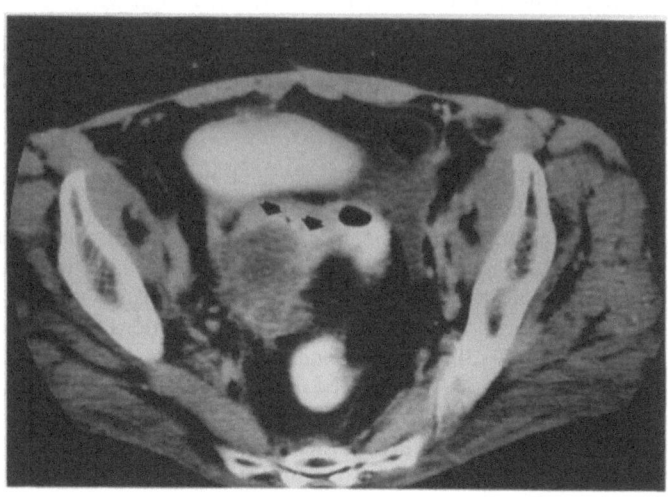

Fig. 13.12. Sigmoid cancer *(arrows)*

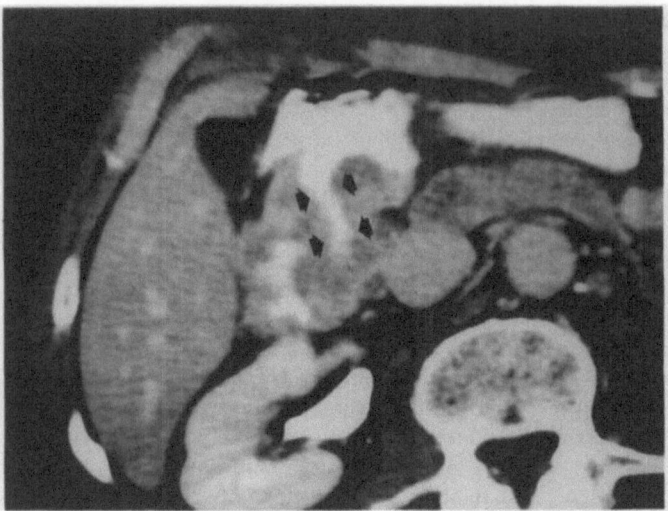

Fig. 13.13. Cancer of the hepatic flexure: concomitant transrectal opacification revealed the extent of the tumor and the colonic stenosis *(arrows)*

most difficult segments to study with CT. Tumoral spread outside of the wall, into the perirectal fat, is not satisfactorily evidenced by CT unless the scans are perpendicular to the longitudinal axis of the colon or rectum. Diffuse mesenteric infiltration by colon carcinoma may be seen as a mass, ascites, or adenopathies around the origin of the superior mesenteric artery.

Rectal cancer can spread to the pelvic muscles, the genital organs, and the urinary tract. Bone involvement is encountered only in very advanced disease. Malignant infiltration of adjacent structures can generally be affirmed when CT scans reveal enlargement or direct destruction of an organ by the tumor. Obliteration of the fat plane between the tumor and an organ is generally insufficient to affirm invasion.

Nodal involvement is rarely overlooked by CT. The threshold for definition of malignancy is nodal enlargement of 1 or 1.5 cm (Balthazar et al. 1988; Freeny et al. 1986; Rifkin 1987; Thompson et al. 1986).

Complications of colorectal carcinomas are well analyzed by CT. Retroperitoneal abscess, for example, is easily recognized by CT regardless of the location of the primary tumor (Maglinte and Pollack 1983). Whereas perforation is not always clinically evident, CT can

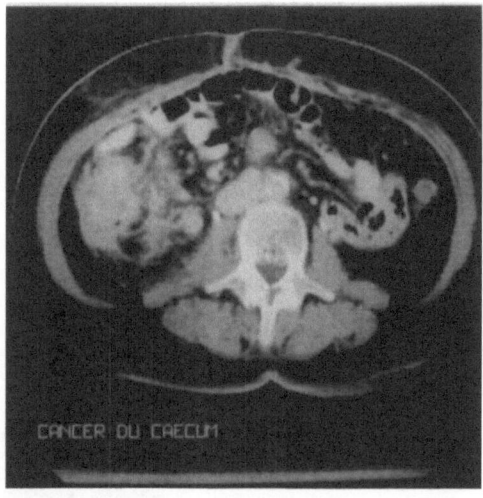

CANCER DU CAECUM

Fig. 13.14. Bulky cecal cancer infiltrating the peritoneal fat and lymph node metastases

readily demonstrate a mass with an abscess as a fluid-density collection, or a mass with inflammatory pericolonic or perirectal modifications (Hulnick et al. 1987). Intussusception has a characteristic appearance when mesenteric fat is identified between the bowel loops.

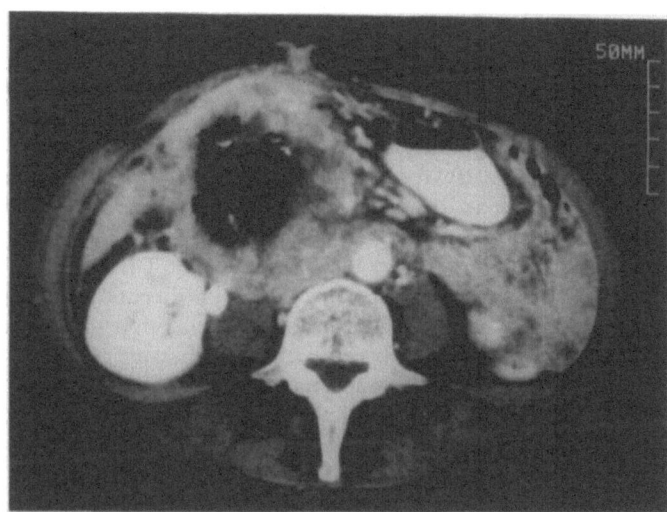

Fig. 13.15. Extensively necrotic bulky cancer of the right colon causing intra- and retroperitoneal infiltration

Table 13.2. CT staging of colorectal cancer: classification system of Thoeni et al. (1981)

Stage I	Intraluminal mass without thickening of colon wall
Stage II	Thickened colon wall (more than 5 mm) or pelvic mass without invasion of adjacent structures or extension to pelvic sidewalls
Stage IIIA	Thickened colon wall or pelvic mass with invasion of adjacent structures but not pelvic sidewalls or abdominal wall
Stage IIIB	Thickened colon wall or pelvic mass extending to pelvic sidewalls and/or abdominal wall without distinct metastases
Stage IV	Metastatic disease with or without local abnormality

13.2.3.3 Problems for Differential Diagnosis with CT

Exploration of the rectosigmoid is frequently unsatisfactory in very thin or very muscular subjects (Meyer et al. 1983). Furthermore, a tumor cannot be distinguished from an inflammatory process. There are no CT features of colonic or rectal masses suggestive of adenocarcinoma rather than another tumor, and in particular another neoplasm. The problems for analysis of the colonic wall and detection of adenopathies are discussed in Section 13.2.3.4.

A perirectal halo is not necessarily a sign of inoperability; such haloes may represent inflammation or tumoral infiltration, and are sometimes seen with operable lesions after radiotherapy. The exact significance of this perirectal halo is unclear; it may correspond to an inflammatory reaction, an edematous reaction, or a tumoral process in the fibrous rectal fascia (Adalsteinsson et al. 1985).

Certain technical and topographic problems can also create difficulties:

- A biopsy taken less than 1 week before CT may cause an inflammatory reaction, leading to an increase in the density of the peritumoral fat, simulating perirectal extension.
- Use of a large amount of air with a rectal transducer may result in overestimation of perirectal growth, secondary to compression of the perirectal space by the rectum and increased attenuation of the perirectal structures.
- Poor analysis of tumor relationships with the prostate, bladder, and vagina, particularly when the cancer lies in the anterior portion of the lower rectum (Adalsteinsson et al. 1985).

13.2.3.4 Value of CT

Owing to the problems encountered with CT, in particular for analysis of the colon wall and detection of adenopathies, some authors do not feel that CT is useful for preoperative local staging (Freeny et al. 1986; Thompson et al. 1986). This opinion is not shared by other investigators (Balthazar et al. 1988; Gothlin et al. 1987; Van Waes et al. 1983).

Overall, the value of CT for diagnosis of colorectal adenocarcinoma is between 47.5% and 77.1% (Freeny et al. 1986; Thompson and Halvorsen 1987). Staging is correct for 60%–70% of cases in the rectum and for 64% of cases in the colon (Adalsteinsson et al. 1985; Balthazar et al. 1988). Globally, stages A, B, and C are poorly evaluated. Stage D lesions are always correctly assessed, and CT-demonstrated abnormalities therefore have a high probability of corresponding to neoplastic involvement. For example, involvement of the posterior peritoneal reflection towards the adjacent muscles allows affirmation of the inoperability of a colonic cancer (Solomon et al. 1988).

In the literature, colorectal tumors are reportedly correctly visualized in 69%–85% of cases (Balthazar et al. 1988; Freeny et al. 1986; Rifkin et al. 1986). Balthazar et al. (1988) emphasized the necessity of satisfactory colorectal preparation, as tumor visualization rose from 68% for a non-prepared colon to 95% for a clean colon. For perirectal involvement, CT has a sensitivity between 55% and 70% (Balthazar et al. 1988; Freeny et al. 1986; Rifkin et al. 1986; Thompson et al. 1986) and a specificity of 80.6% (Freeny et al. 1986). The value of CT for the diagnosis of lymph node metastases is very low, between 23% and 35% for most authors (Freeny et al. 1986; Rifkin et al. 1986; Thompson et al. 1986), although in the series of Balthazar et al. (1988) it reached 73%.

Some controversy exists concerning the frequency of understaging and overstaging for rectal carcinoma. Understaging is frequent for Adalsteinsson et al. (1985), Freeny et al. (1986), and Thompson et al. (1986). For Gothlin et al. (1987), overstaging does occur but there are no false-negative errors. CT findings may allow interstitial implant radiation therapy to be offered to patients with well-differen-

tiated stage A or B1 rectal cancers. These two stages have a very low risk of nodal involvement, especially when the tumor is a differentiated histologic type (Morson 1966).

13.2.3.5 Hepatic Metastases

CT has a value of 76%–94% for detection of hepatic metastases (Freeny et al. 1986). In addition to conventional pre- and postcontrast scans after venous opacification with an iodinated water-soluble contrast medium, several techniques improve the sensitivity of CT: delayed scans, arterial portography, use of EOE-13 (Matsui et al. 1987; Reed et al. 1986).

On conventional precontrast CT scans, most metastases are less dense than the normal adjacent tissue and are relatively well circumscribed. Occasionally, hepatic metastases are isodense or even denser than the liver (because of calcifications or intratumoral hemorrhage). Extensively necrotic tumors may exceptionally mimic a cyst; CT scans cannot analyze the tumoral wall with the same fine detail as ultrasonography. Although metastases are usually hypodense before contrast medium injection, the percentage of isodense forms is hard to determine. Injection of a contrast medium improves the detection of some metastases but may actually mask others. Complete examination including both pre- and postcontrast scans is thus essential. When diagnosis remains uncertain, the complementary techniques mentioned above should be used (arterial injection, use of emulsions).

The differential diagnoses for CT findings include other tumoral pathologies (hepatoma, lymphoma, benign tumor, nodular hyperplasia rather than cavernous hemangioma) and irregular steatosis. In this last pathology, the islands of normal parenchyma appear hyperdense, and the normal liver tissue cannot always be distinguished from a metastasis. When CT studies are limited to preoperative hepatic workups, searches must be made for mesenteric and portal adenopathies, even though these lesions are not always well demonstrated by CT.

13.2.3.6 Other Imaging Techniques

Magnetic Resonance Imaging (MRI). Preoperative staging of colorectal cancer patients with MRI has not yet proven superior to CT because problems persist for analysis of perirectal and nodal involvement (Butch et al. 1986). Nevertheless, the three-dimensional imaging possibilities of MRI should permit better exploration of the sigmoid region. The technical improvements provided by MRI for liver studies improves the value of hepatic examination, and current results are similar to or slightly better than CT (Glazer et al. 1986; Hamm et al. 1987; Reinig et al. 1987; Stark et al. 1987). In a certain number of cases, MRI allows better differentiation of cavernous hemangioma from hepatic metastases.

Other Imaging Techniques. Preoperative intravenous urography has been supplanted by ultrasonography, which can demonstrate urinary stasis, and CT, which can visualize the ureter (Tartter and Steinberg 1986). Hepatic scintigraphy had a sensitivity of 78% and a specificity of 82% in the review by Oren et al. (1986). Exclusive hepatic angiography no longer has any indications for diagnosis of hepatic metastases; by contrast, it can be coupled with CT to improve detection of hepatic metastases (injection into the hepatic artery or superior mesenteric artery). It is useful for analysis of hepatic arterial vascularization prior to surgical implantation of a pump for chemotherapy. Techniques using lipiodol emulsions are also currently employed for the diagnosis of hepatic metastases. Pelvic angiography can serve as a therapeutic vector for intra-arterial chemotherapy for inoperable tumors or locoregional disease recurrences.

13.2.3.7 Imaging Examinations Included in Pretherapy Workups

Discovery of a colonic or rectal cancer requires accurate examination of the entire colon for synchronous lesions and searches for metastases. Colonoscopy is indispensable because this examination is the best means for detecting small synchronous lesions (cancer or, more often, polyps). Barium enema examination is particularly useful for rectal cancers. The distance between a rectal tumor and the anal canal is measured more accurately by a profile view after barium enema examination than by endoscopy (Frager et al. 1987; Waneck et al. 1984). In addition, when colonoscopy is incomplete and does not include the cecum for example, barium enema examination can complete the search for synchronous lesions.

In addition to biologic tests (CEA, liver function tests), pretherapy disease staging may include sonoendoscopy for better analysis of the wall and detection of adenopathies, in particular in the rectum. Transrectal ultrasound allows selection of the best surgical procedure (anterior resection or abdominoperineal resection) by evaluating the distance between the tumor and the anal sphincter, the upper and lower limits of the tumor, and the relationships with the levator ani muscle, the lower pelvic muscle, and neighboring organs (Hildebrandt and Feifel 1985). Routine CT examination is not indispensable for small tumors, and abdominal ultrasonography may be sufficient for preoperative searches for hepatic metastases.

When a bulky tumor prevents satisfactory transrectal ultrasound examination, CT can provide interesting data. Adalsteinsson et al. (1985) found CT valuable for determining the resectability of rectal tumors considered inoperable by clinical criteria. For Freeny et al. (1986), preoperative CT is primarily useful for detection of hepatic metastases. CT can also be used in place of preoperative urography (Clark et al. 1984). At present, though, preoperative CT is basically a second-line procedure performed as a function of sonoendoscopic findings or for large tumors not amenable to surgery initially.

Regardless of the stage of a colorectal cancer, a chest X-ray is indispensable.

13.3 Post-therapy Follow-up

Patients who undergo curative surgery require follow-up because of the possibility of recurrence and metachronous lesions. Between 30% and 40% of all patients treated with a curative intent relapse within 5 years, and half of these recurrences appear in the first 18 months (Gastrointestinal Tumor Study Group 1984; Grabbe and Winkler 1985; Polk and Spratt 1971). The 17%–23% of abnormalities detected by follow-up endoscopic examinations are essentially polyps (Mosnier 1985; Unger and Wanebo 1983); these recurrent lesions are discovered at all periods of follow-up and in all locations. For Unger and Wanebo (1983), polyps are eight times more frequent than metachronous cancers, but this incidence is disputed by other authors. Reilly et al. (1982), for an average follow-up period of under 4 years, found a 7.7% rate of new cancers whereas such lesions were noted in 20% of cases by Weber et al. (1986). The risk of metachronous cancerous lesions appears to rise markedly in the 2nd decade following the first colorectal cancer (Morson 1984).

13.3.1 Post-therapy Follow-up Examinations

In patients not treated in a curative manner who have residual tumor, the examination technique that provided the most precise pretherapy workup serves as the baseline procedure; for bulky lesions, it is usually CT. Likewise, for surveillance of the liver, the first-line imaging technique is that used in the pretherapy workup.

Owing to the risks of recurrence and metachronous lesions, follow-up of patients who have undergone curative treatment takes place at several levels. After abdominoperineal resection, physical examination is aimed at detecting superficial local recurrence in the form of perineal nodules; these nodular lesions are easier to demonstrate in women by digital vaginal examination. Recurrence on a coloanal anastomosis and those rare cases of superficial parietal relapses can also be detected by physical examination.

Besides liver function tests (transaminases, alkaline phosphatases, gamma glutamyl peptidase), CEA assays are the major biologic test. Despite the numerous false-negative and false-positive errors (34% overall for Sandler et al. 1984; average 24% false-negative errors in a review of the literature), CEA appears more useful than other biochemical markers such as CA 19-9 and TPA for the follow-up of treated patients. The elevated error rate makes serial assays mandatory: once a month or every three months the first two years and every 3 or 6 months thereafter. Elevation of the CEA level is determined over three successive assays (two assays if the concentration is twice the normal level). This attitude increases the predictive value of CEA for diagnosis of recurrence (Attiyeh and Stearns 1981; Beart and O'Connell 1983; Lavin et al. 1981; Martin et al. 1981; Wanebo et al. 1978).

Colorectal endoscopy is recommended every 6 months for the first 2 years after resection. Barium studies are a second-line procedure performed as a function of endoscopic findings. Sonoendoscopy can accurately detect postresection perianastomotic recurrence. After abdominoperineal resection, baseline CT or MRI studies are recommended within 4 months of surgery; thereafter, surveillance consists in an examination every 6 months for 2 years, then once a year the following years (Freeny et al. 1987; Thompson et al. 1986). Liver follow-up examinations are based on ultrasonography or CT. A chest X-ray is required every 6 months because half of all nonhepatic metastases occur in the lungs (Polk and Spratt 1971).

While this type of follow-up strategy should facilitate early detection of recurrences, its benefit for improving patient survival is not yet certain. Diagnosis of a metachronous polyp allows polypectomy, thereby preventing development of a new colorectal cancer, but systematic searches for recurrent disease have not yet proved beneficial. No large series have yet shown an improvement in patient survival after resection of a local recurrence, but early diagnosis of a clinically silent recurrence may increase the indications for surgery (Buhler et al. 1984). By contrast, the diagnosis of hepatic metastases at a sufficiently early stage allows resection and prolonged survival.

It must nevertheless be remembered that detection of a recurrent tumor or a metastasis requires a complete workup: 60% of all recurrences combine at least two of the following abnormalities: local recurrence, hepatic metastases, lung metastases. For Sugarbaker et al. (1971), only 24.3% of all intra-abdominal recurrences are solitary and metastases are solitary in only 15% of cases.

13.3.2 Anterior Resection

Although local follow-up of patients treated by resection is managed essentially by endoscopy, this technique must not be used alone because it does not always detect early recurrence. Disease recurrence at the anastomotic site occurs in 1.7%–7% of patients; perianastomotic recurrences are more frequent: 10%–15% (Malcolm et al. 1981; McDermott et al. 1985; Mosnier and Guivarc'h 1987; Olson et al. 1980; Pihl et al. 1981; Russell et al. 1984). Even small, perianastomotic recurrence may be evidenced by sonoendoscopy, whereas the sensitivity of CT is poorer for this type of lesion. Iliac and retroperitoneal node recurrence occurs in only 1%–3% of patients (McDermott et al. 1985).

Along with CEA determinations, which have a postresection sensitivity of 61% for diagnosis of recurrence (Deveney and Way 1984), sonoendoscopy, barium enema, and CT are the main techniques employed for postoperative follow-up. Sonoendoscopy normally shows regular wall thickening corresponding to postoperative fibrosis. Sonographic identification of an early recurrence can be difficult; any wall irregularity within postoperative thickening must be considered suspicious, and requires a repeat examination 3 months later (Fig. 13.16). Biopsy under sonoendoscopic guidance is not yet possible, and proof of malignant evolution must be obtained. Surgical anastomosis by means of a circular suture clip generally causes regular thickening at the site of the colorectal anastomosis. These images normally regress with time, often asymmetrically (Mosnier et al. 1987). These features allow sonographic diagnosis of anastomotic and perianastomotic recurrences with a good degree of sensitivity. Barium enema examination has a sensitivity of 75%–88% for detecting recurrent disease after resection (Chen et al. 1987; Detry et al. 1984). CT has a value of 61% (Dveeney and Way 1984), with a sensitivity of 69% for Chen et al. (1987). Owing to its high cost and limited sensitivity, CT cannot be recommended for routine surveillance of patients who have undergone resection (Figs. 13.17–13.22). Use of indium-111 anti-

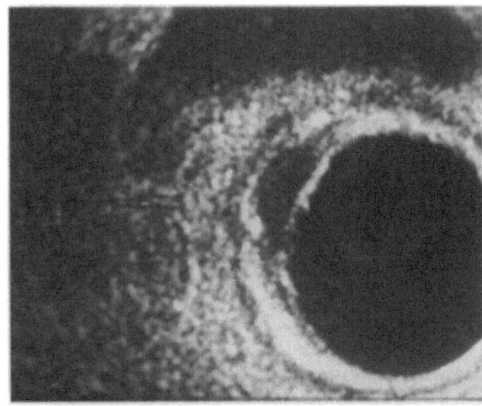

Fig. 13.16. Rectal sonoendoscopy: follow-up examination after resection of a rectal cancer revealed very superficial recurrence at the anastomotic site. (Courtesy of Dr. Valette, Lyons, France)

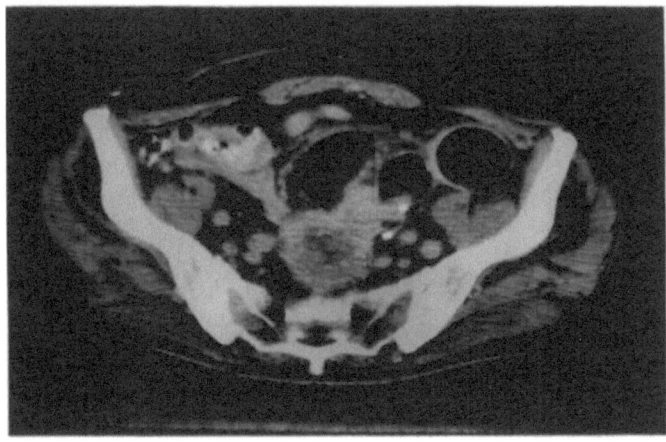

Fig. 13.17. Recurrent sigmoid cancer after resection

CEA monoclonal antibody reportedly allows differentiation of fibrosis and recurrences (Abdel-Nabi et al. 1987).

13.3.3 Abdominoperineal Resection

Estimates of recurrence after abdominoperineal resection vary between 1% and 30% (Phillips et al. 1984; Pihl et al. 1981; Wilking et al. 1985). Postoperative radiotherapy appears to markedly reduce the frequency of recurrences. The incidence of relapses after abdominoperineal resection varies according to the author. In addition to serial CEA assays, CT is used to search for local recurrence. The value of CT for diagnosis of recurrence after abdominoperineal resection is 87% for Thompson et al. (1986). Preliminary reports on MRI reveal that this technique may supplant CT in the not too distant future.

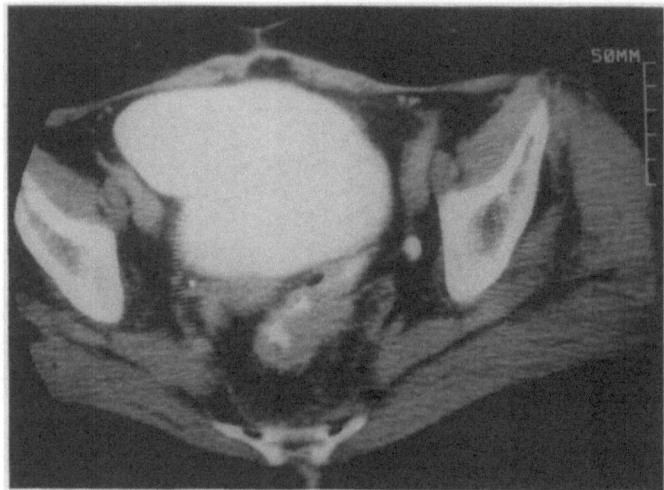

Fig. 13.18. Recurrent sigmoid cancer after resection

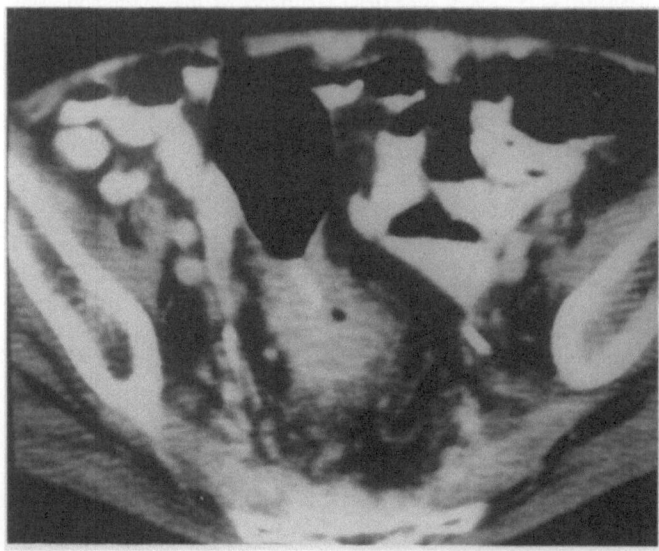

Fig. 13.19. Recurrent sigmoid cancer after resection

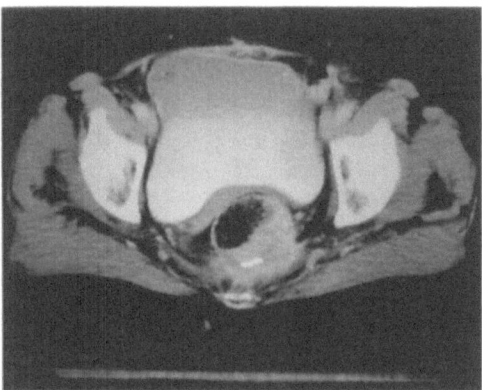

Fig. 13.20. Recurrence at the site of anastomosis of a rectal cancer

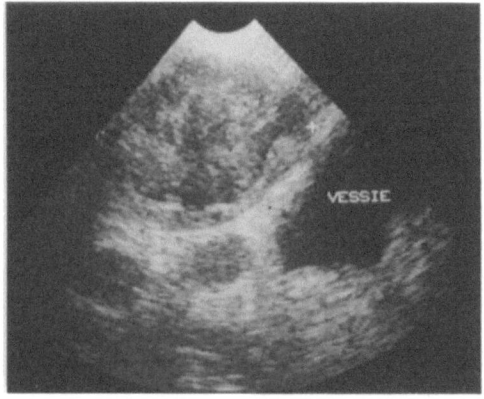

Fig. 13.22. Postresection sonogram of a large recurrence of a cecal cancer which manifested clinically as a mass in the right iliac fossa (73 mm between the *two crosses; VESSIE,* bladder)

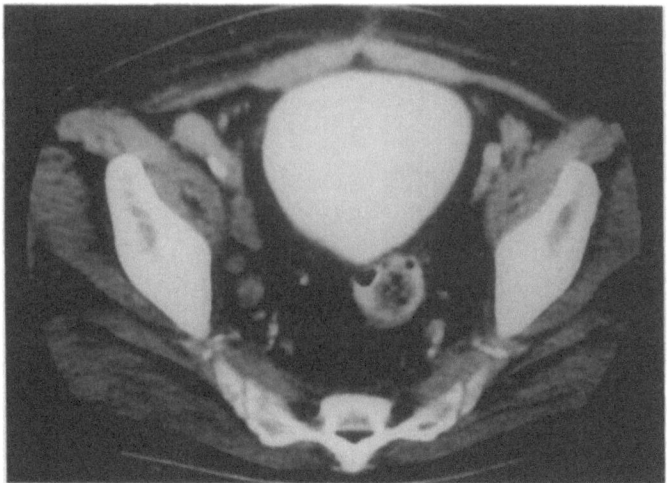

Fig. 13.21. Metastatic pelvic lymph nodes in a patient who underwent resection for colonic cancer. Endoscopic examination failed to detect any abnormality. The recurrence was solely nodal

The normal appearance after abdominoperineal resection varies greatly (Figs. 13.23–13.26). Absence of a postoperative mass is considered rare by Adalsteinsson et al. (1987) but was fairly common for Kelvin et al. (1983). Adalsteinsson et al. (1987) described several possible CT images: no postoperative mass or several fibrous bands, symmetrical presacral mass with distinct margins, large flat presacral mass, asymmetrical or excentric presacral mass, rounded presacral mass with a central low-density area.

When a presacral mass exists, it is visible on the first follow-up examination performed less than 4 months after surgery; this mass usually regresses in size, although to varying degrees, and appears better separated from the sacrum, with sharper borders. Reactive changes following surgery may regress to varying degrees, often creating a thin, transverse crescentic shape or sliver (Kelvin et al. 1983). A presacral mass appears more common after radiotherapy than in the absence of irradiation (Adal-

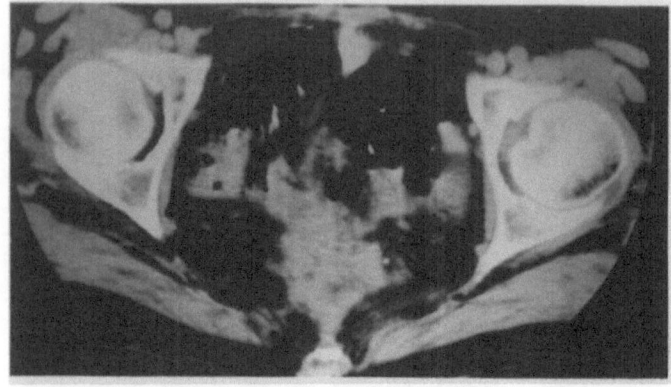

Fig. 13.23. Normal CT appearance after abdominoperineal resection

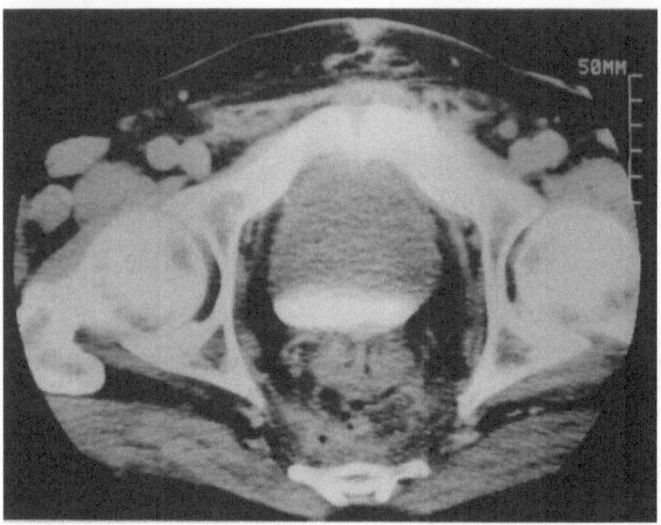

Fig. 13.24. Normal appearance after abdominoperineal resection. Follow-up examination 1 month after surgery

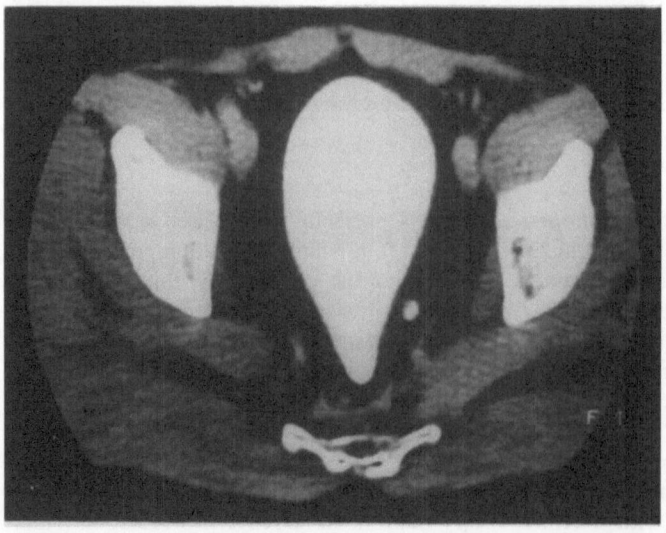

Fig. 13.25. Normal CT follow-up examination 2 years after abdominoperineal resection. Symmetrical, concave presacral fibrosis

steinsson et al. (1987); such masses are more frequent in men than in women because the uterus and vagina are mobile, and can fall back into a posterior position whereas the prostate cannot be displaced backwards (Fig. 13.27).

Owing to the variability of postoperative appearances, baseline CT studies less than 4

months after surgery are justified for reference purposes. Outside of invasion of the surrounding pelvic muscles or adjacent organs, there are no pathognomonic features of disease recurrence (Butch et al. 1985). A solid mass infiltrating the adjacent structures or a mass with liquid necrosis or gas may be observed. The latter type of image may correspond to recurrent disease, an abscess, or post-therapy necrosis. In our experience, even if there is no baseline CT examination, a biconcave appearance is not indicative of recurrence (Figs. 13.28–13.31).

CT-guided fine-needle (20-22 gauge) biopsy under local anesthesia with the patient in the prone position is an excellent means to confirm recurrence. Any presacral mass associated with an elevation in CEA, any mass of recent onset, and any pre-existent mass that increases in size are indications for biopsy (Thompson et al. 1986) (Figs. 13.32-13.34).

MRI may soon supplant CT. Results with systems operating at 0.26 T (Johnson et al. 1987) up to 1.5 T (Krestin et al. 1988) indicate that fibrosis can be distinguished from recurrent lesions. Using a 1.5-T machine, Krestin et al. (1988) obtained a signal intensity ratio of 1.4 ± 0.9 for fibrosis versus 3.6 ± 0.9 for T2-weighted images (1500/100). Study of the relaxation time T1 on a 0.26-T unit revealed a notable difference between fibrosis (average

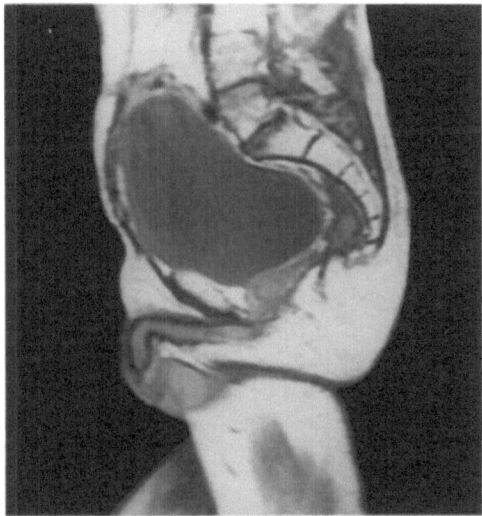

Fig. 13.26. Normal MRI image after abdominoperineal resection. (Courtesy of Dr. Masselot, Villejuif, France)

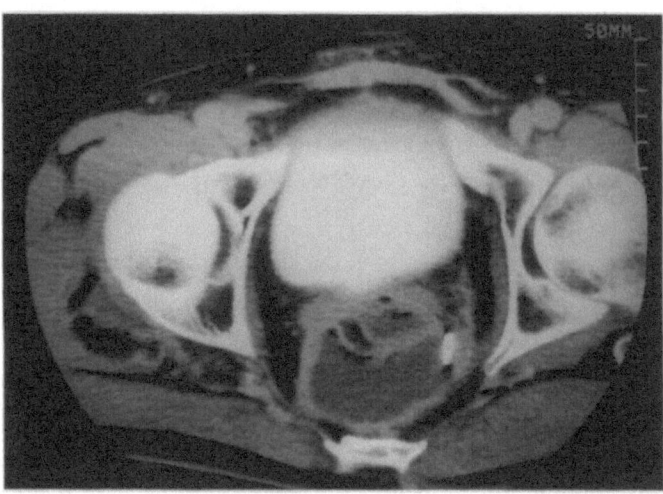

Fig. 13.27. Postoperative complication (abscess) after abdominoperineal resection

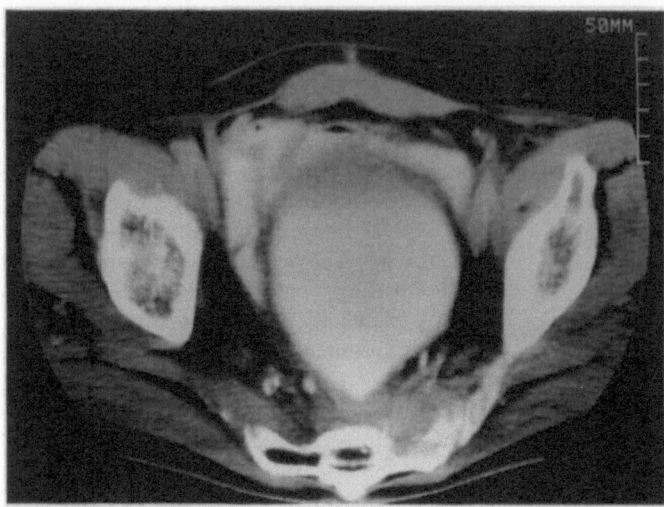

Fig. 13.28. Tumoral recurrence causing lysis of the left aspect of the sacrum after abdominoperineal resection of a rectal cancer

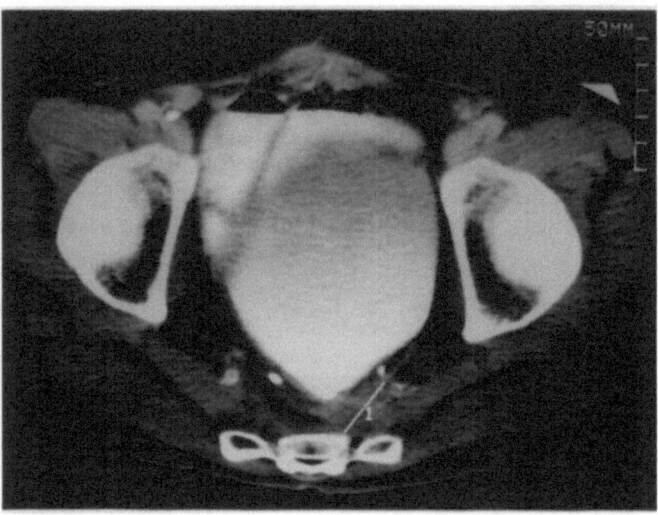

Fig. 13.29. Small (3 cm; *line 1*) recurrence discretely lateralized to the left, after abdominoperineal resection

458 ms) and cancer (average 817 ms) (Johnson et al. 1987). More recent studies (Ebner et al. 1988) have demonstrated that up until 6 months, fibrosis presents an increased signal intensity relative to muscle in T2-weighted images, making it difficult to distinguish early fibrosis from recurrent tumor. By 1 year, a significant decrease is noted in signal intensity on T2-weighted images: this makes it possible to differentiate fibrosis from recurrent tumor. For deLange et al. (1989), the signal intensity of malignant recurrent lesions was indistinguishable from benign lesions (benign inflammatory mass, edematous tissue). Moss (1989) is thus undoubtedly correct in stating that more comprehensive studies are required to

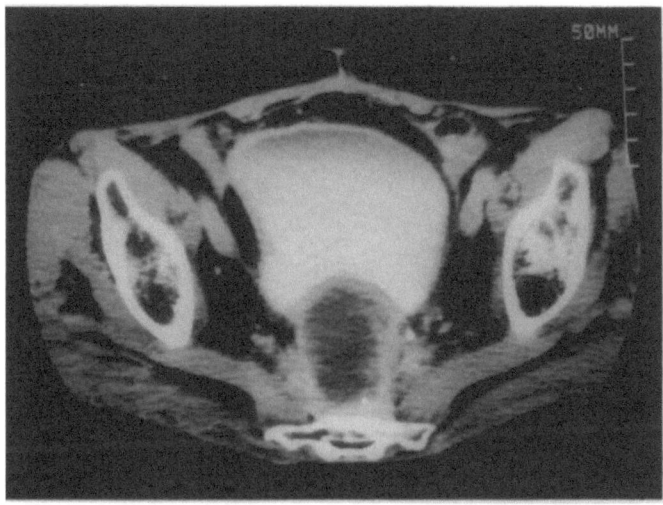

Fig. 13.30. Necrotic presacral recurrence associated with small peripheral adenopathies after abdominoperineal resection for rectal cancer. No bladder invasion

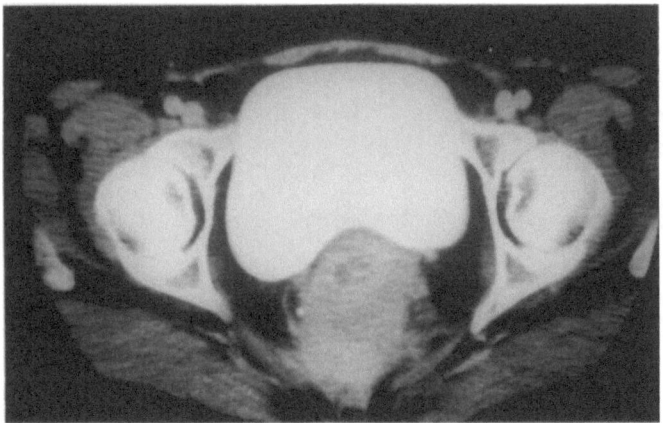

Fig. 13.31. Recurrence after abdominoperineal resection, with extension into the posterior aspect of the uterus

obtain valid answers about the role of the different imaging techniques for the diagnosis of recurrent colorectal cancer.

As mentioned earlier, discovery of a local recurrence necessitates a search for metastases, especially in the liver and lungs, before deciding on the therapeutic strategy.

13.3.4 Pelvic Exenteration

Posterior pelvic exenteration is sometimes curative for rectal cancer. The rectum, anus, uterus, vagina, and adnexa are removed but bladder is left in place and a colostomy is created. In certain cases, a myocutaneous neovagina is created. Pan and Shirkhoda (1987) described the features after pelvic exenteration as follows: nearly constant presacral thickening, less often a focal liquid collection or gas

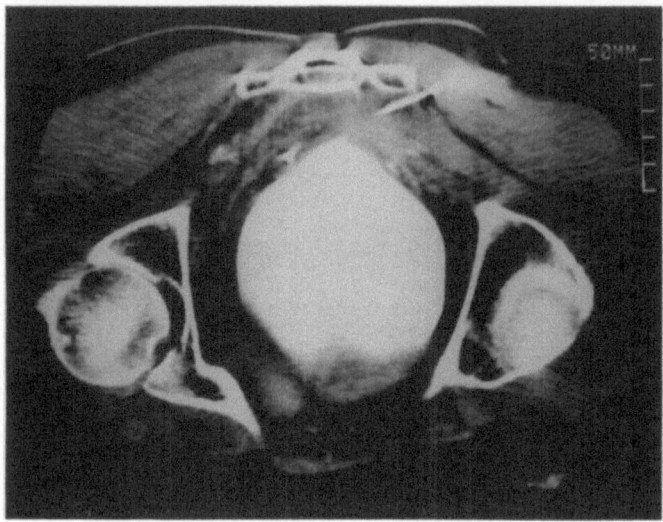

Fig. 13.32. Biopsy of a presacral recurrence after abdominoperineal resection. Biopsy was performed under local anesthesia after CT localization of the lesion with the patient in the prone position

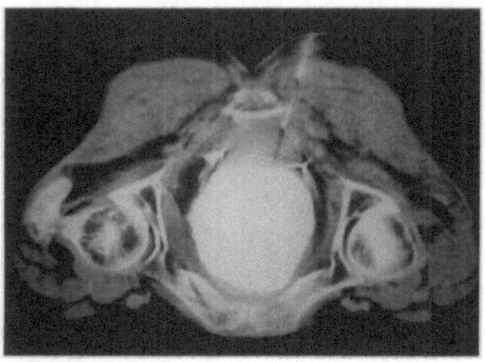

Fig. 13.33. CT-guided aspiration biopsy of a recurrent colorectal cancer after abdominoperineal resection

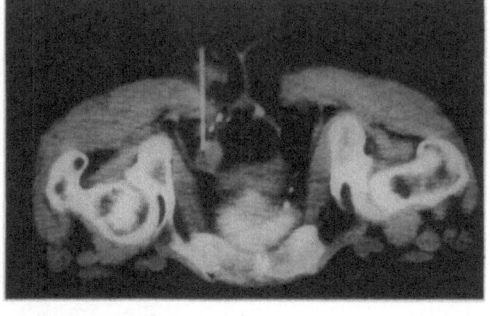

Fig. 13.34. Small nodular recurrence (15 mm long axis) after abdominoperineal resection for rectal cancer

collection at the apex of the neovagina. Lymphocysts have been reported. Diagnosis of recurrence is based on the same findings as for abdominoperineal resection, and merits CT-guided aspiration biopsy.

13.3.5 Hepatic Metastases

After resection of hepatic metastases, imaging studies are required to evaluate regeneration of the liver left in place and to search for any new hepatic metastases. For Hughes et al. (1986), 43% of recurrences after hepatic resection occur in the liver while 31% occur in the lungs. Sonographic examination may be hampered by overlying intestinal gas and satisfactory exploration of the remaining liver is not always possible. For this reason, CT often proves more effective. In addition, like scintigraphy, CT allows more precise determination of lesion size than ultrasound.

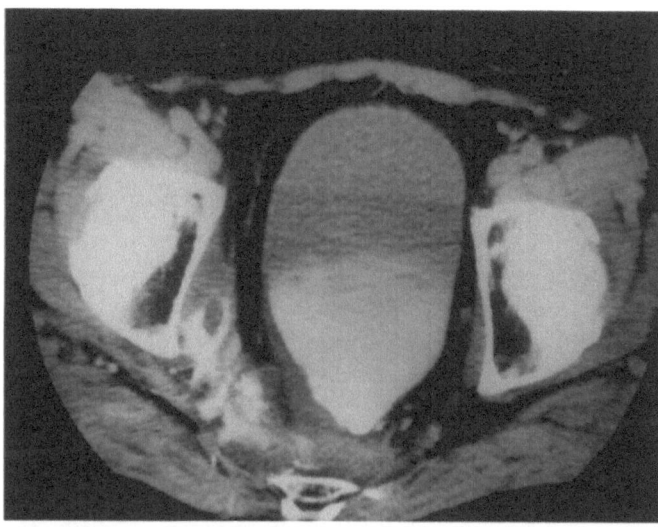

Fig. 13.35. Intra-arterial chemotherapy for recurrent rectal cancer treated by abdominoperineal resection. Accurate positioning of the catheter tip was verified by CT, by injecting contrast medium through the catheter to opacify the recurrence. Repeated intra-arterial chemotherapy cycles failed to significantly slow down the unfavorable disease course. Note the tumoral infiltration of the bladder wall

13.3.6 Non-curative Treatment

Surgery is often limited to a bypass procedure, and patients are offered complementary treatments based on external beam irradiation, coupled or not with chemotherapy (Fig. 13.35). As mentioned earlier, surveillance generally relies on CT studies; ultrasonography is the primary technique for liver follow-up.

CT improves lesion localization for planning external beam radiotherapy. With CT, as with other techniques (except MRI), the efficacy of treatment is difficult to evaluate other than by modifications in lesion size (Fig. 13.36). There are no changes in tissue density indicating whether a tissue is fibrous or tumoral, and contrast enhancement is not of sufficient value to solve this problem. Progression of a residual tumor commonly produces obstructive phenomena demonstrated by abdominal plain films; CT can then generally reveal an increase in tumor size. Hepatic metastases can be followed up by ultrasonography. We recommend use of the following criteria for surveillance purposes (Bruneton et al. 1988):

- Number of metastases (especially if fewer than 5).
- Diameter of the largest lesion, if it does not exceed 7 cm. When the lesion is larger, at least two other lesions, must also be measured.
- The large axis of the right liver, measured on the right mammary line, and the large axis of the left liver measured on the midline. These are the only two measurements useful for evaluating diffuse disease.

13.4 Screening for Colorectal Cancer

Although this book is devoted to the imaging of gastrointestinal tract tumors, the severity and prevalence of colorectal cancers have prompted us to conclude this chapter with a discussion of screening for colorectal adenocarcinomas. Not all authors agree on the best technique, and only fecal occult blood tests appear suitable for mass screening purposes (Winawer 1983).

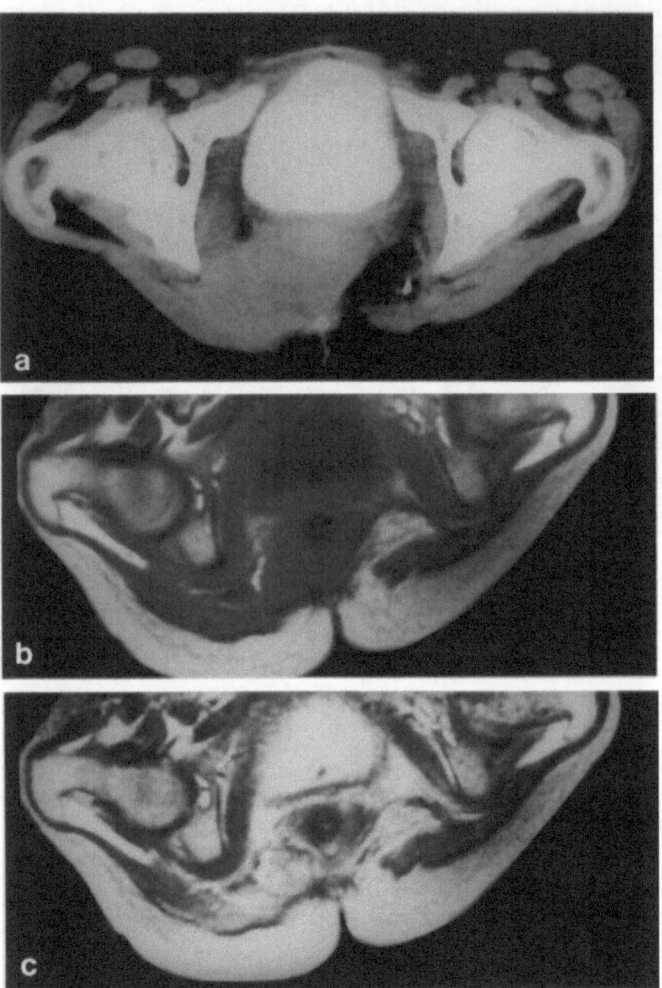

Fig. 13.36a-c. Comparison of CT and MRI for diagnosis of recurrent colorectal cancer. **a** CT easily revealed better the large recurrence, which extends towards the gluteus maximus muscles. T1 and T2 MRI sequences: the T2 sequence is shows the recurrence better and allows differentiation of the noninvaded structures **(b, c)**. (Courtesy of Prof. Masselot, Villejuif, France)

13.4.1 Occult Fecal Blood Tests

Fecal occult blood tests are positive in 2.8% of cases for Cummings et al. (1984). Hemorrhoids are the most common cause of rectal bleeding, but colorectal cancers account for 0.12%-0.35% of cases while adenomas represent 1.02%-1.05% of positive tests (Fugita et al. 1986; Hardcastle et al. 1986). The predictive value of fecal occult blood tests for diagnosis of a neoplasm is 18%-50.9% (Sontag et al. 1983; Winawer and Sherlock 1982); most of these cancers are early lesions (60%-80% are stage A or B) (Cummings et al. 1984; Sontag et al. 1983; Winawer and Sherlock 1982). A positive fecal occult blood test usually prompts colonoscopy in search of a neoplasm (Stroehlein et al. 1984) or DCBE; for Feczko and Halpert (1985), DCBE demonstrates 92% of polyps and all cancers.

13.4.2 High-risk Patients

In Europe and the United States, one-tenth of the population over 45 years of age can be estimated to have one or more colorectal polyps. It is uncertain whether screening really reduces the mortality of colorectal cancer, and this highlights the need for additional controlled studies (Kelvin and Maglinte 1987). Even so, several risk groups can be defined. Overall, three targets can be used for risk identification:

- Rectal bleeding, though usually of non-tumoral origin, warrants a complete colorectal workup.
- Fecal occult blood tests: use in mass screening programs, as mentioned earlier, permits treatment of patients at an early stage.
- Awareness of antecedents which can help evaluate each patient's risk.

While all individuals of both sexes over 40 years can be considered at risk for colorectal cancer, average-risk individuals must be distinguished from high-risk subjects. Average-risk individuals are those with long-standing ulcerative colitis (at least 7 years), patients with a history of adenoma or colorectal cancer, patients with gynecologic cancers (breast, uterus, ovary), and patients with a family history of cancer (standard risk multiplied by 5) (Faivre and Bader 1987). For these patients, three strategies can be used: DCBE, proctosigmoidoscopy (although limited to 60 cm) associated with DCBE, or colonoscopy from the outset (Maglinte et al. 1983). High-risk individuals are those subjects with a family history of colorectal polyposis (preventive colectomy is usually offered because of the inevitable development of colorectal cancer) and the familial colon cancer syndrome (50% risk of cancer). These individuals require very close follow-up based essentially on colonoscopy, which may be replaced periodically by less sensitive examinations such as DCBE.

13.5 References

Abdel-Nabi HH, Schwartz AN, Higano CS, Wechter DG, Unger MW (1987) Colorectal carcinoma: detection with indium-111 anticarcinoembryonic-antigen monoclonal antibody ZCE-025. Radiology 164: 617–621

Adalsteinsson B, Glimelius B, Graffman S, Hemmingsson A, Pahlman L (1985) Computed tomography in staging of rectal carcinoma. Acta Radiol [Diagn] (Stockh) 26: 45–55

Adalsteinsson B, Pahlman L, Hemmingsson A, Glimelius B, Graffman S (1987) Computed tomography in early diagnosis of local recurrence of rectal carcinoma. Acta Radiol 28: 41–47

Adloff M, Arnaud JP (1985) Amputation secondaire du rectum pour récidive néoplastique après résection rectale. Expérience personnelle portant sur 11 cas. Chirurgie 111: 156–162

Agarwal N, Ulahannan MJ, Mandile MA, Cayten CG, Pitchumoni CS (1986) Increased risk of colorectal cancer following breast cancer. Ann Surg 203: 307–310

Araujo Teixeira AM, Carvalho de Sousa J, Gomes A, Bernardo J, Amendoeira I, Simoes MS, Serrao D (1985) Le cancer du rectum. Etude clinique, anatomopathologique et facteurs de survie. Chirurgie 111: 180–188

Astler VB, Coller FA (1954) The prognostic significance of direct extension of carcinoma of the colon and rectum. Ann Surg 139: 846–851

Attiyeh FF, Stearns MW (1981) Second-look laparotomy based on CEA elevations in colorectal cancer. Cancer 47: 2119–2125

Baillet F (1987) Traitement radiothérapique complémentaire après examen des cancers du recutm. Ann Gastroenterol Hepatol (Paris) 23: 299–303

Baker SR, Alterman DD (1985) False-negative barium enema in patients with sigmoid cancer and coexistent diverticula. Gastrointest Radiol 10: 171–173

Bartram CI, Hall-Craggs MA (1987) Interventional colorectal endoscopic procedures: residual lesions on follow-up double-contrast barium enema study. Radiology 162: 835–838

Balthazar EJ, Megibow AJ, Hulnick D, Naidich DP (1988) Carcinoma of the colon: detection and preoperative staging by CT. AJR 150: 301–306

Beart RW, O'Connell MJ (1983) Postoperative follow-up of patients with carcinoma of the colon. Mayo Clin Proc 58: 361–363

Beckman EN, Gathright JB, Ray JE (1984) A potentially brighter prognosis for colon carcinoma in the third and fourth decades. Cancer 54: 1478–1481

Beggs I, Thomas BM (1983) Diagnosis of carcinoma of the colon by barium enema. Clin Radiol 34: 423–425

Behbehani A, Sakwa M, Ehrlichman R, Maguire P, Friedman S, Steele GD, Wilson RE (1985) Colorectal carcinoma in patients under age 40. Ann Surg 202: 610-614

Bell DA, Carr CP, Szyfelbein WM (1986) Fine needle aspiration cytology of focal liver lesions. Results obtained with examination of both cytologic and histologic preparation. Acta Cytol (Baltimore) 30: 397-402

Berardi RS, Chen HP, Lee SS (1986) Squamous cell carcinoma of the colon and rectum. Surg Gynecol Obstet 163: 493-496

Beynon J, McMortensen NJ, Foy DMA, Channer JL, Virjee J, Goddard P (1986) Endorectal sonography: laboratory and clinical experience in Bristol. Int J Colorect Dis 1: 212-215

Bismuth H, Castaing D (1987) Operative ultrasound of the liver and biliary ducts. Springer, Berlin Heidelberg New York London Paris Tokyo

Boulis-Wassif S (1983) Ten years experience with a ...ultimodality treatment of advanced stages of rectal cancer. Cancer 52: 2017-2024

Boulis-Wassif S, Gerard A, Loygue J, Camelot D, Buyse M, Duez N (1984) Final results of a randomized trial on the treatment of rectal cancer with preoperative radiotherapy alone or in combination with 5-Fluorouracil, followed by radical surgery. Trial of the European Organization on Research and Treatment of Cancer. Gastrointestinal Tract Cancer Cooperative Group. Cancer 53: 1811-1818

Boulos PB, Cowin AP, Karamanolis DG, Clark CG (1985) Diverticula, neoplasia, or both? Early detection of carcinoma in sigmoid diverticular disease. Ann Surg 202: 607-609

Brekkan A, Kjartansson P, Tulinius H, Sigvaldason H (1983) Diagnostic sensitivity of X-ray examination of the large bowel in colorectal cancer. Gastrointest Radiol 8: 363-365

Bronen RA, Glick SN, Teplick SK (1984) Diffuse lymphoid follicles of the colon associated with colonic carcinoma. AJR 142: 105-109

Bruneton JN, Drouillard J, Mathieu D (1988) Les métastases hépatiques. Aspects échographiques, tomodensitométriques et en IRM. Feuill Radiol 28: 39-47

Buhler H, Seefeld U, Deyhle P, Buchmann P, Metzger U, Ammann R (1984) Endoscopic follow-up after colorectal cancer surgery. Early detection of local recurrence? Cancer 54: 791-793

Butch RJ, Wittenberg J, Mueller PR, Simeone JF, Meyer JE, Ferrucci JT (1985) Presacral masses after abdominoperineal resection for colorectal carcinoma: the need for needle biopsy. AJR 144: 309-312

Butch RJ, Stark DD, Wittenberg J, Tepper JE, Saini S, Simeone JF, Mueller PR, Ferrucci JT (1986) Staging rectal cancer by MR and CT. AJR 146: 1155-1160

Butler J, Attiyeh FF, Daly JM (1986) Hepatic resection for metastases of the colon and rectum. Surg Obstet Gynecol 162: 109-113

Chawla SK, Marcelo JY, Lopresti P, Chawla K (1986) Synchronous cancers of the colon and rectum: report of eight cases. Am J Gastroenterol 81: 1065-1067

Chen YM, Ott DJ, Wolfman NT, Gelfand DW, Karsteadt N, Bechtold RE (1987) Recurrent colorectal carcinoma: evaluation with barium enema examination and CT. Radiology 163: 307-310

Clark J, Carter B, Smith TJ (1984) The use of computerized tomography scan in the staging and follow-up study of carcinoma of the rectum. Surg Gynecol Obstet 159: 335-342

Coppa GF, Eng K, Ranson JHC, Gouge TH, Localio A (1985) Hepatic resection for metastatic colon and rectal cancer. An evaluation of preoperative and postoperative factors. Ann Surg 202: 203-208

Cummings KM, Michalek A, Mettlin C, Mittelman A (1984) Screening for colorectal cancer using the Hemoccult II stool Guaiac slide test. Cancer 53: 2201-2205

Daniell HW (1986) More advanced colonic cancer among smokers. Cancer 58: 784-787

Deixonne B, Lopez FM (1987) Operative ultrasonography during hepatobiliary and pancreatic surgery. Springer, Berlin Heidelberg New York London Paris Tokyo

De Lange EE, Fechner RE, Wanebo HJ (1989) Suspected recurrent rectosigmoid carcinoma after abdominoperineal resection: MR imaging and histopathologic findings. Radiology 170: 323-328

De Mascarel A, Coindre JM, De Mascarel I, Trojani M, Maree D, Hoerni B (1981) The prognostic significance of specific histologic features of carcinoma of the colon and rectum. Surg Gynecol Obstet 153: 511-514

Detry R, Van Heuverzwyn R, Mahieu P, Kestens PJ (1984) Diagnostic des récidives tumorales après traitement curatif des cancers recto-sigmoïdiens. Acta Gastroenterol Belg 67: 370-375

Deveney KE, Way LW (1984) Follow-up of patients with colorectal cancer. Am J Surg 148: 717-722

Di Candio G, Mosca F, Campatelli A, Cei A, Ferrari M, Basolo F (1987) Endosonographic staging of rectal carcinoma. Gastrointest Radiol 12: 289-295

Doutre LP, Perissat J, Dost C, Albalat F (1982) Les récidives pelvi-périnéales après amputation du rectum pour cancer. A propos de 23 observations. J Chir (Paris) 119: 91-96

Dowling K, Watne A, Foshag L, Vargish T (1985) Management of nonfamilial adenomatous polyps and colon cancers. Surgery 98: 684-688

Dukes CE (1929) The spread of cancer of the rectum. Br J Surg 17: 643-648

Dukes CE (1932) The classification of cancer of the rectum. J Pathol 35: 323-332

Dukes CE, Bussey HJ (1958) The spread of rectal cancer and its effect on prognosis. Br J Cancer 12: 309-320

Ebner F, Kressel HY, Mintz MC, Carlson JA, Cohen EK, Schiebler M, Gefter W, Axel L (1988)

Tumor recurrence versus fibrosis in the female pelvis: differentiation with MR imaging at 1.5T. Radiology 166: 333-340

Eisenberg B, Decosse JJ, Harford F, Michalek J (1982) Carcinoma of the colon and rectum: the natural history reviewed in 1704 patients. Cancer 49: 1131-1134

Faivre J, Bader JP (1987) Le dépistage des cancers colorectaux: une cause nationale. Ann Gastroenterol Hepatol (Paris) 23: 351-352

Faivre J, Gouget N, Martin F, Michiels R, Cabanne F, Klepping C (1979) Incidence des cancers colorectaux dans une population bien définie de 450000 habitants. Gastroenterol Clin Biol 3: 815-820

Feczko PJ, Halpert RD (1985) Reassessing the role of radiology in Hemoccult screening. AJR 146: 697-701

Fork FT, Lindstrom C, Ekelund G (1983) Double contrast examination in carcinoma of the colon and rectum. A prospective clinical series. Acta Radiol [Diagn] (Berl) 2: 177-188

Fortner JG, Silva JS, Golbey RB, Cox EB, Maclean BJ (1984a) Multivariate analysis of a personal series of 247 consecutive patients with liver metastases from colorectal cancer. I. Treatment by hepatic resection. Ann Surg 199: 306-316

Fortner JG, Silva JS, Cox EB, Golbey RB, Gallowitz H, Maclean BJ (1984b) Multivariate analysis of a personal series of 247 patients with liver metastases from colorectal cancer. II. Treatment by intrahepatic chemotherapy. Ann Surg 199: 317-324

Frager DH, Frager JD, Wolf EL, Beneventano TC (1987) Problems in the colonoscopic localization of tumors: continued value of the barium enema. Gastrointest Radiol 12: 343-346

Freeny PC, Marks WM, Ryan JA, Bolen JW (1986) Colorectal carcinoma evaluation with CT: preoperative staging and detection of postoperative recurrence. Radiology 158: 347-353

Freeny PC, Marks WM, Ryan JA, Bolen JW (1987) Computed tomography of colorectal carcinoma: preoperative staging and detection of recurrence. Sem Ultrasound, CT, and MR 8: 432-445

Fujita M, Nakano Y, Ohta J, Taguchi T (1986) Mass screening for colorectal cancer by testing fecal occult blood. Cancer 57: 2241-2245

Gabriel WB, Dukes C, Bussey HJ (1935) Lymphatic spread in cancer of the rectum. Br J Surg 23: 395-413

Gastrointestinal Tumor Study Group (1984) Adjuvant therapy of colon cancer. Results of a prospectively randomized trial. N Engl J Med 310: 737-743

Gingold BS, Mitty WF, Tadros M (1983) Importance of patient selection in local treatment of carcinoma of the rectum. Am J Surg 145: 293-296

Glazer GM, Aisen AM, Francis IR, Gross BH, Gives JW, Ensminger WD (1986) Evaluation of focal hepatic masses: a comparative study of MRI and CT Gastrointest Radiol 11: 263-268

Gothlin JH, Lerner RM, Gadeholt G, Sischy B, Hinson J (1987) CT staging of early rectal carcinoma. Gastrointest Radiol 12: 253-256

Grabbe E, Winkler R (1985) Local recurrence after sphincter-saving resection for rectal and rectosigmoid carcinoma. Value of various diagnostic methods. Radiology 155: 305-310

Greenstein AJ, Heimann TM, Sachar DB, Slater G, Aufses AH (1986) A comparison of multiple synchronous colorectal cancer in ulcerative colitis, familial polyposis coli, and de novo cancer. Ann Surg 203: 123-128

Guernelli N, Briccoli A (1985) La récidive pelvi-périnéale après amputation du rectum pour cancer. Ann Gastroenterol Hepatol (Paris) 21: 343-346

Halvorsen TB (1986) Site distribution of colorectal adenocarcinomas. A retrospective study of 853 tumours. Scand J Gastroenterol 21: 973-978

Hamm B, Wolf KJ, Felix R (1987) Conventional and rapid MR imaging of the liver with Gd-DTPA. Radiology 164: 313-320

Hardcastle JD, Armitage NC, Chamberlain J, Amar SS, James PD, Balfour TW (1986) Fecal occult blood screening for colorectal cancer in the general population. Results of a controlled trial. Cancer 58: 397-403

Hermanek P, Sobin LH (1987) TNM. Classification of malignant tumours. Springer, Berlin Heidelberg New York London Paris Tokyo

Hildebrandt U, Feifel G (1985) Preoperative staging of rectal cancer by intrarectal ultrasound. Dis Colon Rectum 28: 42-46

Hughes KS et al (1986) Resection of the liver for colorectal carcinoma metastases: a multi-institutional study of patterns of recurrence. Surgery 100: 278-284

Hulnick DH, Megibow AJ, Balthazar EJ, Gordon RB, Surapenini R, Bosniak MA (1987) Perforated colorectal neoplasms: correlation of clinical, contrast enema, and CT examinations. Radiology 164: 611-615

Hunter GJ, Willson SA, Chapman M (1983) Necrotic carcinoma of the colon. Clin Radiol 34: 297-299

Johnson CD, Carlson HC, Taylor WF, Weiland LP (1983) Barium enemas of carcinoma of the colon: sensitivity of double- and single-contrast studies. AJR 140: 1143-1149

Johnson H, Carstens R (1986) Anatomical distribution of colonic carcinomas. Interracial differences in a community hospital population. Cancer 58: 997-1000

Johnson LP, Rivkin SE (1985) The implanted pump in metastatic colorectal cancer of the liver. Risk versus benefit. Am J Surg 149: 595-598

Johnson RJ, Jenkins JPR, Ischerwood I, James RD, Schofield PF (1987) Quantitative magnetic resonance imaging in rectal carcinoma. Br J Radiol 60: 761-764

Johnson WR, McDermott FT, Hugues ESR, Pihl EA, Milne BJ, Price AB (1983) Carcinoma of the colon and rectum in inflammatory disease of the disease. Surg Gynecol Obstet 156: 193–197

Kaibara N, Koga S, Jinnai D (1984) Synchronous and metachronous malignancies of the colon and rectum in Japan with special reference to a co-existing early cancer. Cancer 54: 1870–1874

Kelvin FM, Gardiner R (1987) Clinical imaging of the colon and rectum. Raven, New York

Kelvin FM, Gardiner R, Vas W, Stevenson GW (1981) Colorectal carcinoma missed on double contrast barium enema study: a problem in perception. AJR 137: 307–313

Kelvin FM, Maglinte DDT (1987) Colorectal carcinoma: a radiologic and clinical review. Radiology 164: 1–8

Kelvin FM, Korobkin M, Heaston DK, Grant JP, Akwari O (1983) The pelvis after surgery for rectal carcinoma: serial CT observations with emphasis on nonneoplastic features. AJR 141: 959–964

Kerber GW, Frank PH (1984) Carcinoma of the small intestine and colon as a complication of Crohn disease: radiologic manifestations. Radiology 150: 639–645

Kewenter J, Jensen J, Boijsen M, Lycke G, Tylen U (1987) Perception errors with double-contrast enema after a positive Guaiac test. Gastrointest Radiol 12: 79–82

Kirklin JW, Dockerty MB, Waugh JM (1949) The role of the peritoneal reflection in the prognosis of carcinoma of the rectum and sigmoid colon. Surg Gynecol Obstet 88: 326–331

Konishi F, Muto T, Takahashi H, Itoh K, Kanazawa K, Morioka Y (1985) Transrectal ultrasonography for the assessment of invasion of rectal carcinoma. Dis Colon Rectum 28: 889–894

Kramann B, Hildebrandt U (1986) Computed tomography versus endosonography in the staging of rectal carcinoma: a comparative study. Int J Colorect Dis 1: 216–218

Krestin GP, Steinbrich W, Friedmann G (1988) Recurrent rectal cancer: diagnosis with MR imaging versus CT. Radiology 168: 307–311

Labrosse H, Frieh JP, Berard P, Guillemin G (1983) Complications révélatrices du cancer du rectum. Etude rétrospective à propos d'une série de 557 néoplasmes rectaux opérés. Ann Chir 37: 405–410

Langevin JM, Nivatvongs S (1984) The true incidence of synchronous cancer of the large bowel. A prospective study. Am J Surg 147: 330–333

Lavin PT, Day J, Holyoke ED, Mittelman A, Chu TM (1981) A statistical evaluation of baseline and follow-up carcinoembryonic antigen in patients with resectable colorectal carcinoma. Cancer 47: 823–826

Lee TK, Barringer M, Myers RT, Sterchi JM (1982) Multiple primary carcinomas of the colon and associated extracolonic primary malignant tumors. Ann Surg 195: 501–507

Lefall LSD (1981) Colorectal cancer. Prevention and detection. Cancer 47: 1170–1172

Lev R, Grover R (1981) Precursors of human colon carcinoma: a serial section study of colectomy specimens. Cancer 47: 2007–2015

Le Treut YP, Bozon-Verduraz E, Sabiani P, Maillet B, Bricot R (1986) L'exérèse élargie des cancers fixés du côlon. Etude rétrospective de 44 cas. J Chir (Paris) 123: 402–406

Linos DA, O'Fallon WM, Thilstle JL, Kurland LT (1982) Cholelithiasis and carcinoma of the colon. Cancer 50: 1015–1019

Lockhart-Mummery JP (1927–1928) Two hundred cases of cancer of the rectum treated by perineal excision. Br J Surg 14: 110–124

Maglinte DDT, Pollack HM (1983) Retroperitoneal abscess: a presentation of colon carcinoma. Gastrointest Radiol 8: 177–181

Maglinte DDT, Keller KJ, Miller RE, Chernish SM (1983) Colon and rectal carcinoma: spatial distribution and detection. Radiology 147: 669–672

Malcolm AW, Perencevich HP, Olson RM, Hanley JA, Chaffey JT, Wilson RE (1981) Analysis of recurrence patterns following curative resection for carcinoma of the colon and rectum. Surg Gynecol Obstet 152: 131–136

Margulis AR, Thoeni RF (1988) The present status of the radiologic examination of the colon. Radiology 167: 1–5

Martin EW, Cooperman M, Carey LC, Minton JP (1980) Sixty second-look procedures indicated primarily by rise in serial carcinoembryonic antigen. J Surg Res 28: 389–394

Martin EW, James KK, Hurtubise PE, Catalano P, Minton JP (1977) The use of CEA as an early indicator for gastrointestinal tumor recurrence and second-look procedures. Cancer 39: 440–446

Matsui O, Takashima T, Kadoya M, Suzuki M, Hirose J, Kameyama T, Choto S, Konishi H, Ida M, Yamaguchi A, Izumi R (1987) Liver metastases from colorectal cancers: detection with CT during arterial portography. Radiology 165: 65–69

McDermott FT, Hughes ESR, Pihl E, Johnson WR, Price AB (1985) Local recurrence after potentially curative resection for rectal cancer in a series of 1008 patients. Br J Surg 72: 34–37

Meyer JE, Dosoretz DE, Gunderson LL, Stark P, Kopans DB (1983) CT evaluation of locally advanced carcinoma of the distal colon and rectum. J Comput Assist Tomogr 7: 265–267

Midiri G, Amanti C, Benedetti M, Campisi C, Santeusanio G, Castagna G, Peronace L, Du Tondo U, Di Paola M, Pascal RR (1985) CEA tissue staining in colorectal cancer patients. A way to improve the usefulness of serial serum CEA evaluation. Cancer 55: 2624–2629

Miller TL, Skucas J, Gudex D, Listinsky C (1987) Bowel cancer characteristics in patients with regional enteritis. Gastrointest Radiol 12: 45–52

Mir-Madjlessi SH, Farmer RG, Easley KA, Beck GJ (1986) Colorectal and extracolonic malignancy in ulcerative colitis. Cancer 58: 1569–1574

Moertel CG, O'Fallon JR, Go VLW, O'Connell MJ, Thynne GS (1986) The preoperative carcino-embryonic antigen test in the diagnosis, staging, and prognosis of colorectal cancer. Cancer 58: 603-610

Mohiuddin M, Derdel J, Marks G, Kramer S (1985) Results of adjuvant radiation therapy in cancer of the rectum. Cancer 55: 350-353

Morson BC (1966) Factors influencing the prognosis of early cancers of the rectum. Proc R Soc Med 59: 607-608

Morson BC (1984) The evolution of colorectal carcinoma. Clin Radiol 35: 425-431

Mosnier H (1985) Surveillance à long terme des malades opérés de cancers colorectaux. Ann Gastroenterol Hepatol (Paris) 21: 351-353

Mosnier H, Guivarc'h M (1987) Intérêt d'une surveillance locorégionale après intervention curative pour cancer du rectum ou du sigmoïde. Ann Gastroenterol Hepatol (Paris) 23: 15-18

Mosnier H, Outters F, Roullett Audy JC, Guivarc'h M (1987) Technique et pièges de l'échographie endo-rectale dans les tumeurs du rectum. Ann Gastroenterol Hepatol (Paris) 23: 321-327

Moss AA (1989) Imaging of colorectal carcinoma. Radiology 170: 308-310

Nakamura GJ, Schneiderman LJ, Klauber MR (1984) Colorectal cancer and bowel habits. Cancer 54: 1475-1477

Newland RC, Chapuis PH, Pheils MT, MacPherson JG (1981) The relationship of survival to staging and grading of colorectal carcinoma: a prospective study of 503 cases. Cancer 47: 1424-1429

Niederhuber JE, Ensminger W, Gyves J, Thrall J, Walker S, Cozzi E (1984) Regional chemotherapy of colorectal cancer metastatic to the liver. Cancer 53: 1336-1343

Odone V, Chang L, Caces J, George SL, Pratt CB (1982) The natural history of colorectal carcinoma in adolescents. Cancer 49: 1716-1720

Olson RM, Perencevich NP, Malcolm AW, Chaffey JT, Wilson RE (1980) Patterns of recurrence following curative resection of adenocarcinoma of the colon and rectum. Cancer 45: 2969-2974

Oren JW, Folse R, Kraudel KL, Lewis DB (1986) The preoperative liver scan and surgical decision-making in patients with colorectal cancer. Am J Surg 151: 452-456

Pahlman L, Adalsteinsson B, Glimelius B, Lindgren PG, Scheibenpflug D (1984) Ultrasound in pre-operative staging of rectal tumours. Acta Radiol [Diagn] (Stockh) 25: 489-494

Pan G, Shirkhoda A (1987) Pelvic exenteration: role of CT in follow-up. Radiology 164: 665-670

Papillon J, Mayer M, Chassard JL, Bobin JY (1983) Cancer du rectum: perspectives nouvelles de la radiothérapie dans le traitement conservateur. Bull Cancer (Paris) 70: 323-328

Parturier-Albot M, Albot G (1985): "De Novo" carcinoma or early rectal carcinoma. Incidence and diagnosis. Ann Gastroenterol Hepatol (Paris) 21: 231-237

Patt YZ, Peters RE, Chuang VP, Wallace S, Claghorn L, Mavligit G (1985) Palliation of pelvic recurrence of colorectal cancer with intra-arterial 5-Fluorouracil and Mitomycin. Cancer 56: 2175-2180

Petrelli NJ, Barcewicz PA, Evans JT, Ledesma EJ, Lawrence DD, Mittelman A (1984) Hepatic artery ligation for liver metastasis in colorectal carcinoma. Cancer 53: 1347-1353

Phillips RKS, Hittinger R, Blesovsky L, Fry JS, Fielding L (1984) Local recurrence following "curative" surgery for large bowel cancer. II. The rectum and rectosigmoid. Br J Surg 71: 17-20

Pihl E, Hughes ESR, Mc Dermott FT, Price AB (1981) Recurrence of carcinoma of the colon and rectum on the anastomotic suture line. Surg Gynecol Obstet 153: 495-496

Polk HC, Spratt JS (1971) Recurrent colorectal carcinoma: detection, treatment and other considerations. Surgery 69: 9-23

Price J, Metreweli C (1988) Ultrasonographic diagnosis of clinically non-palpable primary colonic neoplasms. Br J Radiol 61: 190-195

Putzki H, Student A, Jablonski M, Heymann H (1987) Comparison of the tumor markers CEA, TPA, and CA 19-9 in colorectal carcinoma. Cancer 59: 223-226

Rao BN, Pratt CB, Fleming ID, Dilawari RA, Green AA, Austin BA (1985) Colon carcinoma in children and adolescents. Cancer 55: 1322-1326

Ramming KP, Juillard G, Parker R, Eilber F (1986) Management of carcinoma of the rectum and anus without abdominoperineal resection. Am J Surg 152: 16-20

Reed WP, Haney PJ, Elias EG, Whitley NO, Forsthoff C, Brown S (1986) Ethiodized oil emulsion enhanced computerized tomography in the preoperative assessment of metastases to the liver from the colon and rectum. Surg Gynecol Obstet 162: 131-136

Reilly JC, Rusin LC, Theuerkauf FJ (1982) Colonoscopy: its role in cancer of the colon and rectum. Dis Colon Rectum 25: 532-538

Reinig JW, Dwyer AJ, Miller DL, White M, Frank JA, Sugarbaker PH, Chang AE, Domman JL (1987) Liver metastasis detection: comparative sensitivities of MR imaging and CT scanning. Radiology 162: 43-47

Rich T, Gunderson LL, Lew R, Galdibini JJ, Cohen AM, Donaldson G (1983) Patterns of recurrence of rectal cancer after potentially curative surgery. Cancer 52: 1317-1329

Rich TA, Weiss DR, Mies C, Fitzgerald TJ, Chaffey JT (1985) Sphincter preservation in patients with low rectal cancer treated with radiation therapy with or without local excision or fulguration. Radiology 56: 527-531

Rifkin MD (1987) Endorectal ultrasound of the rectal wall. Semin Ultrasound CT MR 8: 424-431

Rifkin MD, Marks GJ (1985) Transrectal US as an adjunct in the diagnosis of rectal and extrarectal tumors. Radiology 157: 499–502

Rifkin MD, Wechsler RJ (1986) A comparison of computed tomography and endorectal ultrasound in staging rectal cancer. Int J Colorect Dis 1: 219–223

Rifkin MD, McGlynn ET, Marks G (1986) Endorectal sonographic prospective staging of rectal cancer. Scand J Gastroenterol 21 (Suppl 123): 99–103

Rifkin MD, Ehrlich SM, Marcks G (1989) Staging of rectal carcinoma: prospective comparison of endorectal US and CT. Radiology 170: 319–322

Rose DP, Boyar AP, Wynder EL (1986) International comparisons of mortality rates for cancer of the breast, ovary, prostate, and colon, and per capita food consumption. Cancer 58: 2363–2371

R....n P, Fireman Z, Figer A, Ron E (1986) Colorectal tumor screening in women with a past history of breast, uterine, or ovarian malignancies. Cancer 57: 1235–1239

Russell AH, Tong D, Dawson LE, Wisbeck W (1984) Adenocarcinoma of the proximal colon. Sites of initial dissemination and patterns of recurrence following surgery alone. Cancer 53: 360–367

Russell AH, Pelton J, Reheis CE, Wisbeck WM, Tong DY, Dawson LE (1985) Adenocarcinoma of the colon: an autopsy study with implications for new therapeutic strategies. Cancer 56: 1446–1451

Safford KL, Spebar MJ, Rosenthal D (1981) Review of colorectal cancer in patients under age 40 years. Am J Surg 142: 767–769

Saitoh N, Okui K, Sarashima H, Suzuki M, Arai T, Nunomura M (1986) Evaluation of echographic diagnosis of rectal cancer using intrarectal ultrasonic examination. Dis Colon Rectum 29: 234–242

Salmon RJ, Guillet JL, Vige P, Durand JC, Fenton J, Mathieu G, Rousseau J, Pilleron JP (1983) Cancers opérables du rectum: radiothérapie pré-opératoire. Etude rétrospective de 192 cas traités à l'Institut Curie. Bull Cancer (Paris) 70: 429–433

Sandler RS, Freund DA, Herbst CA, Sandler DP (1984) Cost effectiveness of postoperative carcinoembryonic antigen monitoring in colorectal cancer. Cancer 53: 193–198

Shamsuddin AM, Kato Y, Kunishima N, Sugano H, Trump BF (1985) Carcinoma in situ in nonpolypoid mucosa of the large intestine. Report of a case with significance in strategies for early detection. Cancer 56: 2849–2854

Sibilly A, Jung F, Gelot JM, Neidhardt J, Anselm Y (1980) Linites plastiques colorectales primitives. Revue de la littérature. A propos de trois cas personnels. Ann Chir 34: 409–414

Silverstein F, Kimmey M, Martin R, Haggitt R, Mack L, Moss A, Franklin D (1986) Ultrasound and the intestinal wall: experimental methods. Scand J Gastroenterol 21 (Suppl 123): 34–40

Simpson WC, Mayo CW (1939) The mural penetration of the carcinoma cell in the colon: anatomic and clinical study. Surg Gynecol Obstet 68: 872–877

Sischy B (1982) The place of radiotherapy in the management of rectal adenocarcinoma. Cancer 50: 2631–2637

Siskind BN, Burrell MI (1986) Intraluminal meniscoid ulcer of the colon: an unusual sign of malignancy. Gastrointest Radiol 11: 251–253

Skucas J, Spataro RF, Cannucciari DP (1982) The radiographic features of small colon cancers. Radiology 143: 335–340

Slater G, Greenstein AJ, Gelernt I, Kreel I, Bauer J, Aufses AH (1985) Distribution of colorectal cancer in patients with and without ulcerative colitis. Am J Surg 149: 780–782

Slater GI, Haber RH, Aufses AH Jr (1986) Changing distribution of carcinoma of the colon and rectum. Surg Gynecol Obstet 158: 216–218

Solomon A, Bar-Ziv J, Stern D (1988) Staging cecal and ascending colon carcinoma with computed tomography. Gastrointest Radiol 13: 152–154

Sontag SJ, Durczak C, Aranha GV, Chejfec G, Frederick W, Greenlee HB (1983) Fecal occult blood screening for colorectal cancer in a Veterans Administration hospital. Am J Surg 145: 89–94

Stark DD, Wittenberg J, Butch RJ, Ferrucci JT (1987) Hepatic metastases: randomized, controlled comparison of detection with MR imaging and CT. Radiology 165: 399–406

Steinberg SM, Barkin JS, Kaplan RS, Stablein DM (1986a) Prognostic indicators of colon tumors. The Gastrointestinal Tumor Study Group experience. Cancer 57: 1866–1870

Steinberg SM, Barwick KW, Stablein DM (1986b) Importance of tumor pathology and morphology in patients with surgically resected colon cancer. Findings from the Gastrointestinal Tumor Study Group. Cancer 58: 1340–1345

Stevenson GW, Goodacre R, Jackson R, Ragbeer M, Rowland R (1984) Dysplasia to carcinoma transformation in ulcerative colitis. AJR 143: 108–110

Stroehlein JR, Goulston K, Hunt RH (1984) Diagnostic approach to evaluating the cause of a positive fecal occult blood test. Cancer 34: 148–157

Sugarbaker PH, Gianola FJ, Dwyer A, Neuman NR (1987) A simplified plan for follow-up of patients with colon and rectal cancer supported by prospective studies of laboratory and radiologic test results. Surgery 102: 79–87

Tartter PI, Steinberg BM (1986) The role of preoperative intravenous pyelogram in operations performed for carcinoma of the colon and rectum. Surg Gynecol Obstet 163: 65–69

Tepper JE (1983) Radiation therapy of colorectal cancer. Cancer 51: 2528–2534

Thoeni RF, Moss AA, Schnyder P, Margulis AR (1981) Detection and staging of primary rectal and rectosigmoid cancer by computed tomography. Radiology 141: 135–138

Thompson WM, Halvorsen RA (1987) Computed tomographic staging of gastrointestinal malignancies. Part II. The small bowel, colon, and rectum. Invest Radiol 22: 96–105

Thompson WM, Halvorsen RA, Foster WL, Roberts L, Gibbons R (1986) Preoperative and postoperative CT staging of rectosigmoid carcinoma. AJR 146: 703–710

Thorson AG, Christensen MA, Davis SJ (1986) The role of colonoscopy in the assessment of patients with colorectal cancer. Dis Colon Rectum 29: 306–311

Tio TL, Tytgat GNJ (1986) Comparison of blind transrectal ultrasonography in assessing rectal and perirectal diseases. Am J Gastroenterol 21 (Suppl 123): 104–111

Toman R, Gregor O, Pastorova J, Drnkova V (1982) Clinical and epidemiological study of colorectal cancer. Am Gastroenterol Hepatol 18: 321–324

Triboulet JP, Piette F, Bergoend H, Lagache G (1981) Dermatomyosite et cancer colique. Revue de la littérature à propos d'un cas. Ann Chir 36: 287–292

Unger SW, Wanebo HJ (1983) Colonoscopy: an essential monitoring technique after resection of colorectal cancer. Am J Surg 145: 71–76

Van Waes PFGM, Koehler PR, Feldberg MAM (1983) Management of rectal carcinoma: impact of computed tomography. AJR 140: 1137–1142

Vobecky J, Leduc C, Devroede G (1984) Sex differences in the changing anatomic distribution of colorectal carcinoma. Cancer 54: 3065–3069

Wagner JS, Adson MA, Van Heerden JA, Adson MH, Ilstrup DM (1984) The natural history of hepatic metastases from colorectal cancer. A comparison with resective treatment. Ann Surg 199: 502–508

Wanebo HJ, Stearns M, Schwartz MK (1978) Use of CEA as an indicator of early recurrence and as a guide to a second look procedure in patients with colorectal cancer. Ann Surg 188: 481–493

Waneck R, Lechner G, Jantsch H, Kovats E, Schiessel R (1984) Lateral distant view for improved accuracy in locating rectal tumors. AJR 142: 519–523

Wang KY, Kimmey MB, Nyberg DA, Mack LA, Haggitt RC, Shuman WP, Franklin DW, Silverstein FE (1987) Colorectal neoplasms: accuracy of US in demonstrating the depth of invasion. Radiology 165: 827–829

Weber CA, Deveney KE, Pellegrini CA, Way LW (1986) Routine colonoscopy in the management of colorectal carcinoma. Am J Surg 152: 87–92

Wilking N, Herrera L, Petrelli NJ, Mittelman A (1985) Pelvic and perineal recurrences after abdominoperineal resection for adenocarcinoma of the rectum. Am J Surg 150: 561–563

Winawer SJ (1983) Detection and diagnosis of colorectal cancer. Cancer 51: 2519–2524

Winawer SJ, Sherlock P (1982) Surveillance for colorectal cancer in average-risk patients, familial high-risk groups, and patients with adenomas. Cancer 50: 2609–2614

Wolmark N, Wieand HS, Rockette HE, Fisher B, Glass A, Lawrence W, Lerner H, Cruz AB, Volk H, Shibata H, Evans J, Prager D et al (1983) The prognostic significance of tumor location and bowel obstruction in Dukes' B and C colorectal cancer. Findings from the NSABP clinical trials. Ann Surg 198: 743–752

Wolmark N, Fisher B, Wieand HS, Henry RS (1984a) The prognostic significance of preoperative carcinoembryonic antigen levels in colorectal cancer. Results from NSABP clinical trials. Ann Surg 199: 375–382

Wolmark N, Fisher ER, Wieand HS, Fisher B (1984b) The relationship of depth of penetration and tumor size to the number of positive nodes in Dukes' C colorectal cancer. Cancer 53: 2707–2712

Wolmark N, Fisher B, Wieand HS (1986) The prognostic value of the modifications of the Dukes' C Class of colorectal cancer. An analysis of the NSABP clinical trials. Ann Surg 203: 115–122

Wright HK, Higgins EF (1982) Natural history of occult right colon cancer. Am J Surg 143: 169–170

Wu WC, Gelfand DW, Ott DJ, Gilliam JH (1982) Water-soluble contrast enema as an aid to colonoscopy. AJR 138: 357–358

Zinkin LD (1983) A critical review of the classifications and staging of colorectal cancer. Dis Colon Rectum 26: 37–43

14 Cancer of the Anal Canal*

Cancer of the anus, a pathology of elderly individuals, consists essentially of epidermoid carcinomas located in the anal canal. Lesions of the anal margin are considered skin cancers. Systematic biopsy of all atypical anal lesions is an effective strategy for correct diagnosis. Because sonoendoscopy has not yet become a routine procedure, the role of imaging techniques remains limited, and they are therefore discussed in the sections on diagnosis and post-therapy follow-up.

14.1 Epidemiology

Anal cancers are 50 times less frequent than large bowel carcinomas (Singh et al. 1981), with an annual incidence of 2 per 100 000 population. There is a marked female-to-male predominance of 3 to 1; patient age at diagnosis ranges between 50 and 70 years. While the role of premalignant lesions remains unclear, epithelial dysplasia and leukoplakia have been observed. Patients with Crohn's disease are at increased risk for anal cancer (multiplied by 10 for Serota et al. 1981). Transitional forms have been found between condylomata and verrucous carcinoma. No risk factors have actually been identified, however, and neither infectious pathologies nor anal fistulae appear to promote these neoplasms.

14.2 Pathogenesis

14.2.1 Gross Features

Three forms have been described: (a) a dumb-bell-shaped, exophytic tumor with a superior

---

* Written in collaboration with A. Geoffray.

rectal prolongation, narrowing at the pectinate level, and an inferior anal prolongation; (b) ulceration with a peripheral rim, similar to rectal adenocarcinoma; (c) a concentric infiltrating lesion causing stenosis of the anal canal. In the literature review of Eschwege et al. (1987), the frequency by location was as follows: anorectal zone (59.6%), intra-anal canal (24.2), ano-cutaneous junction (16.2%). At diagnosis, 51% of the tumors measured less than 3 cm in the series of Beahrs and Wilson (1976), and only 26% were larger than 5 cm.

14.2.2 Histology

Epidermoid cancers comprise two major histologic subgroups although they have similar presentations, modes of spread, and patterns of recurrence (Sayuyers 1972; Schneider and Schulte 1981). Squamous cell carcinomas, composed of keratin-producing cells, usually originate below the pectinate line. By contrast, cloacogenic carcinomas (also referred to as basaloid or transitional cell tumors) are non-keratinizing, epithelial tumors believed to derive from remnant embryonic cloacal cells at or just below the pectinate line. Occasionally, both of these histologic forms are associated. Small cell carcinoma (Bowman et al. 1984) and mucinous adenocarcinoma (Jones and Morson 1984) are two other rare epithelial neoplasms of the anal canal.

14.2.3 Mode of Spread

Anal carcinomas may invade the submucosa, then the muscularis (especially the internal sphincter), and finally the perianal fat. Anal carcinomas are rarely circumferential but proximal extension can occur into the rectum.

Anteriorly, regional spread occurs towards the rectovaginal septum in women and towards the ureter and the prostate in men; posteriorly, spread occurs towards the sacrum, and laterally towards the ischiorectal fossae. Dissemination along the lymphatic pathways follows a hypogastric route into the retroperitoneal lymph nodes and the inguinal region. Metastases, though rare, may occur in the liver, lungs, and brain.

14.2.4 Histoprognosis

The possible prognostic differences between squamous cell carcinoma and cloacogenic carcinoma remain controversial. For Bowman et al. (1984), cloacogenic carcinomas have a worse prognosis than squamous cell carcinomas.

Several staging systems have been developed, including the TNM classification (Table 14.1) and Dukes' classification adapted for the anus (Dukes and Galvin 1956):

Stage A   Epithelial and subepithelial tumor
Stage B   Involvement of the muscle and adjacent tissues:
　　B1   Invasion of the internal sphincter
　　B2   Invasion of the external sphincter
　　B3   Invasion of the adjacent pelvic tissues
Stage C   Regional lymph node involvement
Stage D   Unresectable tumor or metastasis

14.3 Clinical Features

Cancer of the anal canal not only has a misleading appearance, but can also present numerous different features. Biopsies are therefore essential for all atypical lesions that do not respond to symptomatic treatment. Rectal bleeding, the main presenting complaint, is much more common than pain or a sensation of an anal mass.

Cancers of the anal margin may present as large, readily visible ulcerations or exophytic tumors. Occasionally, the benign appearance of the lesions (suggesting hemorrhoids or condylomata) masks the actual cancer. Typical advanced cancers of the anal canal may present

Table 14.1. TNM classification of anal canal cancers. (From Hermanek and Sobin 1987)

T - Primary tumor

TX	Primary tumor cannot be assessed
T0	No evidence of primary tumor
Tis	Carcinoma in situ
T1	Tumor 2 cm or less in greatest dimension
T2	Tumor more than 2 cm but not more than 5 cm in greatest dimension
T3	Tumor more than 5 cm in greatest dimension
T4	Tumor of any size invades adjacent organ(s), e. g. vagina, urethra, bladder [involvement of the sphincter muscle(s) *alone* is not classified T4]

N - Regional lymph nodes

NX	Regional lymph nodes cannot be assessed
N0	No regional lymph node metastasis
N1	Metastasis in perirectal lymph node(s)
N2	Metastasis in unilateral internal iliac and/or inguinal lymph node(s)
N3	Metastasis in perirectal and inguinal lymph nodes and/or bilateral internal iliac and/or inguinal nodes

M - Distant metastasis

MX	Presence of distant metastasis cannot be assessed
M0	No distant metastasis
M1	Distant metastasis

as an ulcerating, exophytic tumor (40%), a nodular infiltrating lesion responsible for stenosis (40%), or a polypoid growth (20%) (Eschwege et al. 1987). Existence of an apparently banal inflammatory condition often masks the malignancy.

Digital rectal examination for determination of the extent of endorectal spread must be completed by a biopsy. Physical examination should include searches for enlarged perirectal nodes (which are often better evaluated under general anesthesia) and inguinal adenopathies (which can be biopsied under local anesthesia). For Singh et al. (1981), 50% of patients already have nodal involvement at the time of diagnosis.

14.4 Imaging (Figs. 14.1, 14.2)

Although not not yet widely used for local disease workups of anal cancer, endosonography or blind transrectal ultrasound (with a rotative

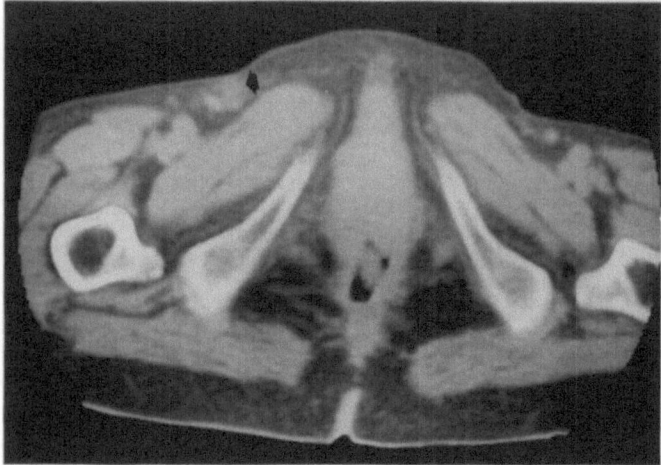

Fig. 14.1. Cancer of the anal canal infiltrating the perianal fat, associated with a right inguinal adenopathy *(arrow)*

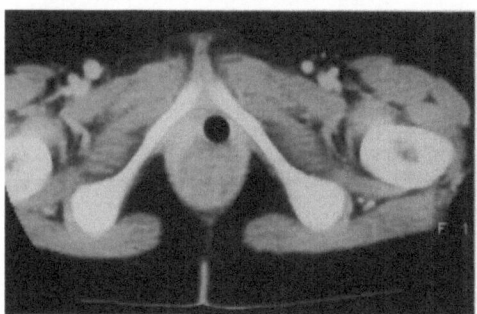

Fig. 14.2. Bulky cancer of the anal canal infiltrating the posterior wall of the vagina (tampon can be visualized in the vagina)

or linear transducer) will probably become the examination techniques of choice in the next few years because they can accurately determine lesion size and evaluate the depth of penetration, as for rectal lesions. Endorectal sonography is especially useful for detecting perirectal adenopathies. Exploration of the inguinal region with a high-frequency transducer is a useful complement to physical examination. Barium enema examinations may reveal a plaque-like contour in the most distal rectum (squamous cell carcinomas) or a submucosal appearance (cloacogenic neoplasms) (Cohan et al. 1985). Large lesions obviously corresponding to T3 or T4 tumors are a good

indication for CT, which can easily detect concomitant pelvic and para-aortic adenopathies. Disease staging must include evaluation of possible metastatic spread to the liver (sonography or CT), lungs, or skeleton.

14.5 Treatment

14.5.1 Radiotherapy

Irradiation with a curative intent may be given by either external beam therapy or a radiocurietherapy association. European authors reserve such therapy for stage T1 and T2 tumors, because delivery of more than 70 Gy results in loss of sphincter function. Palliative radiation therapy may be combined with chemotherapy and a colostomy. Interstitial radiotherapy is systematically completed by inguinocrural irradiation (Rousseau et al. 1979). Endocurietherapy may be performed with five to seven iridium-192 interstitial implants, which deliver 15-20 Gy. In European series, survival at 3 years is 80% for stage T1 and T2 tumors (Eschwege et al. 1987). Depending on tumor size, sphincter preservation is possible for 30%-80% of patients.

14.5.2 Surgery

Surgical management consists in abdomino-perineal resection; adenopathies are managed by external or deep iliac inguinal node resection.

14.5.3 Therapeutic Options

Not all authors agree on the use of exclusive radiotherapy for T1 and T2 tumors, even though this method gives satisfactory results. If postradiation results are deemed insufficient, abdominoperineal resection can be performed as palliative treatment; this is especially true for T4 tumors. Inguinal adenopathies (less than N2) are managed by local irradiation; N3 adenopathies are treated with radiotherapy and surgery. Enlarged inferior mesenteric and superior hemorrhoidal nodes are removed during abdominoperineal resection. By contrast, external and internal iliac dissection during abdominoperineal resection is too radical a procedure and has an unacceptably high morbidity.

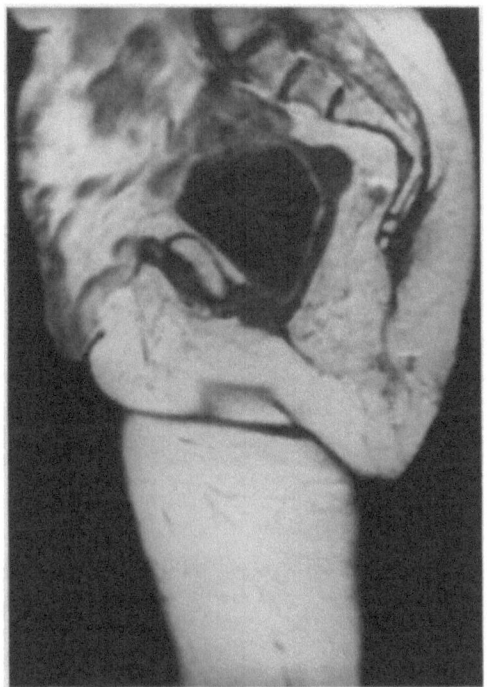

Fig. 14.3. Postirradiation fibrosis after treatment for anal canal cancer. (Courtesy of Prof. Masselot, Villejuif, France)

14.5.4 Post-therapy Follow-up (Figs. 14.3–14.6)

Postirradiation complications consist mainly of fecal incontinence because of sphincter destruction; rectovaginal fistulae are less common. The recurrence rate ranges between 24% and 62% (Bowman et al. 1984; Frost et al. 1984; Singh et al. 1981). For Frost et al. (1984), treatment of recurrent lesions results in a prognosis of 26% at 5 years.

Diagnosis of recurrent disease can be hampered by radiation-induced sequellae. Although soft tissue thickening subsequent to radiotherapy can make interpretation difficult, CT scans are a useful adjunct to physical examination. The usually symmetrical nature of postradiation fibrosis permits differentiation from tumoral lesions.

Disease recurrences after abdominoperineal resection are similar to relapses of colorectal cancer (see Chap. 13), consisting of a presacral mass, with or without genitourinary extension. Owing to the very variable character of this mass in treated patients (in particular those who have undergone complementary irradiation), CT is advisable during the first 4 months after surgery, as after resection for rectal cancer (Cohan et al. 1985). CT can visualize enlarged inguinal and pelvic lymph nodes, involvement of the gluteal muscles, extension to the genital and urinary tracts, retroperitoneal adenopathies, and liver metastases.

14.6 Conclusion

Carcinoma of the anal canal is a rare, but curable tumor whose frequently misleading clinical appearance can delay diagnosis. Imaging techniques, and especially endorectal ultrasound using appropriate transducers, should improve patient staging, in particular through better evaluation of the nodal involvement which is very frequent at the time of diagnosis.

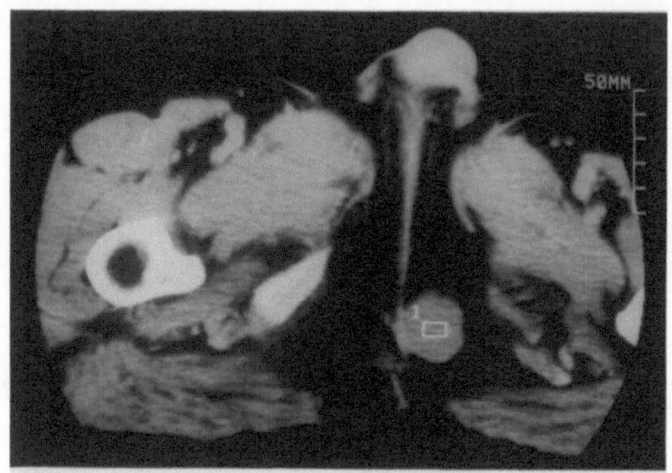

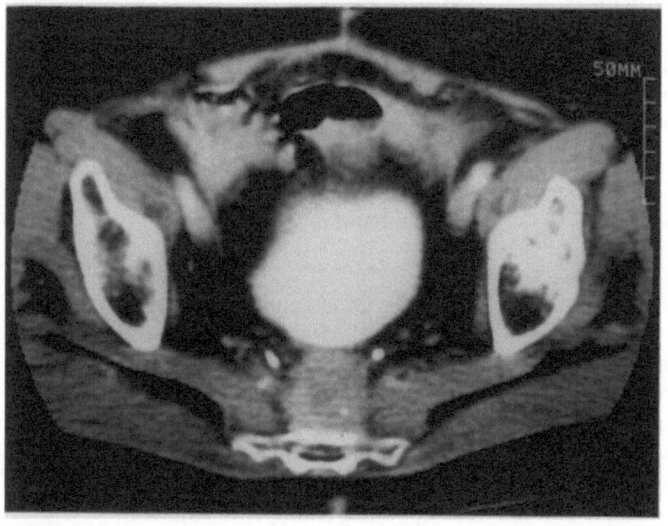

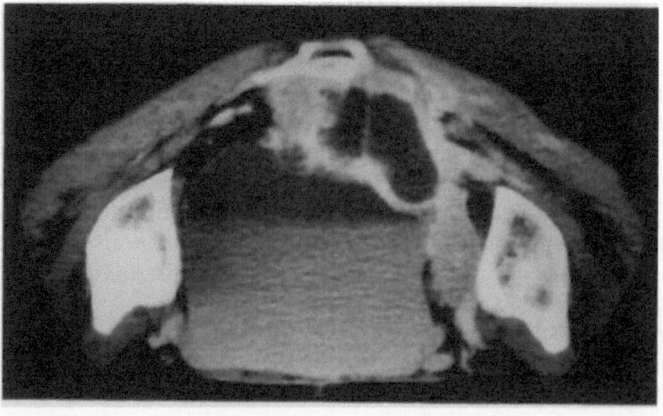

◀ **Fig. 14.4** *(above)*. Recurrence of an anal canal cancer (density 42 HU in square 1)

Fig. 14.5 *(middle)*. Recurrence of an anal canal cancer after abdominoperineal resection

Fig. 14.6 *(below)*. Extensive recurrence of an anal canal cancer treated by abdominoperineal resection. The recurrence has caused lytic destruction of the lower left edge of the sacrum. Associated iliac adenopathies. Examination was performed with the patient in the prone position prior to aspiration biopsy

14.7 References

Beahrs OH, Wilson SM (1987) Carcinomas of the anus. Ann Surg 184: 422–428

Bowman BM, Moertel CG, O'Connell MJ, Scott M, Weiland LH, Beart W, Gunderson LL, Spencer RJ (1984) Carcinoma of the anal canal: a clinical and pathologic study of 188 cases. Cancer 54: 114–125

Cohan RH, Silverman PM, Thompson WM, Halvorsen RA, Baker ME (1985) Computed tomography of epithelial neoplasms of the anal canal. AJR 145: 569–573

Dukes CE, Galvin C (1956) Colloid carcinoma arising within fistulae in the anorectal region. Ann R Coll Surg Engl 18: 246–261

Eschwege F, Chavy A, Cope R, Gerard JP, Lasser P, Parc R, Potet F, Rougier P (1987) Cancer de l'anus. In: Zeitoun P (ed) Cancers digestifs. Flammarion, Paris, pp 192–210

Frost DB, Richards PC, Montague ED, Giacco GG, Martin RG (1984) Epidermoid cancer of the anorectum. Cancer 53: 1285–1293

Hermanek P, Sobin LH (1987) TNM. Classification of malignant tumours. Springer, Berlin Heidelberg New York London Paris Tokyo

Jones EA, Morson BC (1984) Mucinous adenocarcinoma in anorectal fistulae. Histopathology 8: 279–292

Rousseau J, Mathieu G, Fenton J (1979) Résultats et complications de la radiothérapie des épithéliomas du canal anal. Etude de 128 cas traités de 1956 à 1970. Gastroenterol Clin Biol 3: 207–208

Sayuyers JL (1972) Squamous cell cancer of the perianus and anus. Surg Clin North Am 52: 935–941

Schneider TC, Schulte WJ (1981) Management of carcinoma of anal canal. Surgery 90: 729–734

Singh R, Nime R, Mittelman A (1981) Malignant epithelial tumors of the anal canal. Cancer 48: 411–415

15 Leiomyosarcoma*

Leiomyosarcomas are malignant tumors that arise from the muscular coat of the alimentary tract, and particularly from the muscularis externa. Sarcomatous degeneration of benign leiomyomas has been postulated, but such occurrences are undoubtedly very rare (Palmer 1948; Shepherd 1950), and most leiomyosarcomas are probably malignant from the outset.

At diagnosis, most gastrointestinal leiomyosarcomas are large, multinodular hypervascular tumors adherent to the adjacent organs; hemorrhagic and necrotic changes are common, with possible development of cavities communicating with the intestinal lumen.

These usually slowly-growing tumors can spread by local infiltration, intraperitoneal implants, and hematogeneous dissemination to the liver, lungs, and skeleton. Lymphatic spread is uncommon (Skandalakis et al. 1960; Starr and Dockerty 1955).

Histologically, these tumors present a great diversity of pathologic features, which can sometimes render diagnosis of malignancy very difficult. Leiomyosarcomas are composed of interlacing fascicles of spindle-shaped cells with eosinophilic cytoplasm and oval nuclei; these cells interdigitate with the normal muscle tissue, which is gradually destroyed. All intermediate grades exist between low-grade and highgrade malignancy tumors. Low-grade tumors have abundant stroma, with interlacing, organized cell bundles resembling leiomyoma; although leiomyosarcomas are characterized by greater cellularity and hypervascularity, correct diagnosis can be difficult. The best histologic indicator of malignancy is the mitotic count, even though the course of certain histologically benign-appearing tumors is complicated by development of metastases. In high-grade leiomyosarcomas, the cell bundles appear disorganized, they exhibit marked pleomorphism, and the mitotic count is over 10 per high-power field (Chiotasso and Fazio 1982).

15.1 Esophagus

15.1.1 General Features

Leiomyosarcomas are six to ten times less frequent than leiomyomas, the most common esophageal tumor (Ala-Kulju and Salo 1987; Baker and Good 1955; Kostiainen et al. 1973), and represent fewer than 0.5% of all esophageal malignancies (Balthazar 1981; Berk et al. 1971; Itai and Shimazu 1978; Rainer and Brus 1965). Histologically, whereas leiomyomas are almost constantly intramural and very rarely ulcerated, leiomyosarcomas are often intraluminal, and one-third of cases present ulceration. Multiple tumors are infrequent (Johnston et al. 1953) and calcifications are rarely reported (Itai and Shimazu 1978).

The frequency of sites within the esophagus (upper third 19.2%, middle third 31.3%, lower third 49.5%) is similar to the distribution of leiomyomas (Alcantara et al. 1986; Balthazar 1981; Becour 1984; Bruneton et al. 1981; Lombardo and Lattanzio 1985). By contrast, these two tumor types differ by size, as leiomyosarcomas are often over 5 cm in diameter at the time of diagnosis (Table 15.1).

Associated neoplasms reported in patients with esophageal leiomyosarcomas include gastric leiomyosarcoma (Howard 1902), head and neck cancer (Bruneton et al. 1981), and especially epidermoid esophageal cancer (Rella et al. 1965); this last malignancy was a finding in 8.5% of the 82 cases of leiomyosarcoma reviewed by Becour (1984).

---

* Written in collaboration with C. Balu-Maestro.

Endoscopic biopsy is nearly always positive because of the usually polypoid nature of esophageal leiomyosarcomas (Partyka et al. 1981). When problems persist for affirming malignancy, the mitotic count appears the best diagnostic element. As for leiomyosarcomas in other sites, degeneration of an esophageal leiomyoma has not yet been demonstrated (Becour 1984).

In the literature, mean patient age at diagnosis is 58 years, and males predominate (61% for Becour 1984). The presenting symptoms summarized in Table 15.2 correspond to the review of 62 cases. Whereas leiomyomas are sometimes asymptomatic, leiomyosarcomas always caused symptoms, essentially dysphagia (85.6%) and weight loss (51.5%). By contrast, upper gastrointestinal bleeding is less common

Table 15.1. Diameter (230 cases) and barium findings (214 cases) for gastrointestinal leiomyosarcomas

	Esophagus	Stomach	Small intestine	Colon/rectum
Diameter	(24 cases)	(98 cases)	(51 cases)	(57 cases)
<5 cm	16.6%	6.1%	23.6%	7.1%
5–10 cm	50.1%	28.6%	37.2%	56.5%
>10 cm	33.3%	64.3%	39.2%	36.8%
Barium findings	(24 cases)	(104 cases)	(56 cases)	(30 cases)
Intraluminal	62.5%	17.3%	23.2%	40%
Intramural	12.5%	23.1%	17.8%	33.3%
Subserosal	20.9%	48.1%	51.7%	10%
Dumbbell	4.1%	10.6%	7.8%	16.7%
Ulceration	29.1%	56.7%	21.4%	60%
Negative	–	0.9%	30.3%	–

Table 15.2. Clinical symptoms of gastrointestinal leiomyosarcoma (499 cases)

	Esophagus (62 cases)	Stomach (127 cases)	Small intestine (150 cases)	Colon/rectum (160 cases)
Pain	24.2%	47.2%	66.6%	36.8%
Bleeding or anemia	8%	59.8%	56.6%	44.3%
Weight loss	51.4%	24.4%	13.3%	13.1%
Dysphagia	85.6%	1.6%	–	–
Palpable mass	–	32.3%	46.7%	25.6%
Weakness	–	9.4%	6%	7.5%
Obstruction	–	–	16%	5%
Asymptomatic	–	1.6%	–	1.8%

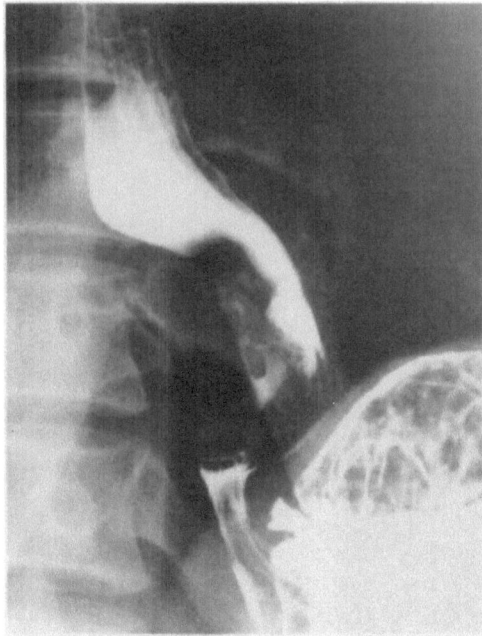

Fig. 15.1. Leiomyosarcoma of the lower third of the esophagus

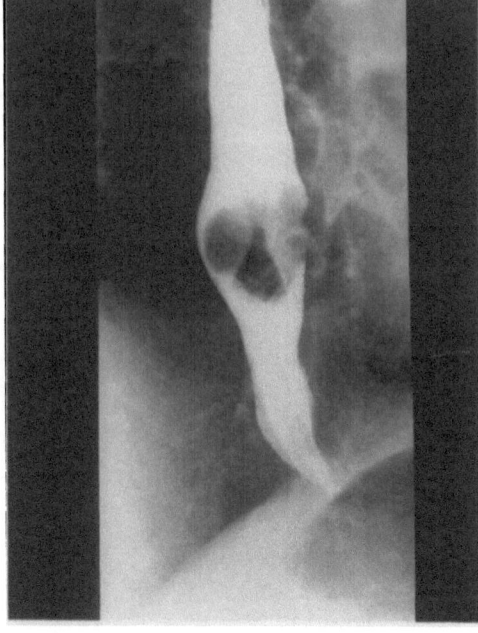

Fig. 15.2. Polypoid leiomyosarcoma of the esophagus

with esophageal leiomyosarcomas than with such lesions elsewhere in the gastrointestinal tract.

Fiberoptic endoscopy is diagnostic owing to the generally intraluminal nature of these lesions (78.2% for Becour 1984). Infiltrating and subserosal lesions are rare, but create problems for endoscopy, which will only demonstrate the normal-appearing mucosa. It is in these relatively rare cases that other techniques such as sonoendoscopy and CT play major roles.

Although leiomyosarcomas have a better prognosis than carcinoma, too few cases have been reviewed to permit true evaluation (Sweet et al. 1956). However, involvement of local or regional lymph nodes is almost constant, and 28.6% of patients have liver metastases at the moment of diagnosis. The longest survivals have been obtained after surgical resection. In his literature review, Becour (1984) cited a mean postoperative survival of 27.5 months. Radiotherapy and chemotherapy have only secondary roles.

15.1.2 *Imaging* (Figs. 15.1–15.4)

Routine chest X-rays reveal esophageal leiomyosarcomas as a posterior mediastinal opacity in 36.8% of cases. These tumors can lead to fistulization and formation of a lung abscess

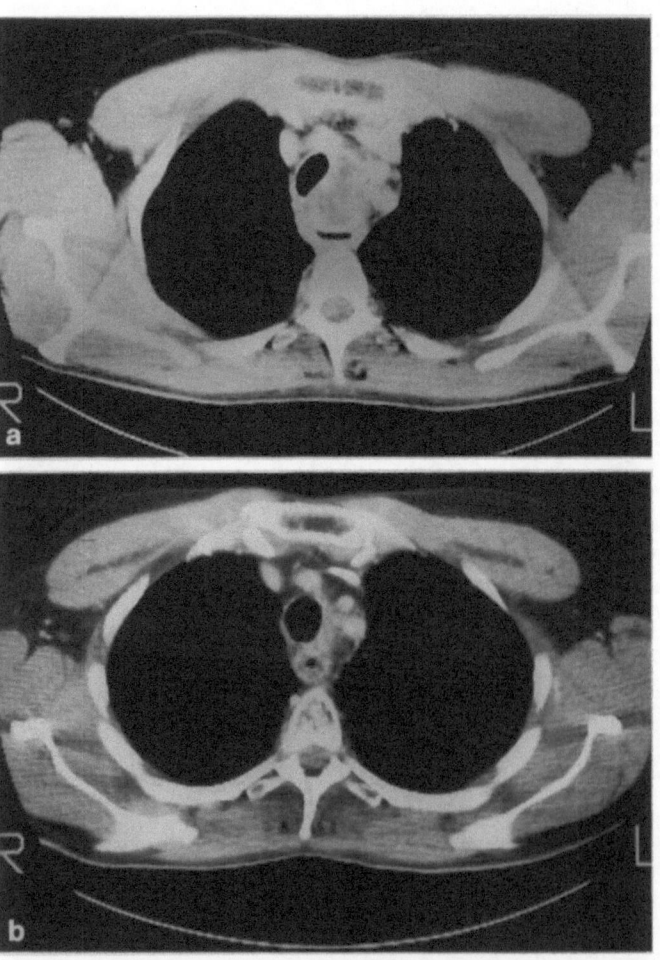

Fig. 15.3 a, b. CT study of a leiomyosarcoma of the esophagus: pretherapy study revealed a 4-cm long tumoral mass **(a)**. After irradiation, the tumor regressed **(b)**

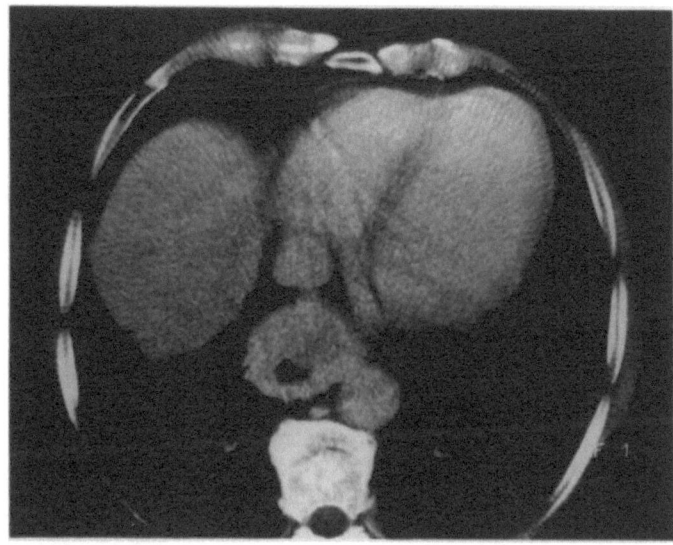

Fig. 15.4. Leiomyosarcoma of the lower third of the esophagus, without peripheral extension towards the rest of the mediastinum

(Lipschlutz and Fischer 1954). The radiologic features observed on *barium studies* are summarized in Table 15.1. Generally speaking, leiomyomas tend to be intramural and smaller than 10 cm in diameter; leiomyosarcomas, in contrast, are bulky and only rarely entirely intramural (only 12.5% of the cases reviewed in the literature). Moreover, tumoral ulceration, demonstrable in over one-quarter of all leiomyosarcomas, is an infrequent complication of leiomyomas. Constrictive lesions have been described on rare occasions (Lombardo and Lattanzio 1985).

Few reports have described the *CT* features of these tumors, which may image as a soft tissue mass, with or without associated mediastinal adenopathy (Balthazar 1981; Becour 1984). For Balthazar (1981), esophageal leiomyosarcomas are *angiographically* avascular.

The usual diagnosis for intraluminal and constrictive lesions, based on the radiographic presentation, is an epidermoid carcinoma; other less commonly entertained diagnoses include carcinosarcoma, a fibrovascular polyp, or a neurogenic tumor. Purely subserosal lesions may suggest a neurogenic tumor or posterior mediastinal lymphadenopathy. Completely intramural lesions usually are initially considered leiomyoma.

Overall, there are no particular radiologic features suggesting the diagnosis of esophageal leiomyosarcoma. Imaging studies, and CT in particular, are indicated primarily to determine the resectability of esophageal malignancies.

15.2 Stomach

15.2.1 General Features

Leiomyosarcoma, which is four to nine times less frequent than leiomyoma in the stomach (Bruneton et al. 1981; Skandalakis et al. 1960), represents 1% of all gastric malignancies (Ming 1973; Philips et al. 1970). Taking all gastric tumors into account, leiomyosarcoma has a higher incidence in children than in adults (Goldthorn and Canizaro 1986).

Leiomyosarcomas are more frequent than leiomyomas in the upper third of the stomach but are less frequent in the antrum. In a review of 82 cases, 36.6% of gastric leiomyosarcomas occurred in the upper third of the stomach, 48.8% in the body of the stomach, and only 14.6% in the gastric antrum (Abbas et al. 1986; Bruneton et al. 1981, 1987; Nauert et al. 1982; Scatarige et al. 1985; Subramanyam et al.

1982). Leiomyosarcomas are often already rather large at diagnosis, probably because they remain clinically latent for long periods. For example, 64.3% of the cases reviewed were over 10 cm long at diagnosis (Table 15.1). Diagnosis of malignancy can be difficult; the gross pathologic appearance may suggest leiomyoma, even when hepatic metastases are present (Megibow et al. 1985). Average patient age at diagnosis is 57 years; there is a very discrete male predominance (54%) (Bruneton et al. 1981).

Gastric leiomyosarcomas are rarely asymptomatic. The friable nature of the slowly-growing tumoral tissue explains the frequency of upper gastrointestinal bleeding; the relative rarity of intraluminal forms explains the habitual absence of obstructive symptoms. Physical examination detects an abdominal mass in one-third of cases (Table 15.1). Acute complications include hemoperitoneum (Ramos and Mitsudo 1984).

Favorable prognostic factors include a tumor diameter smaller than 6 cm, less than 5/25 HpS, mild cellularity, oval form of cells, expansible growth pattern, no metastasis. These

factors are all in favor of a low-grade leiomyosarcoma (Abbas et al. 1986), for which mean survival is 98 months versus only 25 months for high-grade tumors (Evans 1985). Despite the existence of liver metastases, the prognosis for gastric leiomyosarcoma is better than for carcinoma (Skandalakis et al. 1960).

15.2.2 Imaging (Figs. 15.5–15.11)

Plain films may demonstrate gastric leiomyosarcoma as an opacity (14.6% of cases). An

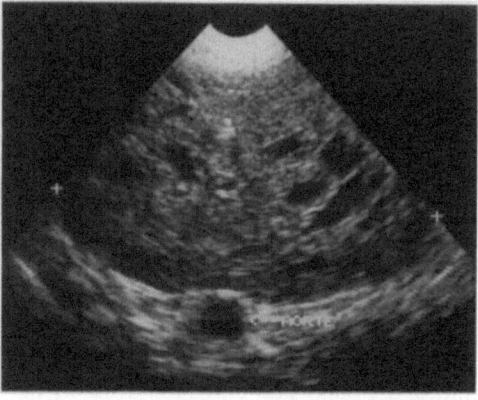

Fig. 15.6. Subserosal gastric leiomyosarcoma: ultrasonography visualized a solid mass with small areas of necrosis (138 mm between the *two crosses*)

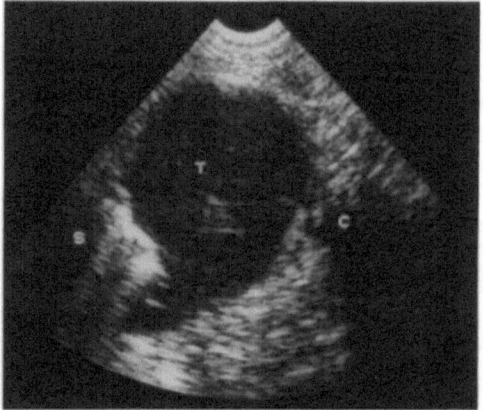

Fig. 15.7. Gastric leiomyosarcoma: ultrasonography of this lesion revealed extensive subserosal growth displacing the transverse colon downwards. *S*, stomach; *T*, tumor; *C*, transverse colon

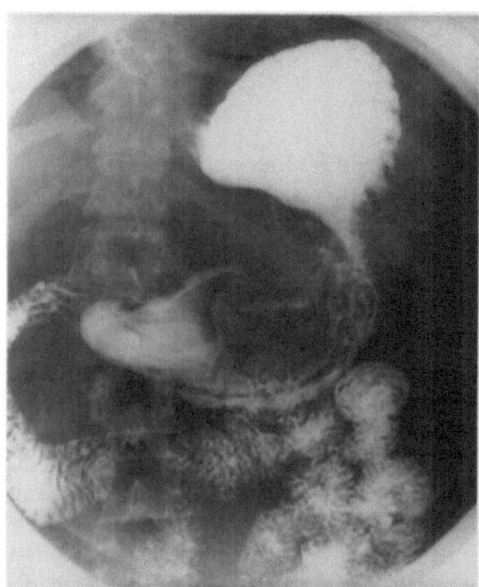

Fig. 15.5. Bulky leiomyosarcoma of the body of the stomach: this ulcerated lesion caused upper gastrointestinal bleeding

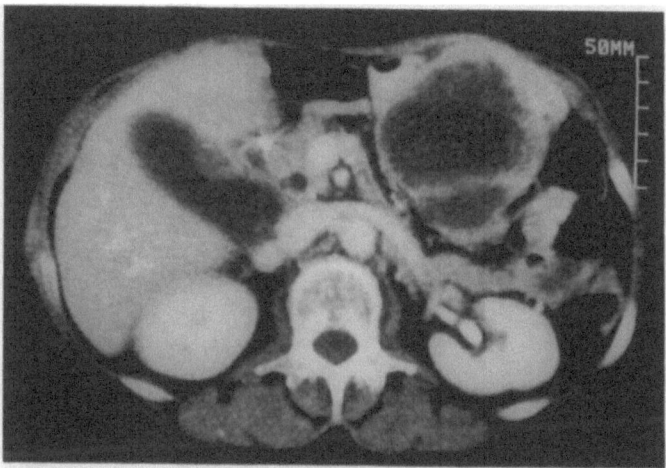

Fig. 15.8. Extensively necrotic recurrence of a gastric leiomyosarcoma

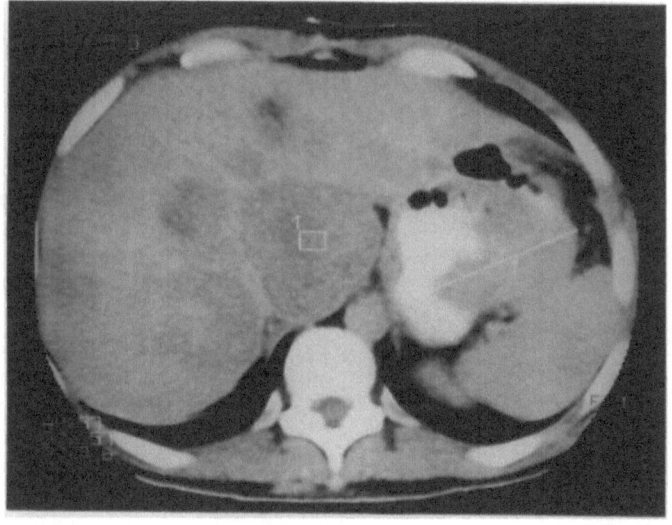

Fig. 15.9. Gastric leiomyosarcoma associated with liver metastases (the long axis of the tumor measured 7 cm, *line 1;* after contrast medium injection, the density of the liver metastases in *square 1* was 57 HU)

air-fluid level due to liquefaction necrosis is seen in 6.7% of cases (Bruneton et al. 1981). *Barium studies* are usually positive because of the often large dimensions of gastric leiomyosarcomas (Table 15.1). As opposed to gastric leiomyomas, which are usually intramural and sometimes ulcerated, gastric leiomyosarcomas are often large and tend to develop subserosally; 56.7% of cases reviewed presented ulcera-

tion (Table 15.1). The often subserosal nature of gastric leiomyosarcomas, aside from those cases where there is a communication between the necrotic tumor and the lumen, is poorly studied by barium explorations; for this type of tumor, ultrasonography and CT provide determinant information. However, barium studies can reveal spread towards the gastric cardia (Nauert et al. 1982).

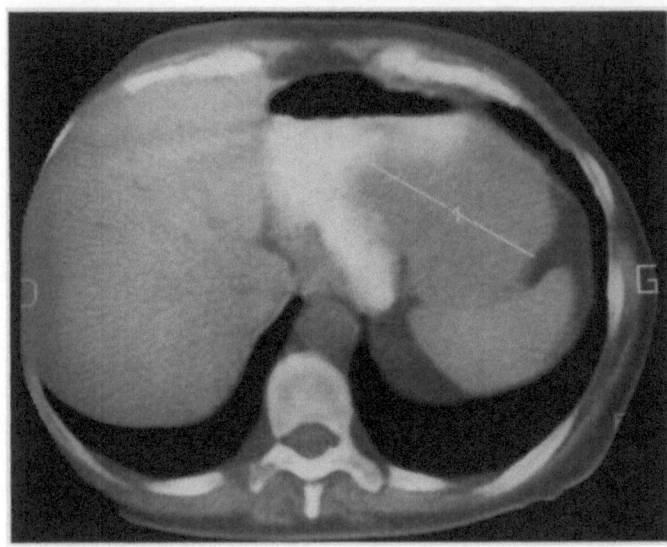

Fig. 15.10. Gastric leiomyosarcoma (8.2 cm long axis, *line 1*)

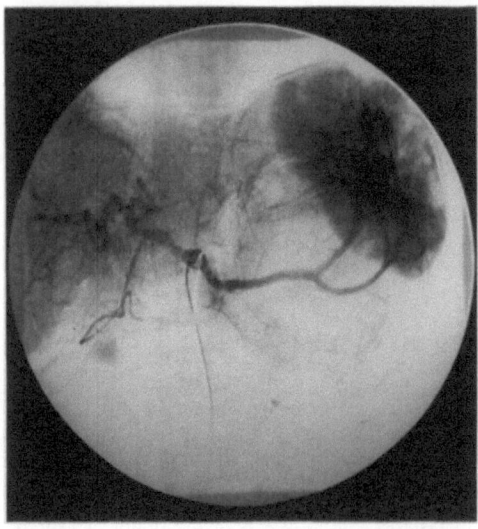

Fig. 15.11. Gastric leiomyosarcoma: angiography revealed very moderate hypervascularity

The *sonographic patterns* of gastric leiomyosarcoma depend on whether or not central necrosis is present. The tumor or the tumoral recurrence is usually a solid mass (Capelle and Leclere 1986; Nauert et al. 1982). However, because these tumors can reach considerable size and because secondary necrotic changes may occur, sonograms may demonstrate an irregular, poorly marginated solid lesion with

large echo-free areas (Nauert et al. 1982; Rodriguez Alvarez et al. 1985; Subramanyam et al. 1982). The liver metastases of gastric leiomyosarcomas are hypoechoic and necrotic (Subramanyam et al. 1982). Ultrasonography can demonstrate extension of a gastric lesion towards the neighboring viscera; in particular, real-time examinations can detect of involvement of the spleen, pancreas, or left kidney (Bruneton et al. 1987). Ultrasound-guided needle biopsy is particularly helpful for subserosal lesions when endoscopy fails to provide determinant information (Scatarige et al. 1985). Follow-up of treated patients can include abdominal ultrasound to search for recurrence and hepatic metastases (Capelle and Leclere 1986).

In fact, ultrasonography is a complement to *CT*, the most effective imaging technique for etiologic diagnosis, workup, and follow-up of gastric leiomyosarcomas. CT is rarely negative, whether for disease workups or patient monitoring. The tumor often images as a solid lesion, although tumoral necrosis and cystic degeneration are common (Bruneton et al. 1987; McLeod et al. 1984; Rodriguez Alvarez et al. 1985). Calcifications are exceptional (Balfe et al. 1981). Necrotic lesions show peripheral enhancement after contrast medium injection (Clark and Alexander 1982). CT completed by ultrasonography can adequately analyze disease spread to adjacent organs, in particular to the pancreas and spleen (Bruneton et al. 1987; Scatarige et al. 1985). Owing to their frequently subserosal nature, the tumor may spread to the mesentery or the omentum (Scatarige et al. 1985). The rarity of adenopathies is an interesting phenomenon (Berg and McNier 1960). Bulky gastric lesions associated with hepatic metastases may occur in the absence of adenopathy; this particular constellation suggests gastric leiomyosarcoma rather than lymphoma. In addition to peritoneal extension, metastasis may occur to the liver, lungs, retroperitoneum, and spleen. Liver metastases are often necrotic; their detection can correct gross diagnosis of an apparently benign, muscular tumor of the stomach.

From a diagnostic standpoint, the habitual absence of adenomegaly suggests a muscular tumor rather than gastric lymphoma. The differential diagnosis for intramural tumors includes leiomyoma or a benign neurogenic tumor. Combined use of ultrasound and CT scans should eliminate the difficulties formerly encountered with barium examinations for depicting the topographic origin of a subserosal gastric lesion. These two techniques should also obviate the need for diagnostic *angiography,* although in 17 reports reviewed in the literature, hypervascularity was a constant finding on the angiograms (Fujii et al. 1972; Granmayeh et al. 1978; Nance and Cohn 1970; Nauert et al. 1982; Sandler et al. 1978).

Overall, like other tumors which grow into the subserosa, gastric leiomyosarcomas have benefitted essentially from CT and ultrasonography. Combined use of these two techniques permits satisfactory diagnosis and follow-up of this type of tumor. Under these conditions, the barium examination, like angiography, no longer appears to have any major indications.

15.3 Small Intestine

15.3.1 General Features

The incidence of leiomyosarcomas and leiomyomas appears similar (Baker and Good 1955). Leiomyosarcoma accounts for 0.2% of all gastrointestinal malignancies (Wilson et al. 1980) and between 9.1% and 15.9% of all malignant intestinal tumors (Awrich et al. 1980; Barclay and Schapira 1983; Chiotasso and Fazio 1982; Goel et al. 1976). The topographic distribution in a review of 181 cases was as follows: duodenum 27.6%, jejunum 38.1%, ileum 33.7%, Meckel's diverticulum 0.6% (Bahnini et al. 1985; Barclay and Schapira 1983; Bruneton et al. 1981; Chiotasso and Fazio 1982; Curran 1986; Levis et al. 1986; Meurisse et al. 1984; Saubier et al. 1981; Subramanyam et al. 1982).

Table 15.1 summarizes the size of these lesions at diagnosis. Multiple intestinal leiomyosarcomas are rare (Bahnini et al. 1985). Associated lesions, though infrequent, may include Crohn's disease (Akwari et al. 1978), celiac disease, or another malignancy (Chiotasso and Fazio 1982).

Mean patient age at diagnosis of intestinal leiomyosarcoma is 56 years; male predominance has been demonstrated (64.7%) (Bruneton et al. 1981). Such tumors are rare in children (El Shafie et al. 1971).

Just as there are no significant differences between the general features of leiomyomas and those of intestinal leiomyosarcomas, their clinical symptoms are also similar (Table 15.2).

In a review of 150 cases, the main presenting symptoms were abdominal pain, bleeding, and an abdominal mass. Obstruction is common (16%). Patients presenting with a fever should be examined for fistulization or perforation (Meurisse et al. 1984). The mean preoperative duration of clinical symptoms is 2 years for Chiotasso and Fazio (1982). Post-treatment follow-up is essential owing to the risks of local recurrence, spread into the peritoneum, and especially hepatic metastases (Capelle and Leclere 1986). Average survival at 5 years ranges from 20% to 50% (Akwari et al. 1978), despite the fact that over one-half of patients undergo palliative surgery. Several prognostic factors have been identified, with a duration of symptoms of more than 1 year, a tumor diameter under 9 cm, and the absence of metastases being favorable factors (Chiotasso and Fazio 1982).

15.3.2 *Imaging* (Fig. 15.12)

Plain abdominal films may be the only examination required before surgery in patients presenting with acute obstruction. Complicated cases may demonstrate air-fluid levels secondary to obstructive phenomena or, less often, to tumoral necrosis (Grosdidier et al. 1970). *Barium contrast studies* were negative in nearly one-third of the cases reviewed (Table 15.1). As for gastric leiomyosarcoma, subserosal lesions predominate. Ulceration is present in 20% of cases. Annular constricting lesions are rare (Levine et al. 1987).

Sonographically, intestinal leiomyosarcomas resemble such lesions in the stomach, although they are generally not as large. The smaller size of intestinal lesions explains the higher frequency of solid lesions (Curran 1986; Levis et al. 1986; Saubier et al. 1981; Subramanyam et al. 1982). Large tumors contain areas of necrosis. The differential diagnosis for ileal lesions in women is ovarian carcinoma.

CT is not always effective in evaluating these tumors and may fail to identify a leiomyosarcoma (nine negative cases out of 31 for McLeod et al. 1984). Small diameter leiomyosarcomas appear solid; bulky lesions exhibit more or less extensive areas of necrosis (Clark and Alexander 1982; Megibow et al. 1985). CT can demonstrate infiltration of the mesentery and the presence of hepatic metastases. Owing

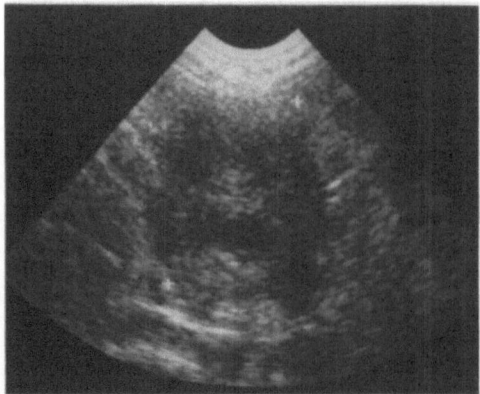

Fig. 15.12. Intestinal leiomyosarcoma: echo-poor lesion with a more echogenic center (45 mm between the *two crosses*)

to the insufficiency of results with barium examinations, but also with CT, *angiography* may still have a notable role to play because these tumors are hypervascular (Megibow et al. 1985; Meurisse et al. 1984; Saubier et al. 1981). Vascularity may appear less marked when there is necrosis, but there are no angiographic features that can rule out a diagnosis of leiomyoma; tumoral margins were well defined in 65% of the 20 cases reviewed (Bonnet et al. 1976; Campbell et al. 1977; Etienne et al. 1971; Granmayeh et al. 1978; Hollender et al. 1972; Jeanpierre 1973; Leone and Bryan 1968; Lombard-Platet et al. 1975; Meyers 1971; Zollikofer et al. 1979). Hepatic metastases of intestinal leiomyosarcoma are hypervascular (Granmayeh et al. 1978).

Overall, recent imaging techniques have not supplanted angiography for excluding a diagnosis of a benign or malignant muscular tumor of the small intestine. However, when intestinal leiomyosarcoma has already been diagnosed, the lesions are usually large enough for visualization by CT.

15.4 Colon and Rectum

15.4.1 *General Features*

Colorectal leiomyosarcoma is extremely rare. Balthazar (1981) cited 150 cases of rectal leiomyosarcomas and only 40 colonic leiomyosarcomas. Compared with the other leiomyosarcomas, colorectal sites account for only one out of every eight cases (Martinez Rodriguez and Garcia Garcia 1986). Rectal leiomyosarcoma represents 0.07%-0.1% of all rectal tumors (Diamante and Bacon 1967; Dukes and Bussey 1947; Khalifa et al. 1986). Lesions tend to occur in the rectum rather than other portions of the colon (Hamlin et al. 1985). The frequency of colorectal lesions in a review of 121 cases was: right colon 16.4%, transverse colon 10.8%, left colon 11.9%, rectum 60.9% (Balthazar 1981; Bruneton et al. 1981; Khalifa et al. 1986; Posen and Bar-Maor 1983; Rao et al. 1984; Stavorovsky et al. 1980; Tristaino and Talpacci 1986).

Mean age at diagnosis of colorectal leiomyosarcoma is 56 years; there is no sex predilection (Bruneton et al. 1981). Colorectal leiomyosarcoma is extremely rare in children (Posen and Bar-Maor 1983).

Clinical manifestations commonly include rectal bleeding, pain, and a palpable abdominal mass (Table 15.2). Diagnosis is commonly made during investigation of a complication (mucosal ulceration, perforation, abscess formation, internal fistula) (Rao et al. 1980). Less frequent symptoms include autoamputation with spontaneous evacuation per anum, acute onset simulating appendicitis, an association with polyposis coli, or prevalent metastatic deposits in the parotid region (De Roo and Vaas 1969; Guisto et al. 1958; MacKenzie et al. 1954; Trygstad 1932; Warkel et al. 1975).

Endoscopy plays an essential role in the diagnosis of rectal leiomyosarcomas (Hamlin et al. 1985) which have a less favorable prognosis than leiomyosarcomas in other sites (Balthazar 1981). Several parameters such as the grade and diameter at diagnosis are of prognostic value. In the review by Khalifa et al. (1986), low-grade leiomyosarcomas had a mean prognosis of 66.7% at 5 years versus only 33.3% for high-grade lesions. Rectal leiomyosarcomas smaller than 3 cm at diagnosis have an average 5-year prognosis of 70% versus 25% for lesions 7 cm or larger.

15.4.2 *Imaging* (Figs. 15.13, 15.14)

Plain films demonstrate intratumoral calcification on rare occasions (Gharemani et al. 1978). Despite the limited number of published reports on *barium studies,* ulcerated intramural and intraluminal lesions appear to be the most frequent (Table 15.1). A constrictive, neoplastic-appearing lesion suggestive of carcinoma is less frequent (Balthazar 1981; Posen and Bar-Maor 1983; Tristaino and Talpacci 1986). Owing to its rarity, colorectal leiomyosarcoma is not identified as such after imaging studies. Few reports have been published concerning the use of *ultrasound, CT,* and *MRI,* and no specific features have been found comparable to those observed in the stomach and small intestine (Capelle and Leclerc 1986; Hamlin et al. 1985; McLeod et al. 1984; Megibow et al. 1985; Tristaino and Talpacci 1986). Because probably malignant rectal tumors are usually considered to be of carcinomatous

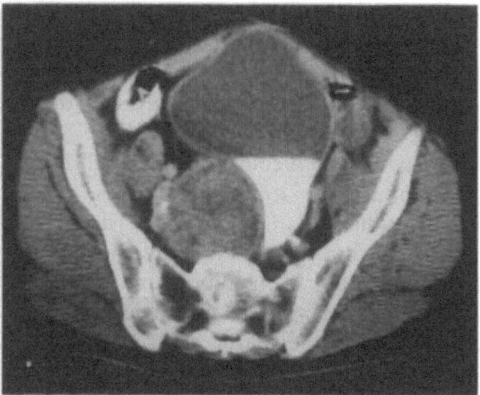

Fig. 15.13. Rectal leiomyosarcoma displacing the bladder anteriorly, associated with right iliac nodal infiltration

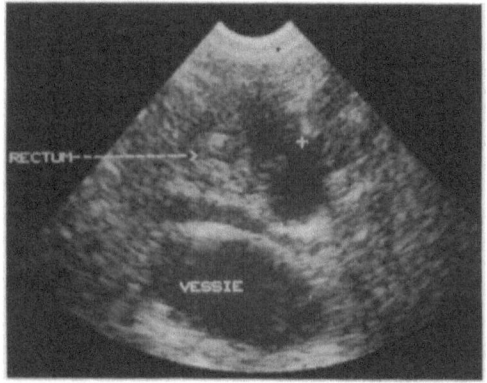

Fig. 15.14. Rectal leiomyosarcoma: ultrasonography performed using a perineal approach allowed visualization of this only slightly echoic tumor (23 mm between the *two crosses*) located on the left edge of the rectum. This lesion remained separate from the seminal vesicles and the bladder *(VESSIE)*

etiology, angiographic studies are rare. For Balthazar (1981), colorectal leiomyosarcoma is only moderately vascular.

15.5 Conclusion

Leiomyosarcoma is less common than leiomyoma in the esophagus and stomach, but appears to occur with at least equal frequency in the small intestine and colorectum. CT can

provide satisfactory disease workups of leiomyosarcomas. For gastric lesions, the diagnosis is suggested by a constellation of bulky
necrotic lesions, hepatic metastases, and the
absence of locoregional adenopathies. Small
diameter leiomyosarcomas in the small intestine are not always demonstrated by CT, and
barium studies are often negative. The hypervascular nature of leiomyosarcoma allows
identification by arteriography, and this technique retains a certain diagnostic value for intestinal leiomyosarcomas.

15.6 References

Abbas JS, Massad M, Mufarrij A, Saksouk F, Ku-
layalat M (1986) Gastric leiomyosarcoma: a clinicopathologic study. Int Surg 71: 176-181

Akwari OF, Dozois RR, Weilano LH, Beahrs OH
(1978) Leiomyosarcoma of the small and large
bowel. Cancer 42: 1375-1384

Ala-Kulju K, Salo JA (1987): Smooth muscle tumors
of the oesophagus. Scand J Thor Cardiovasc Surg
21: 65-68

Alcantara M, Merlo R, Martinez Potenciano JL,
Carrobles JM, Morente M, Cuesta MA, Martinez
Chacon J (1986) Leiomyosarcoma del esofago.
Rev Esp Enferm Apar Dig 70: 161-164

Awrich AE, Irish CE, Vetto RM, Fletcher WS (1980)
A twenty-five years experience with primary malignant tumors of the small intestine. Surg Gynecol Obstet 151: 9-14

Bahnini A, Hakami F, Halleb A, Parc R, Loygue J
(1985) Les leiomyosarcomes de l'intestin grêle. A
propos de 3 cas. J Chir (Paris) 122: 215-220

Baker HL, Good CA (1955) Smooth-muscle tumors
of the alimentary tract. Their roentgen manifestations. AJR 74: 246-255

Balfe DM, Koehler RE, Karstaedt N, Stanley RJ,
Sagel SS (1981) Computed tomography of gastric
neoplasms. Radiology 140: 431-436

Balthazar EJ (1981) Gastrointestinal leiomyosarcoma. Unusual sites: esophagus, colon and porta
hepatis. Gastrointest Radiol 6: 295-303

Barclay THC, Schapira DV (1983) Malignant tumors of the small intestine. Cancer 51: 878-881

Becour F (1984) A propos d'un cas inédit de léiomyosarcome de l'oesophage. Thesis, Université de
Paris-Sud

Berg J, McNier G (1960) Leiomyosarcoma of the
stomach. Cancer 13: 25-33

Berk RN, Scher GS, Bode DF (1971) Unusual tumors of the gastrointestinal tract. AJR 113:
159-170

Bonnet J, Deval V, Boisot B, Rabin A, Terme R, Delorme G (1976) Léiomyome et léiomyosarcome du
duodénum. Ann Radiol (Paris) 19: 663-668

Bruneton JN, Drouillard J, Roux P, Lecomte P, Tavernier J (1981) Leiomyoma and leiomyosarcoma
of the digestive tract. A report of 45 cases and review of the literature. Eur J Radiol 1: 291-300

Bruneton JN, Caramella E, Cazenave P, Birtwisle Y,
Hericord P, Drouillard J (1987) Gastric leiomyosarcoma. Comparative value of barium examinations, ultrasonography and CT scans. Eur J Radiol 7: 160-162

Campbell DR, Mason WF, Fraser DB, Standen JR
(1977) Arteriography in malignant neoplasms of
the bowel. J Assoc Can Radiol 28: 204-207

Capelle J, Leclere J (1986) Récidives abdomino-
pelviennes des léiomyosarcomes. Aspects échographiques à propos de 19 cas. J Radiol 67: 601-
604

Chiotasso PJP, Fazio VW (1982) Prognostic factors
of 28 leiomyosarcomas of the small intestine. Surg
Gynecol Obstet 155: 197-202

Clark RA, Alexander ES (1982) Computed tomography of gastrointestinal leiomyosarcoma. Gastrointest Radiol 7: 127-129

Curran FT (1986) Leiomyosarcoma of the duodenum. Br J Hosp Med 36: 285-286

De Roo T, Vaas F (1969) Leiomyosarcoma of the
transverse and descending colon: two case reports
and review. Am J Gastroenterol 52: 150-156

Diamante M, Bacon HE (1967) Leiomyosarcoma of
the rectum: report of a case. Dis Colon Rectum
10: 347-351

Dukes CE, Bussey HJ (1947) Sarcoma and melanoma of the rectum. Br J Cancer: 1: 30-37

El Shafie M, Spitz L, Ikeda S (1971) Malignant tumors of the small bowel in neonates presenting
with perforation. J Pediatr Surg 6: 62-64

Etienne JP, Delavierre P, Petite JP, Durand H (1971)
Léiomyosarcome de l'oesophage. Sem Hop 47:
1170-1172

Evans HL (1985) Smooth muscle tumors of the gastrointestinal tract. A study of 56 cases followed
for a minimum of 10 years. Cancer 56: 2242-2250

Fujii K, Yamagata S, Suzuki J, Sasaki R, Shoji T,
Makabe M, Memezawa H, Maesawa S (1972) Angiographic features of submucosal tumours of the
stomach. Tohoku J Exp Med 107: 287-299

Ghahremani GG, Meyers MA, Port RB (1978) Calcified primary tumors of the gastrointestinal tract.
Gastrointest Radiol 2: 331-339

Goel IP, Didolkar MS, Elias EG (1976) Primary malignant tumors of the small intestine. Surg Gynecol Obstet 143: 717-719

Goldthorn JF, Canizaro PC (1986) Gastrointestinal
malignancies in infancy, childhood, and adolescence. Surg Clin North Am 66: 845-861

Granmayeh M, Jonsson K, McFarland W, Wallace
S (1978) Angiography of abdominal leiomyosarcoma. AJR 130: 725-730

Grosdidier J, Robert D, Parietti R (1970) Léiomyosarcome du duodénum. Sem Hop 46: 1220-1222

Guisto DF, Thoshinsky MJ, Brizzolara LG (1958)
Leiomyosarcoma of the ascending colon associat-

ed with multiple polyposis. Am J Surg 95: 1007-1010

Hamlin DJ, Petterson H, Wajsman Z, Bland K, Hackett RL (1985) Leiomyosarcoma of the rectum versus prostatic malignancy. Differentiation by magnetic resonance imaging. Fortschr Geb Roentgenstr 143: 482-484

Hollender LF, Otteni F, Thomas M, Bur F (1972) Etude anatomoclinique de 21 tumeurs malignes primitives du jéjunum et de l'iléon. Ann Chir 26: 639-648

Howard WT (1902) Primary sarcoma of esophagus and stomach. JAMA 38: 393-399

Itai Y, Shimazu H (1978) Leiomyosarcoma of the esophagus with dense calcification. Br J Radiol 51: 469-471

Jeanpierre B (1973) Les léiomyomes de l'intestin grêle. Revue générale à propos de deux observations personnelles. Medical thesis, Dijon

Johnston JB, Clagett PT, McDonald JR (1953) Smooth muscle tumours of the oesophagus. Thorax 8: 251-265

Khalifa AA, Bong WL, Rao VK, Williams MJ (1986) Leiomosarcoma of the rectum. Report of a case and review of the literature. Dis Colon Rectum 29: 427-432

Kostiainen S, Virkkula L, Teppo L (1973) Smooth muscle tumors of the esophagus. Scand J Thorac Cardiovasc Surg 7: 98-103

Leone AJ, Bryan CS (1968) Leiomyosarcoma of the small bowel demonstrated by selective inferior mesenteric angiography. J Can Assoc Radiol 19: 126-129

Levine MS, Drooz AT, Herlinger H (1987) Annular malignancies of the small bowel. Gastrointest Radiol 12: 53-58

Levis P, Ragghianti CM, Giovenali E, Falcetto G, Giudici M (1986) Il leiomiosarcoma del piccolo intestino. Presentazione di un caso e considerazioni generali. Minerva Chir 41: 1223-1228

Lipschultz BM, Fischer S (1954) Leiomyosarcomas of the esophagus. Gastroenterology 27: 661-666

Lombard-Platet R, Mathon C, Revelin P, Piulachs J, Boulez P (1975) Les léiomyosarcomes de l'intestin grêle. Lyon Chir 71: 189-193

Lombardo G, Lattanzio M (1985) Leiomyosarcoma dell'esofago. Descrizione di un caso clinico e revisione delle letteratura. Minerva Chir 40: 811-818

MacKenzie DA, McDonald JR, Waugh JM (1954) Leiomyoma and leiomyosarcoma of the colon. Ann Surg 139: 67-75

McLeod AJ, Zornoza J, Shirkhoda A (1984) Leiomyosarcoma: computed tomographic findings. Radiology 152: 133-136

Martinez Rodriguez E, Garcia Garcia J (1986) Tumores leiomiomatosos del tubo digestivo. Factores etiologicos, criterios de malignidad y estudio clinico. Rev Esp Enferm Apar Dig 70: 529-535

Megibow AJ, Balthazar EJ, Hulnick DH, Naidich DP, Bosniak MA (1985) CT evaluation of gastrointestinal leiomyomas and leiomyosarcomas. AJR 144: 727-731

Meurisse M, Wahlen C, Honore P, Dekoster G, Carlier P, Desaive C (1984) Les léiomyosarcomes du duodenum. A propos de trois nouvelles observations. Ann Chir 38: 45-49

Meyers MA (1971) Leiomyosarcoma of the duodenum. Clin Radiol 22: 257-260

Ming S (1973) Tumors of the esophagus and stomach. In: Atlas of tumor pathology, 2nd series, fasc 7. AFIP, Washington, p 224

Nance FC, Cohn I (1970) The management of leiomyosarcoma of the stomach. Surg Clin North Am 50: 1129-1136

Nauert TC, Zornoza J, Ordonez N (1982) Gastric leiomyosarcomas. AJR 139: 291-297

Palmer ED (1948) Leiomyosarcoma of the stomach with particular reference to the gastroscopic picture. Am J Dig Dis 15: 84-87

Partyka EK, Sanowski RA, Kozarek RA (1981) Endoscopic diagnosis of a giant esophageal leiomyosarcoma. Am J Gastroenterol 75: 132-134

Phillips JC, Lindsay JW, Kendall JA (1970) Gastric leiomyosarcoma: roentgenologic and clinical findings. Am J Dig Dis 15: 239-246

Posen JA, Bar-Maor JA (1983) Leiomyosarcoma of the colon in an infant. A case report and review of the literature. Cancer 52: 1458-1461

Rainer GW, Brus R (1965) Leiomyosarcoma of the esophagus; review of the literature and report of 3 cases. Surgery 58: 343-350

Rao BK, Kapur MM, Roy S (1980) Leiomyosarcoma of the colon: a case report and review of the literature. Dis Colon Rectum 23: 184-190

Ramos SM, Mitsudo S (1984) Hemoperitoneum secondary to exogastric leiomyosarcomas and leiomyoblastomas. Am J Gastroenterol 79: 637-641

Rella AJ, Farell JT, Comer JV (1965) Concurrent leiomyosarcoma and squamous cell carcinoma of the esophagus. NY State J Med 65: 1254-1256

Rodriguez Alvarez JL, Garcia Campos F, Menendez Sanchez J, Ratia Gimenez T, Perez Mora N (1985) Leiomiosarcoma gastrico. Rev Esp Enferm Apar Digest 67: 437-444

Sandler MA, Ratanaprakarn S, Madrazo L (1978) Ultrasonic findings in intramural exogastric lesions. Radiology 128: 189-192

Saubier EC, Lemmens L, Partensky C, Allantaz F (1981) Léiomyosarcome du duodénum. A propos d'une observation et revue de la littérature. J Chir (Paris) 118: 473-481

Scatarige JL, Fishman EK, Jones B, Cameron JL, Sanders RC, Siegelman SS (1985) Gastric leiomyosarcoma: CT observations. J Comput Assist Tomogr 9: 320-327

Shepherd JA (1950) Perforation of leiomyosarcoma of the stomach. Br J Surg 37: 479-481

Skandalakis JE, Gray SW, Shepard D (1960) Smooth muscle tumors of the stomach. Int Abstr Surg 110: 209-226

Starr GF, Dockerty MB (1955) Leiomyomas and leiomyosarcomas of small intestine. Cancer 8: 101–111

Stavorovsky M, Jaffa AJ, Papo J, Baratz M (1980) Leiomyosarcoma of the colon and rectum. Dis Colon Rectum 23: 249–254

Subramanyam BR, Balthazar EJ, Raghavendra BN, Madamba MR (1982) Sonography of exophytic gastrointestinal leiomyosarcoma. Gastrointest Radiol 7: 47–51

Sweet RH, Soutter L, Tejada C (1956) Muscle wall tumours of oesophagus. J Thorac Surg 91: 3–23

Tristaino B, Talpacci A (1986) In tema di leiomiosarcoma del colon. Revisione della letterature e presentazione di un caso. Minerva Chir 41: 1515–1520

Trygstad R (1932) A case of leiomyosarcoma of the cecum. Am J Cancer 16: 662–664

Warkel RL, Stewart JB, Temple AJ (1975) Leiomyosarcoma of the colon: report of a case and analysis of the relationship of histology to prognosis. Dis Colon Rectum 18: 501–506

Zollikofer CL, Castaneda-Zuniga WR, Nath PH, Amplatz K (1979) Angiographic appearance of leiomyoma of the small intestine: report of two cases. Cardiovasc Radiol 2: 131–134

16 Lymphomas*

Malignant lymphomas of the gastrointestinal tract have been the subject of numerous recent studies aimed at defining the imaging appearances of these rare entities, and in particular the non-Hodgkin's lymphomas (NHL). Owing to the submucosal origin of the disease, even deep biopsies performed with state-of-the-art techniques are not always diagnostic. This explains the continued importance of imaging studies, especially because therapeutic approaches have evolved. For example, surgery is no longer the treatment of choice for gastric lymphoma, the most frequent gastrointestinal site, with many authors currently advocating radiotherapy and above all chemotherapy. Furthermore, CT now allows improved evaluation of the subdiaphragmatic nodes and the extent of disease within the gastrointestinal tract (Lee et al. 1979).

The radiologic features of gastrointestinal NHL and Hodgkin's disease (HD) must be distinguished because of the differences in their patterns of anatomic distribution and frequency. Nearly one in every 20 cases of NHL is a primary gastrointestinal lesion with a favorable prognosis. In contrast to carcinomas, NHL generally does not elicit a fibroblastic stroma reaction. The resultant large lesions are readily demonstrated radiologically, and, despite the frequent absence of clinical symptoms, their size suggests the correct diagnosis. Both primary and secondary HD are rare. In contrast to NHL, the prognosis is poor because gastrointestinal HD corresponds to stage IV disease from the outset. HD is associated with an intense fibroblastic stroma reaction producing moderately-sized, focal lesions suggestive of carcinoma.

16.1 Non-Hodgkin's Lymphoma

The overall frequency of primary NHL of the gastrointestinal tract has been estimated at 5%–6.2%. The reported incidence for secondary forms is even higher: 15.6%–44%, depending on whether radiologic and clinical data or autopsy series are considered (Freeman et al. 1972; Rosenberg et al. 1961; Schmid et al. 1980).

For Dawson et al. (1961), diagnosis of primary gastrointestinal lymphomas is based on four criteria:

- No enlargement of peripheral or mediastinal lymph nodes.
- Normal white blood cell counts.
- Predominance of the gastrointestinal lesion, with only regional lymph node involvement.
- No liver or spleen involvement.

Primary lymphomas are often considered focal lesions that can be classed in four categories (Musshoff 1977):

Stage I   Submucosal involvement with invasion towards the mucosa
Stage II   Parietal involvement, but no node enlargement
Stage III   Lesions evolving from the entire wall plus associated node enlargement
Stage IV   Generalized disease

The radiologic features of primary and secondary lymphomas are similar, except for colonic sites (Lecomte et al 1980). The prognosis for primary forms, which varies from 30% to 45% survival at 5 years, is thus better than for carcinoma (Brady and Asbell 1979; Sandler 1984).

---

* Written in collaboration with P.J. Valette.

16.1.1 Esophagus

The rarity of esophageal involvement is underscored by the fact that only 15 cases were found in a literature review of 2200 cases of gastrointestinal NHL (Bruneton et al. 1986). NHL of the esophagus represents less than 1% of all gastrointestinal lymphomas (Table 16.1). Dissemination from mediastinal nodes and extension of a gastric lymphoma into the lower third of the esophagus are the most frequent etiologies (Hricak et al. 1980). Clinical symptoms were mentioned for only one-half of the cases reviewed, with dysphagia being cited only 50% of the time.

Nodular masses are the most common radiologic finding: multiple nodules (Fig. 16.1) are more prevalent than polypoid lesions (Agha and Schnitzer 1985; Levine et al. 1985; Perfettini et al. 1985). CT can demonstrate submucosal infiltration and mediastinal involvement (Agha and Schnitzer 1985; Perfettini et al. 1985). These lesions are almost always associated with a similar gastric lesion. The differential diagnoses for nodular lesions include leiomyoma (although NHL is usually more extensive), esophageal varices (but varices tend to have a tortuous appearance), and hematogenous metastases (especially of malignant melanoma). Less frequent findings include large ulcerations (Carnovale et al. 1977; Caruso and Berk 1970; Matsura et al. 1985) and infiltrative processes, which occasionally cause obstructive stenosis. In these last cases, radiologic images can return to normal following radiotherapy.

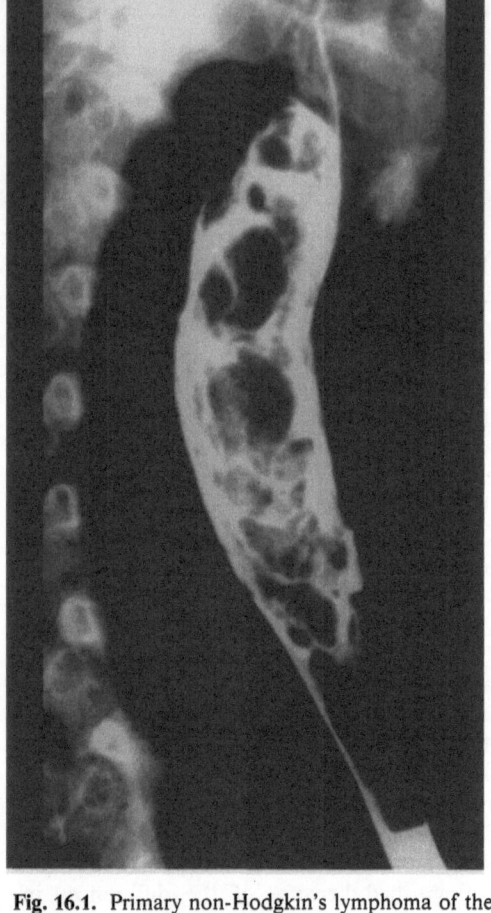

Fig. 16.1. Primary non-Hodgkin's lymphoma of the esophagus: multinodular lesion. (Courtesy of Dr. Schmutz, Strasbourg, France)

Table 16.1. Incidence of gastrointestinal NHL

	Esopha-gus	Stomach	Small intestine	Colon/rectum
Incidence of primary lesions	0.03%	3.9%	1.2%	0.9%
Incidence with respect to other gastrointestinal sites	<1%	50%–70%	35%–70%	15%
Incidence with respect to other malignant tumors	Rare	3%–5%	10%–30%	0.5%

16.1.2 Stomach

The stomach is the most frequent site of gastrointestinal NHL, especially for primary malignancies. For Freeman et al. (1972), gastric sites account for 3.9% of all cases of NHL. Other authors have reported a frequency as high as 6% (Bush and Ash 1969; Privett et al. 1977). Gastric sites predominate among gastrointestinal tract lesions in general, accounting for 48.2%–78.5% of cases (Ehrlich et al. 1968; Loehr et al. 1969; Wang and Peterson 1956). NHL of the stomach represents

Table 16.2. Incidence of clinical symptoms in gastrointestinal NHL

Clinical symptom	Stomach (1100 cases)	Small intestine (700 cases)	Colon/ rectum (400 cases)
Pain	73%	63%	74%
Weight loss	41%	34%	57%
Bleeding	26%	24%	28%
Vomiting	24%	15%	11%
Diarrhea	–	20%	43.6%
Palpable mass	18%	54%	40%
Obstruction	–	15%	22%

Table 16.3. Incidence of barium patterns for gastrointestinal NHL radiologic diagnosis

Radiologic pattern	Stomach (570 cases)	Small intestine (200 cases)	Colon (118 cases)
Ulcerated form	49%	33.5%	3.5%
Tumoral form (>3 cm diameter)	36%	43%	50%
Infiltrating form		53%	
Non-stenosing	22%	33%[a]	25.5%
Stenosing		20%	
Hypertrophic form	19%		
Nodular form (<3 cm diameter)	2%	4.5%	45.5%
Frequency of combined forms	28%	34%	24.5%
Radiologic diagnosis of:			
NHL	13%	30%	0%
Malignancy	77%	20%–50%	50%–70%

[a] Aneurysmal form in 17%.

40%–75% of gastric sarcomas and 3%–5% of all gastric neoplasms (Burgess et al. 1971; Kline and Glatstein 1973; Sandler 1984). In a review of 1100 cases (Bruneton et al. 1986), average patient age was 59 years, and 65% of patients were male. Table 16.2 summarizes the frequencies of clinical symptoms. Dysphagia was rare (2.1% of cases) and associated with lesions of the upper third of the stomach, with or without extension to the esophagus. Perforation occurred in 3.6% of cases. The site of predilection is the antrum (62.7%) (Lecomte et al. 1980b). Owing to the absence of a fibroblastic stroma reaction, lesions attained 10 cm or more in two-thirds of cases (Joseph and Lattes 1966; McNeer and Berg 1959; Menuck 1976; Sherrick et al. 1965).

For a long period, endoscopy and biopsies were disappointing for diagnosis of gastric lymphoma because of the submucosal or necrotic nature of these lesions. The three endoscopic patterns encountered for NHL include diffuse infiltration, ulceration, and polypoid lesions. These patterns have no anatomic correlation and are not correlated with the grade of lymphoma (Taal et al. 1987). Improvement of the accuracy of biopsies requires brush cytology, multiple biopsies (at least ten), and repeated biopsies on the same site to reach the submucosa (Lozowski and Hajdu 1984; Taal et al. 1987). For teams that use such investigative protocols, the sensitivity of endoscopic biopsy is between 44% and 96% (Dragosics et al. 1985; Fork et al. 1985; Spinelli et al. 1980).

Potential associated lesions include chronic gastritis (60% for Brooks and Enterline 1983),

gastric Crohn's disease (Kini et al. 1986), and pseudolymphoma. The endoscopic appearance of this last pathology (also referred to as focal lymphoid hyperplasia or reactive lymphorecticular hyperplasia) often suggests adenocarcinoma (especially an erosive pattern, but also an ulcerative or submucosal nodular pattern). The differential diagnosis for lymphoma may require immunohistologic staining for lymphocytic markers (Lerman-Sagie et al. 1985; Tokunaga et al. 1987). Pseudolymphomas may degenerate into lymphomas (Scoazec et al. 1986; Tokunaga et al. 1987).

The prognosis for gastric NHL is twice as favorable as for gastric cancer: 82% for grade I lesions; 44% for grade II (Brooks et al. 1983). The overall survival rate at 5 years is now over 50% (Remine and Braasch 1986; Sandler 1984; Thorling 1984).

16.1.2.1 Radiologic Features (Figs. 16.2–16.11)

Imaging studies are especially important because of the limitations of endoscopy. Table 16.3 lists the findings for barium studies of 570 cases (Bruneton et al. 1986). The rarity of stenosing tumors in the stomach is related

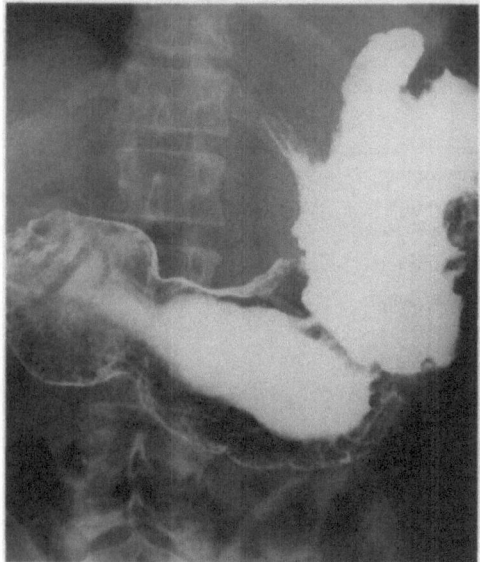

Fig. 16.2. Lymphoma of the upper third of the stomach (infiltrating tumoral lesion)

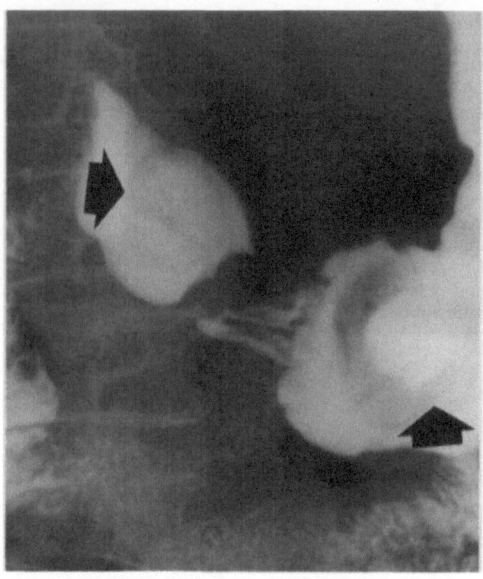

Fig. 16.4. Gastric lymphoma: association of an ulcerated gastric lesion and an ulcerated lesion of the bulb *(arrows)*

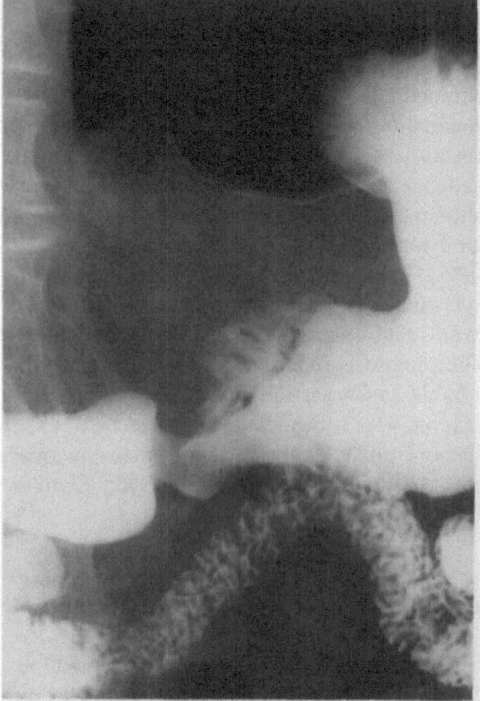

Fig. 16.3. Primary gastric lymphoma: unusual stenosing infiltrating lesion

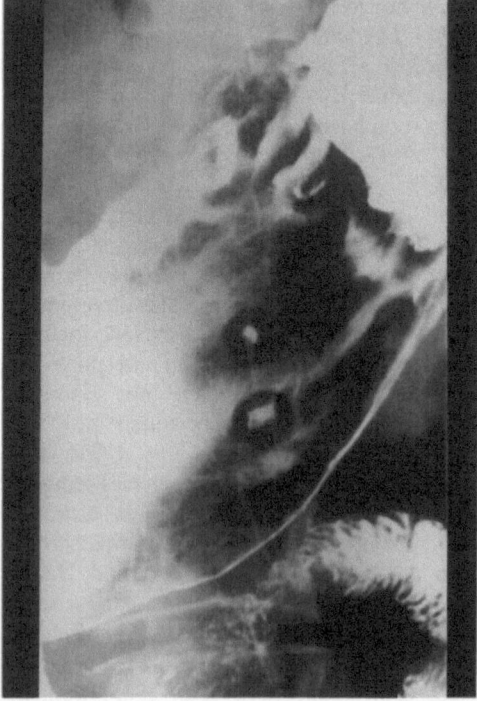

Fig. 16.5. Primary lymphoma of the stomach: multiple ulcerated lesions. (Courtesy of Dr. Schmutz, Strasbourg, France)

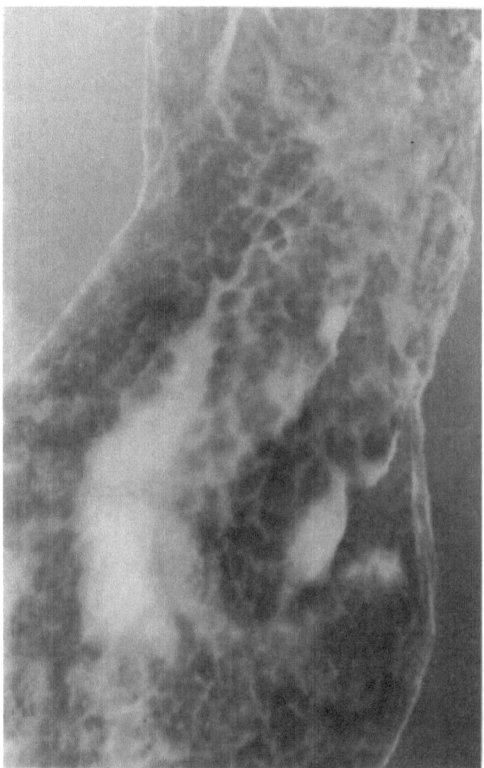

Fig. 16.6. Diffuse submucosal infiltration of the entire stomach: the mucosa was endoscopically normal

to the absence of a fibroblastic stroma reaction. Complex lesions exist in 28% of patients, and 14.7% of them have diffuse gastric disease (Contreary et al. 1980; Green et al. 1979; Hricak et al. 1980). While a lesion in the antrum, the site of predilection, is non-diagnostic in itself, lesion size (10 cm or more) is suggestive of NHL prior to histologic confirmation, even though clinical signs may be minimal. Both Meyers et al. (1975) and Hricak et al. (1980) have cited extragastric extension as another characteristic of the disease. According to Hricak et al. (1980), 10% of cases spread to the distal esophagus; extension to the duodenum is even more frequent (33%). The features of the early or minimal lymphomatous lesions described by Sato et al. (1986) include slight enlargement of folds with a smooth contour suggesting submucosal tumor infiltration and constant ulceration as a unicentral, indefinite shallow depression.

The radiographic features of gastric NHL are helpful for differential diagnosis, because cancer is often hard to exclude solely on the basis of symptoms. Hypertrophic folds are suggestive of benign or diffuse hypertrophy, or Ménétrier's disease (Marshak et al. 1976a). Gastric ulcer is occasionally entertained as a possibility for benign-appearing filling defects.

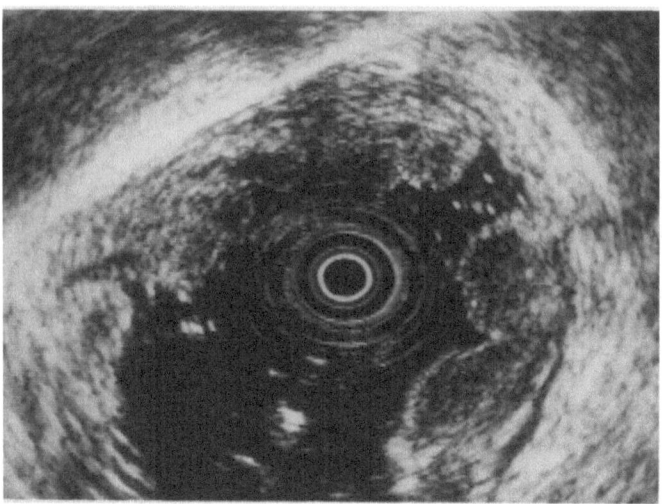

Fig. 16.7. Endosonography of a gastric lymphoma: nodular lesion without extension towards the muscularis propria

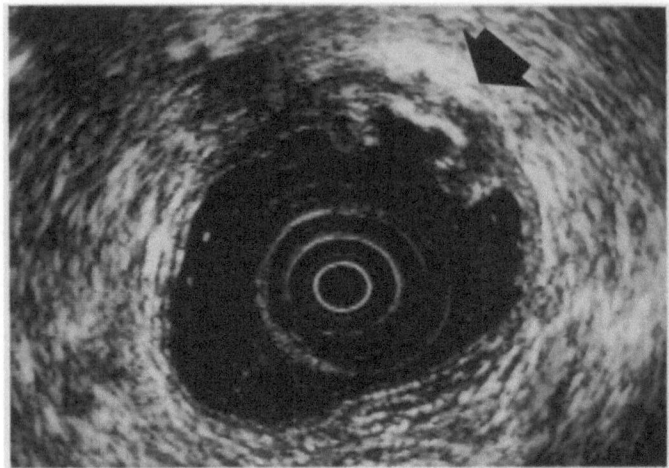

Fig. 16.8. Endosonography of a gastric lymphoma: ulceration with thick borders destroying the gastric wall *(arrow)*

Nodular lesions, often contiguous to a tumoral mass, may suggest other gastric sarcomas (Calenoff 1972; Salmela and Kohler 1969). Benign lymphoid hyperplasia can resemble gastric NHL both clinically and radiologically. Of the AIDS patients explored by barium studies, 84% had multiple, diffuse lesions (Wall et al. 1986). Most of these abnormalities have an infectious etiology (*Candida albicans,* herpes, cytomegalovirus), but associations of Kaposi's sarcoma and lymphoma have also been reported (Dworkin et al. 1985; Frager et al. 1986). The radiographic patterns of uncomplicated AIDS can resemble those of lymphoma (for example, a multinodular pattern).

Barium studies have a diagnostic accuracy of 77% for malignant tumors and 13% for lymphoma. In very large series, the lymphoma detection rate has even reached 56%. Barium follow-up examinations of patients with gastric lymphoma treated by radiotherapy and/or chemotherapy may demonstrate a return to normal without scar tissue formation (Krudy et al. 1983), tumor regression with development of a benign or malignant ulcer (Fox et al. 1984), stenosing lesions with appearance of linitis plastica (Libshitz et al. 1985), ulceration, or tumoral perforation.

Ultrasonography offers several advantages (Salem and Hiltz 1978; Lorenz et al. 1987; Yeh

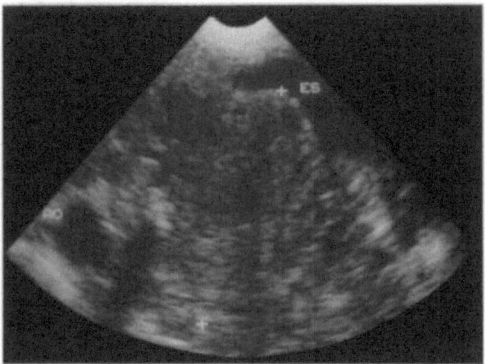

Fig. 16.9. Gastric lymphoma: ultrasonography demonstrated a solid mass displacing the gastric lumen anteriorly. *ES,* stomach; *AO,* aorta (85 mm between the *two crosses*)

and Rabinowitz 1981): detection of gastric wall thickening (corresponding to submucosal infiltration) as a solid, but very hypoechoic or even fluid pattern and detection of celiomesenteric and retroperitoneal adenopathies during disease staging. Sonoendoscopy allows more precise workups because it can demonstrate localized or extensive hypoechoic infiltration and thickening of the gastric wall or a polypoid pattern (Bolondi et al. 1987). Staging is better because sonoendoscopy accurately analyzes the various layers of the gastric wall (Tio et al. 1986).

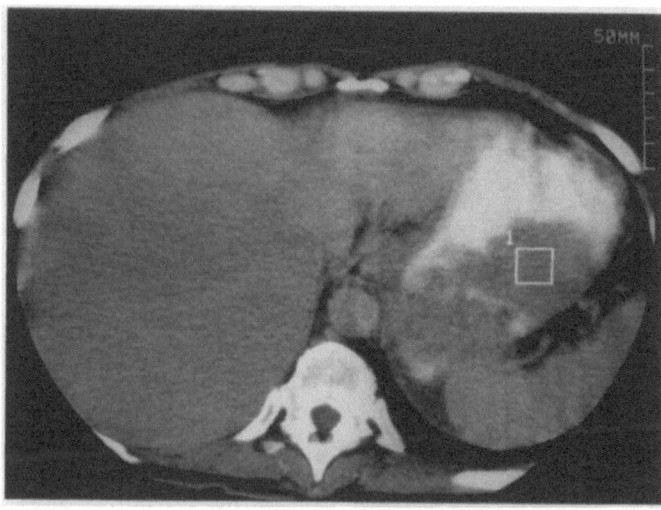

Fig. 16.10. Gastric lymphoma: solid lesion (58 HU in *square 1*) infiltrating the body of the stomach. Scans did not demonstrate any nodal enlargement

CT is the technique of choice for pretherapy staging of gastric lymphoma. Infiltration of the gastric wall is well visualized by CT, even though this pattern is not specific (Balfe et al. 1981; Brown et al. 1982; Buy and Moss 1982; Lorenz et al. 1987; Megibow 1986; Stetter et al. 1984; Yeh and Rabinowitz 1981). CT is less sensitive than barium studies for detection of small lesions (Megibow 1986). CT findings for gastric lymphoma include thickening (2–8 cm) of over half the stomach wall, focal parietal thickening, and ulcerated polypoid masses. Pre- and post-therapy perforation can be identified on CT scans as a fluid collection associated with a lymphomatous mass or an abscess, but never free intraperitoneal air (Megibow 1986). Although gastric wall thickening is nonspecific, certain signs suggest lymphoma rather than adenocarcinoma: sharp definition of the outer contour of the mass, presence of retroperitoneal adenopathies, greater wall thickening than with adenocarcinoma.

Gastric NHL can thus be diagnosed by barium contrast radiography completed by CT or ultrasonography, keeping in mind the following general features:

- Radiological lesions at least 10 cm in diameter in over two-thirds of cases.
- Lack of correlation between often discrete clinical symptoms and large radiologic lesions.
- Rarity of stenosing forms.
- Frequency of complex forms, which may spread to the esophagus and especially to the duodenum.

16.1.3 Small Intestine

The second most frequent site of gastrointestinal NHL is the small intestine (Table 16.1) (Contreary et al. 1980; Freeman et al. 1972; Green et al. 1979; Jones et al. 1973; Novak et al. 1979). Multiple gastrointestinal disease sites are common, and 35%–50% of all patients with gastrointestinal lymphoma have intestinal lesions. Primary NHL accounts for 10%–40% of all intestinal neoplasms (O'Rourke et al. 1986), and is the most common intestinal tumor in children (Goldthorn and Canizaro 1986). A significant geographic factor has been identified, particularly in the Far East, where intestinal lesions are the most common primary gastrointestinal NHL as well as the most frequent malignancy of the small intestine (Al Mondhiry 1986; Cooper and Read 1985).

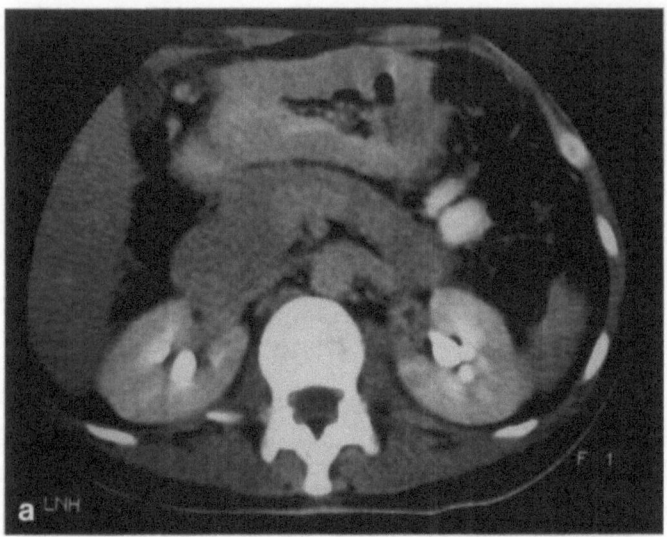

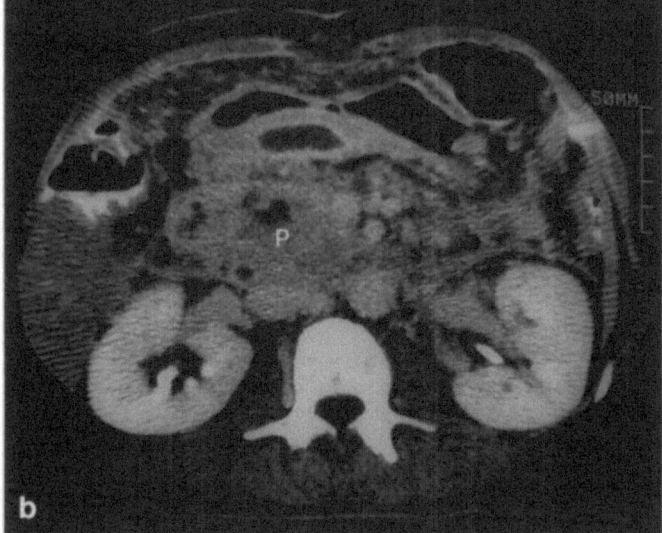

Fig. 16.11a, b. CT study of the relationships of gastric lymphomas with neighboring organs. **a** Thickening of the entire gastric antrum without invasion of the adjacent structures (particularly the pancreas). **b** Lymphomatous infiltration of the posterior aspect of the stomach associated with nodal involvement and especially infiltration of the head of the pancreas *(P)*

16.1.3.1 General Features

The general characteristics of intestinal NHL were drawn from a review of some 700 cases in the literature (Bruneton et al. 1986). Average patient age was 47 years; 57% of patients were male. Table 16.2 lists the associated clinical symptoms. The palpable mass noted in 54% of patients corresponded either to the lymphomatous lesion itself or to stasis above the tumor causing obstruction. Obstruction occurred in 15% of patients, perforation in 14.5% (Contreary et al. 1980), and malabsorption in 7% (Cupps et al. 1969; Fu and Perkin 1972; Green et al. 1979; Isaacson et al. 1979; Loehr et al. 1969). Lymphoma is a rare complication of celiac disease (Cooper and Read 1985; Skinner 1985). Intestinal lymphoma has also been reported as a complication of AIDS (Steinberg et al. 1985).

Burkitt's lymphoma, which generally affects persons under the age of 30, is invariably accompanied by symptoms which include diarrhea and malabsorption. The entire small intestine is involved, although the terminal ileum is often spared. The gastrointestinal tract is affected much more frequently by Burkitt's lymphoma than by other forms of NHL. Most lesions occur in the ileum (68%), but both the jejunum (38%) and duodenum (12%) can be affected (Cupps et al. 1969; Dunnick et al. 1979; Loehr et al. 1969; Nassar et al. 1978).

Multiple disease sites in different segments (18%) or in the same segment (16%) of the small intestine occur in 34% of patients (Lecomte et al. 1980a). Lesions exceed 5 cm in over 77% of cases; smaller lesions correspond to focal stenosing lesions or multinodular disease.

Although the overall prognosis for primary NHL of the intestine is comparable to that for gastric lymphomas, association with an immunoproliferative disease carries a poor prognosis (Bush and Ash 1969; Vessal et al. 1980).

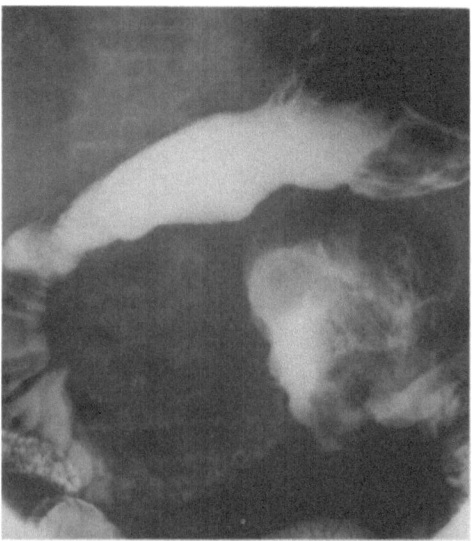

Fig. 16.12. Lymphoma of the duodenojejunal flexure (pseudoaneurysmal lesion)

16.1.3.2 Radiographic Features
(Figs. 16.12–16.15)

Table 16.3 lists the frequencies of radiologic features based on 200 cases in the literature (Bruneton et al. 1986). Infiltrating forms represent over one-half of all cases (53%). Owing to the absence of a fibroblastic stroma reaction, the lumen is generally dilated by tumoral infiltration. Constricting lesions are less common. The most frequent radiologic findings are nonconstricting lesions with thickened folds, occasionally with a pseudonodular appearance or loss of the mucous membrane pattern, or with a classic aneurysmal appearance (17%). Aneurysmal forms are suggestive of NHL. Radiologically, these lesions have been compared to a length of garden hose whose supra- and subjacent segments seem normal (Norfray et al. 1973). Aneurysmal lesions can reach considerable dimensions. The distal loop cannot be opacified until relatively late in the examination owing to the large dimensions of the lesion and the loss of peristaltic capacity. Lu-

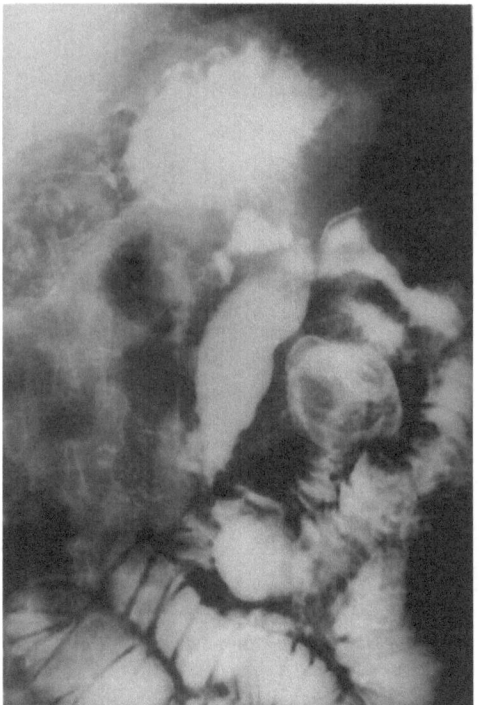

Fig. 16.13. Non-stenosing, infiltrating jejunal lymphoma

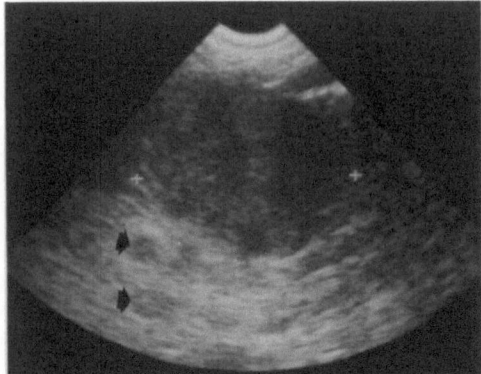

Fig. 16.14. Ultrasound study of a duodenojejunal lymphoma: this solid, partially necrotic (lower edge) lesion was associated with deep nodal infiltration *(arrows)* (75 mm between the *two crosses*)

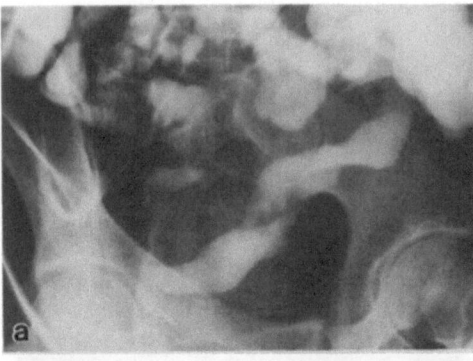

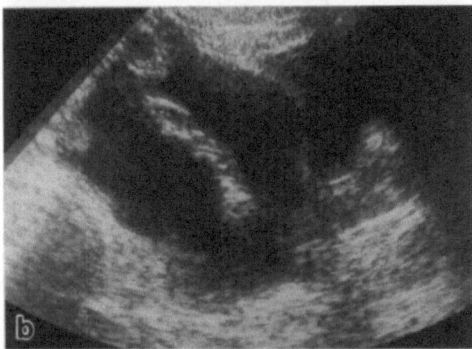

Fig. 16.15a, b. Barium examination of an ileal lymphoma **(a)** and sonographic study **(b)**

men dilatation is variable. The mottled appearance of the barium on early films corresponds to secretions and food particles trapped in the dilated loop. Both segmental dilatation near a fibrous or neoplastic inflammatory zone and scleroderma (which causes dilatation but is characterized by long atonic segments with atrophic connivent valvulae) can be ruled out because of the complete disappearance of the connivent valvulae. In rare instances, however, connective tissue sarcomas have a similar radiologic appearance. Infiltrating growths are an infrequent cause of lumen narrowing: 9.1% of such lesions are constricting multinodular tumors while 10.9% are ulcerative forms associated with loss of mucosal markings. The differential diagnosis for focal lesions is carcinoma (Levine et al. 1987). When large segments of intestine appear involved, confusion is possible with peritoneal carcinosis.

Tumoral lesions, accounting for 43% of intestinal NHL, may present as an extraluminal mass (22.5%), an intramural tumor or intraluminal mass (18%), or a dumbbell tumor (2.5%).

For predominantly extraluminal mesenteric masses, a further distinction is made between nodal forms and sprue. In nodal forms, an extrinsic mass syndrome is created by mesenteric adenopathies which displace the adjacent loops. Sprue patterns, observed in 10.1% of cases (Marshak et al. 1976b), are always clinically signalled by diarrhea; 30% of patients also have steatorrhea. The radiographic features for extraluminal masses include dilated loops with prominent mucosa and signs of flocculation and segmentation. Both intramural and intraluminal forms cause obstruction, and especially intussusception (Greco et al. 1986) owing to their large size (5–7 cm long). Intra-extraluminal (dumbbell) forms are much rarer, but can lead to fistula formation in adjacent loops. Ulcerating lesions (33.5% of cases) are often associated with infiltrating and multinodular forms.

Nodular lesions tend to be multiple and under 3 cm in diameter; they image as numerous filling defects, and the mucosa projects upwards and appears "studded". The lumen is not narrowed by these rare forms, which account for only 4.5% of cases. The differential diagnosis is regional enteritis (Sartoris et al. 1984). Nodular lesions are common in Burkitt's lymphoma (Ramos et al. 1978). Thirty-four percent of the review cases mentioned the simultaneous presence of various combinations of these radiologic forms. Diffuse multinodular disease, which can involve the entire gastrointestinal tract, is extremely rare (Harris et al. 1976; Petzel and Mathea 1972). Tumors generally cause obstruction (9.5% of cases, including 6% for intussusception). The frequencies reported by radiologic studies were lower than those for clinical investigations since barium studies (not even a barium enema) are not always performed when there are clinical symptoms of obstruction. Fistulae, observed in 1.7% of cases, are generally associated with dumbbell tumors. Perforation was noted in 5% of cases. Radiologic exploration of complicated forms was often limited to an abdominal plain film.

Radiologic studies correctly diagnose intestinal malignancy in 20%–50% of cases and lymphoma in 30% (Loehr et al. 1969). Less frequent diagnoses prior to histologic confirmation include regional enteritis (Federman et al. 1963) and polyposis. As for exploration of the stomach, various other techniques have been proposed. *Angiography,* though rarely used, has demonstrated avascular lesions without neovascularity or venous phase abnormalities. This technique currently appears to have no indications for diagnosis of small bowel NHL (Boijsen and Reuter 1966; Lunderquist et al. 1971). By contrast, *CT* is increasingly performed; as for gastric lesions, CT can demonstrate intestinal wall thickening and enlarged mesenteric nodes that suggest the diagnosis of lymphoma (Megibow 1986; Thompson and Halvorsen 1987). Smaller lesions may be diagnosed as Crohn's disease or metastases, especially in the absence of adenopathy (Megibow 1986). The thickened intestinal wall visible on *sonograms* is often very hypoechoic or even cyst-like (Miller et al. 1980). Cavitating masses (aneurysmal pattern) can also be detected by ultrasonography (Hamza et al. 1987).

16.1.4 Colon and Rectum

16.1.4.1 General Features

Primary NHL of the colon and rectum is rare, representing only 0.1% of all cases of NHL (Freeman et al. 1972). Colorectal sites follow gastric and intestinal sites in frequency, and account for an average of 15% of cases (Table 16.1). Lymphoma is exceptional, though, being the cause of only 0.5% of all malignant tumors of the colon and rectum (Zornoza and Dodd 1980). Nearly 400 cases were reviewed to define the general features of colorectal NHL (Bruneton et al. 1986). The average age of patients at diagnosis was 50 years (range 3–82 years) and 64% of patients were male. Patients with primary lesions were generally younger than those with secondary colorectal involvement (Herrmann et al. 1980). The average age of patients with primary ileocecal lesions was much lower (around 30 years).

Table 16.2 summarizes the associated clinical symptoms. Palpable masses, noted in 40% of patients, corresponded either to the tumor itself or to stercoral stasis above a site of stenosis. As for gastric and intestinal NHL, asymptomatic involvement was rare, especially with secondary forms; this is in contradiction to autopsy findings (Okamato et al. 1973). NHL can develop as a complication of hemorrhagic rectocolitis (Wig et al. 1980), while lymphomatous colonic lesions may be complicated by colonic pneumatosis or acute colectasia (O'Connell and Thompson 1978).

The sites of colonic NHL, in decreasing order of frequency, are the cecum (52.5% of cases), rectum (21.2%), right colon (13.8%), left colon (13.5%), and transverse colon (5.6%). Concomitant ileal involvement exists in 38% of patients with primary NHL of the colon (Herrmann et al. 1980; Wychulis et al. 1966).

Except for pseudopolypoid forms, primary lesions have an average diameter of over 5 cm (8 cm for Wychulis et al. 1966). Diffuse, often nodular forms usually range from 2 mm to 2.5 cm. The prognosis for primary lesions (34%–55.2% survival at 5 years) contrasts markedly with the unfavorable outlook for secondary involvement (less than 1 year for all authors) (Herrmann et al. 1980; Wychulis et al. 1966).

16.1.4.2 Radiographic Features
(Figs. 16.16–16.21)

Table 16.3 summarizes the radiographic findings reported in 118 review cases, either alone or in combination. Tumors (intramural or intraluminal, dumbbell, and purely mesenteric forms) predominated (50%). Intraluminal tumors, the most prevalent (30%), are a common cause of obstruction, with or without intussusception, owing to their average size of 5–10 cm. The usual diagnosis for these generally primary tumors based on radiologic findings is carcinoma (O'Connell and Thompson 1978; Taleb et al. 1975). Dumbbell tumors, which account for 19% of cases, are also frequently misdiagnosed as carcinoma. Purely mesenteric forms represent only 1% of cases.

Small intramural or intraluminal nodular lesions represent 45.5% of cases. These often multiple forms can reach 2.5 cm in diameter and be mistaken for ulcerative colitis, Crohn's disease, amebiasis, or pseudomembranous co-

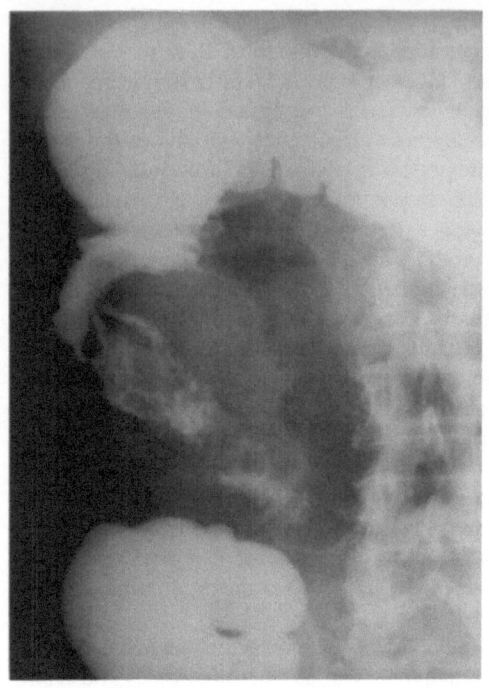

Fig. 16.17. Cecal lymphoma (infiltrating tumor)

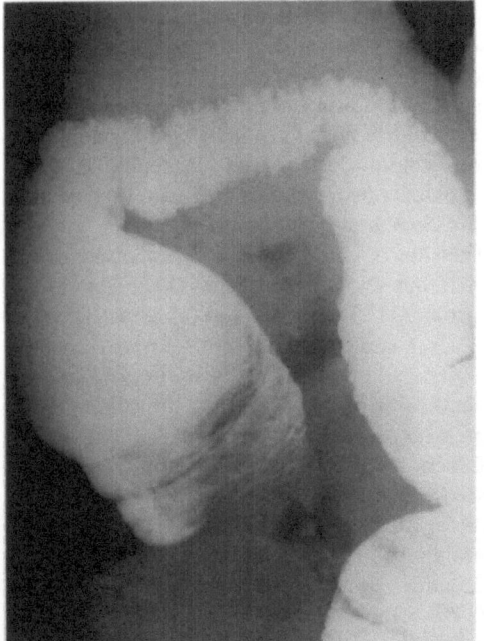

Fig. 16.16. Cecal lymphoma (tumoral lesion)

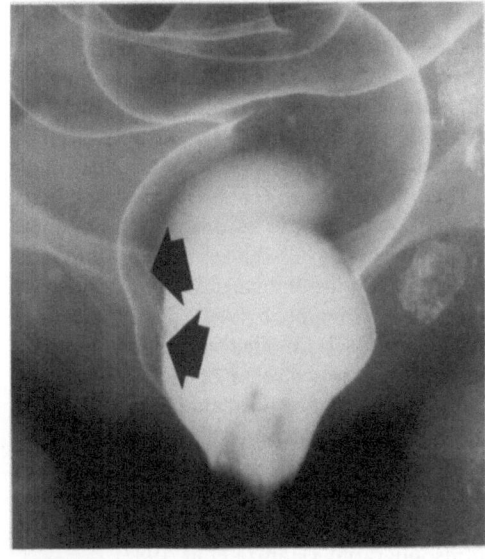

Fig. 16.18. Rectal lymphoma: wall infiltration (arrows) with pelvic adenopathies

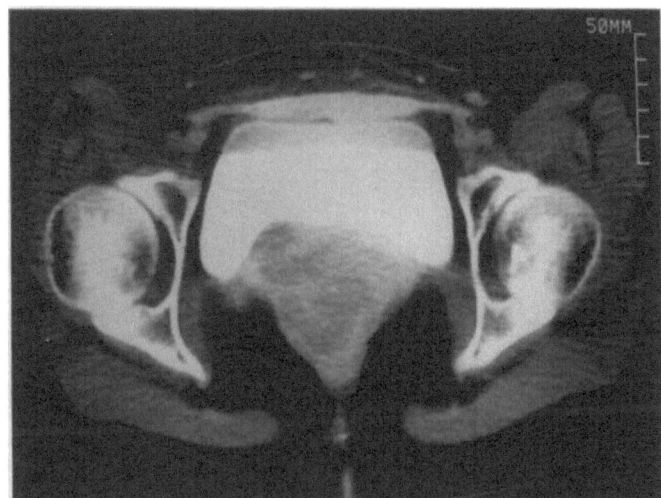

Fig. 16.19. Rectal lymphoma inuading the posterior aspect of the bladder

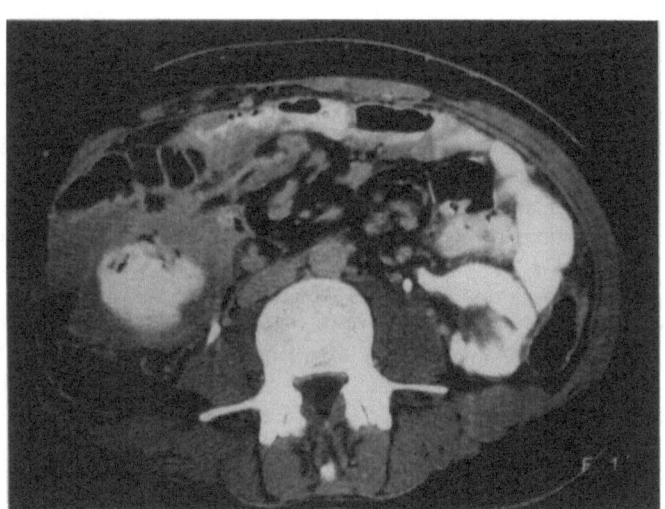

Fig. 16.20. Cecal lymphoma associated with metastatic mesenteric lymph nodes

litis. Smaller lesions may be misdiagnosed as polyposis or lymphoid hypertrophy (Bruneton et al. 1983; De Smet et al. 1976; Richards 1986; Williams et al. 1984).

Diffuse or focal infiltrating disease represents 25.5% of cases. The differential diagnosis is an inflammatory lesion or, when the sigmoid colon is involved, a gynecologic pathology (Zeller et al. 1983). Ulcerating forms are rare in the colon, where they account for only 3.5% of cases. Complex radiologic patterns are observed in 24.5% of patients. In contrast to gastric and intestinal lymphomas, the radiologic features of colonic NHL differ for primary forms (essentially tumors) and secondary involvement (usually multinodular or infiltrating lesions). Infiltrating lesions with thickened folds are the most frequent primary form in the rectum (Taleb et al. 1975). Nodular forms are less common.

Although radiologic studies appear insufficient for the diagnosis of primary colonic or rectal NHL, the occurrence of tumoral forms explains accurate diagnosis of malignancy in 50%-70% of cases.

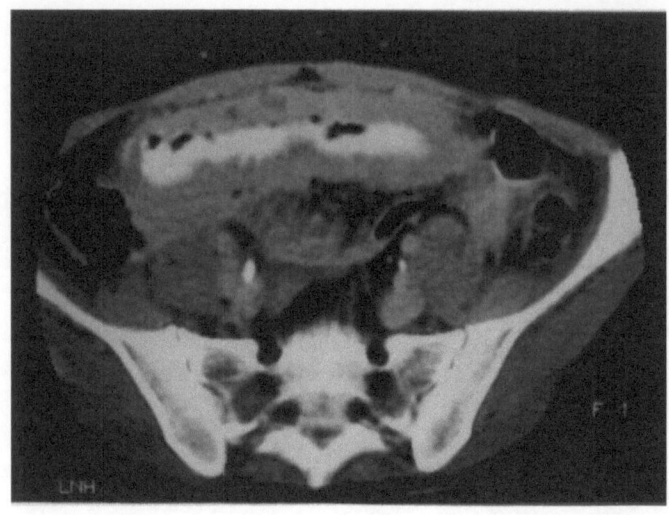

Fig. 16.21. Lymphoma of the transverse colon causing thickening of the entire colon wall in a patient with AIDS

16.2 Hodgkin's Disease

Both primary and secondary gastrointestinal HD are much less frequent than NHL of the gastrointestinal tract. HD represents only 1%-1.7% of all malignant lymphomas of the gastrointestinal tract (Isaacson et al. 1979; Lewin et al. 1978; Aozasa et al. 1985). In the series of Novak and Probst (1973), only 1.2% of all cases of HD concerned gastrointestinal sites. For Portmann et al. (1954), all primary and secondary clinical forms in the gastrointestinal tract accounted for 3.7% of cases.

In addition to the limited involvement of the gastrointestinal tract, HD differs from NHL on a histologic level, since it induces a fibroblastic stroma reaction. Although the resultant lesions are relatively focal, even primary gastrointestinal sites of HD have a poor prognosis because they correspond to stage IV disease. While the rarity of this pathology precludes any general prognostic conclusions, gastrointestinal HD appears to have a less favorable outcome than gastrointestinal NHL.

16.2.1 Esophagus

The esophagus is the least frequent site of gastrointestinal HD (Hoffken et al. 1973; Wood and Coltman 1973). Few reports of primary lesions have been published in the literature (Carnovale et al. 1977; Morrison et al. 1973; Peeples et al. 1979; Shukla and Misra 1979; Trotman et al. 1980). Patients tend to be relatively young (38 years in review cases). Clinical symptoms almost always include dysphagia; weight loss and pain are less common. Totally asymptomatic cases and achalasia are exceptional (Peeples et al. 1979).

As opposed to other gastrointestinal sites of HD, esophageal lesions tend to be large, ranging from 5 to 10 cm in diameter. There do not appear to be any sites of predilection within the esophagus itself. Radiotherapy reportedly always causes a regression in lesion size.

Radiologic findings include esophageal narrowing that is considered malignant before confirmation (Agha and Schnitzer 1985); intramural masses suggesting a benign process, (differential diagnosis leiomyoma or metastasis); and multiple polypoid masses that may appear varicoid. Histologic examination is required to diagnose HD.

16.2.2 Stomach

The general characteristics of gastric HD were defined after the review of 89 literature cases (Bruneton et al. 1986). As indicated in Table 16.4, the stomach is the most common site of gastrointestinal HD (Hoffken et al. 1973; Wood and Coltman 1973). Autopsies

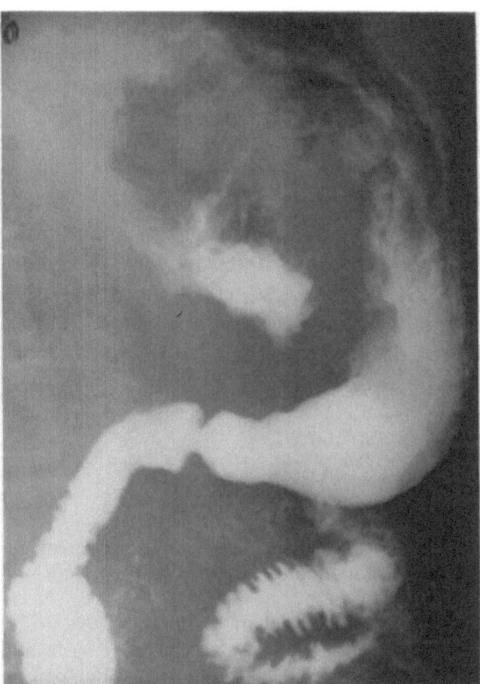

Fig. 16.22. Gastric Hodgkin's disease (ulcerated tumoral syndrome)

Table 16.4. Incidence of gastrointestinal HD

	Esophagus	Stomach	Small intestine	Colon/rectum
Incidence of secondary forms	3.7%	11.4%	5.2%	4.7%
Incidence with respect to NHL	Rare	5.6%	3.3%	Rare
Incidence with respect to other gastrointestinal sites	2%-14.5%	35.8%-50%	24%-35%	13%-27.5%

following generalized lymphoma have demonstrated at least microscopic evidence of gastric involvement in one in every ten cases. HD accounts for 0.5% of all gastric neoplasms and 5.6% of all malignant gastric lymphomas (Kahn et al. 1972; Nicoloff et al. 1963; Sherrick et al. 1965). Common presenting complaints, in decreasing order of frequency, include abdominal pain (67.4% of cases), weight loss (50.6%), anorexia (25.8%), and nausea and vomiting (24.7%).

Lesions are 15 cm or smaller in 71% of cases. The antrum is the site of predilection (55% of cases), but 21% of patients have multiple lesions in the stomach (Portmann et al. 1954). Secondary involvement is often demonstrated radiologically as large folds corresponding to diffuse lesions. The rare primary forms are solitary or multiple tumors which may cause stenosis or ulceration. Histologic confirmation is required to diagnose HD. The diagnosis based solely on radiologic patterns is carcinoma (Fig. 16.22).

16.2.3 Small Intestine

The small intestine is the second most frequent site of gastrointestinal HD after the stomach, yet fewer than 100 cases were reported before 1976. Sixty-six cases were reviewed in the literature (Bruneton et al. 1986). The frequencies are listed in Table 16.4. The average patient age is 49 years (range 22-79 years in review cases), and women are affected more often than men. Clinical symptoms, occurring alone or in combination, include abdominal pain (94% of patients), weight loss (59%), vomiting (41%), diarrhea (35.3%), abdominal mass (29.4%), and bleeding (11.7%). Intestinal HD can complicate steatorrhea or hemorrhagic rectocolitis (Cohen and Canter 1959). The site of predilection is the jejunum (61.6% of cases), followed by the ileum (23%) and the duodenum (15.4%). Lesions are less than or equal to 5 cm in 78% of cases.

The radiologic patterns of intestinal HD include infiltrating forms (58%, 43% of which are stenotic), tumors (58%), and ulcerated lesions (12%). Complex forms occur in 5% of patients, accompanied by obstruction (Cohen and Canter 1959) or signs of intestinal perforation (Edwards 1969). Sixteen percent of patients have multiple intestinal sites. The radiologic appearances of tumors and small stenosing, infiltrating lesions are usually interpreted as carcinoma prior to histologic analysis.

16.2.4 Colon and Rectum

Both primary and secondary HD of the colon and rectum are exceedingly rare, even more so than NHL of these same sites, which is itself infrequent. Only 20 cases affecting the colon were reported before 1970 (Kushelev 1975) and fewer than ten cases involving the rectum were published before 1978 (Laurin 1975). The general features of colonic and rectal HD were defined on the basis of 20 cases in the literature (Bruneton et al. 1986). Table 16.4 summarizes frequency data. The average age of patients at diagnosis was 35 years, and male predominance was noted in the review cases. The most common presenting symptoms, in decreasing order of frequency, are weight loss, bleeding, fever, palpable mass, diarrhea, and pain. The cecum is the site of predilection, being affected more often than either the left colon or the rectum. Barium enemas reveal a higher incidence of infiltrating lesions (stenosing or not) than tumors. Nodular forms are more common than ulcerating lesions in the rectum. Diffuse involvement is exceptional (Dawson et al. 1961), and associations with an ileal lesion are much less common than in NHL (Wig et al. 1980). The rarity of colorectal HD precludes diagnosis solely by radiologic studies.

16.3 Conclusion

Despite the trophism of malignant lymphomas in the gastrointestinal tract, diagnosis of NHL appears possible using the following radiologic criteria:

- Large lesions (10 cm or more in over two-thirds of cases, especially in the stomach)
- A general lack of correlation between vague clinical symptoms and marked radiologic findings.
- The frequency of multiple lesions, present in nearly one-third of cases (different forms in a given gastrointestinal segment or involvement of several different segments).
- The exceptional nature of stenosing lesions owing to the absence of a fibroblastic stroma reaction in NHL.

Diagnosis of NHL is especially important because biopsies are not always conclusive, and patients with gastrointestinal NHL are not always good candidates for surgery. Disease staging should include complete studies of the entire gastrointestinal tract aimed at detecting any associated tumors. By contrast to NHL, both primary and secondary gastrointestinal HD involvement are rare, and always correspond to stage IV lesions. Owing to the absence of a fibroblastic stroma reaction, the radiologic findings are often identical to those of carcinoma.

16.4 References

Agha FP, Schnitzer B (1985) Esophageal involvement in lymphoma. Am J Gastroenterol 80: 412–416

Albin J, Lewis E, Eftekhari F, Shirkhoda A (1987) Computed tomography of rectal and perirectal disease in AIDS patients. Gastrointest Radiol 12: 67–70

Al Mondhiry H (1986) Primary lymphomas of the small intestine: east-west contrast. Am J Hematol 22: 89–105

Aozasa K, Tsujimoto M, Inoue A, Nakagawa K, Hanai J, Kurata A, Nosaka J (1985) Primary gastrointestinal lymphoma. A clinicopathologic study of 102 patients. Oncology 42: 97–103

Balfe DM, Koehler RE, Karstaedt N, Stanley RJ, Sagel SS (1981) Computed tomography of gastric neoplasms. Radiology 140: 431–436

Boijsen E, Reuter SR (1966) Mesenteric angiography in the evaluation of inflammatory and neoplastic disease of the intestine. Radiology 87: 1028–1036

Bolondi L, Casanova P, Caletti GC, Grigioni W, Zani L, Barbara L (1987) Primary gastric lymphoma versus gastric carcinoma: endoscopic US evaluation. Radiology 165: 821–826

Brady LW, Asbell SO (1980) Malignant lymphoma of the gastrointestinal tract. Erskine Memorial Lecture 1979. Radiology 137: 291–298

Brooks JJ, Enterline HT (1983) Primary gastric lymphomas. A clinicopathologic study of 58 cases with long-term follow-up and literature review. Cancer 51: 701–711

Brown BM, Federle MP, Jeffrey RB (1982) Gastric wall thickening and extragastric inflammatory processes: a retrospective CT study. J Comput Assist Tomogr 6: 762–765

Bruneton JN, Thyss A, Bourry J, Bidoli R, Schneider M (1983) Colonic and rectal lymphomas. Report of 6 cases and review of the literature. Fortschr Geb Roentgenstr 138: 283–287

Bruneton JN, Manzino JJ, Caramella E (1986) Gastrointestinal lymphomas. In: Bruneton JN, Schneider M (eds) Radiology of lymphomas. Springer, Berlin Heidelberg New York Tokyo, pp 70-89

Burgess JN, Dockerty MB, Remine WH (1971) Sarcomatous lesions of the stomach. Ann Surg 173: 758-766

Bush RS, Ash CL (1969) Primary lymphoma of the gastrointestinal tract. Radiology 92: 1349-1354

Buy JN, Moss AA (1982) Computed tomography of gastric lymphoma. AJR 859-865

Calenoff L (1972) Gastrointestinal Kaposi's sarcoma: roentgen manifestations. AJR 114: 525-528

Carnovale RL, Goldstein HM, Zornoza J, Dodd GD (1977) Radiologic manifestations of esophageal lymphoma. AJR 128: 751-754

Caruso RD, Berk RN (1970) Lymphoma of the esophagus. Radiology 95: 381-382

Cohen N, Canter JW (1959) Hodgkin's disease of the small intestine. Report of six cases. Am J Dig Dis 4: 361-376

Contreary K, Nance FC, Becker WF (1980) Primary lymphoma of the gastrointestinal tract. Ann Surg 191: 593-598

Cooper BT, Read AE (1985) Small intestinal lymphoma. World J Surg 9: 930-937

Cupps RE, Hodgson JR, Dockerty MB, Adson MA (1969) Primary lymphoma in the small intestine: problems of roentgenologic diagnosis. Radiology 92: 1355-1362

Dawson IMP, Cornes JS, Morson BC (1961) Primary malignant lymphoid tumours of the intestinal tract. Report of 37 cases with a study of factors influencing prognosis. Br J Surg 49: 80-89

De Smet AA, Tubergen DG, Martel W (1976) Nodular lymphoid hyperplasia of the colon associated with dysgammaglobulinemia. AJR 127: 515-517

Dragosics B, Bauer P, Radaszkiewicz T (1985) Primary gastrointestinal non-Hodgkin's lymphomas. A retrospective clinicopathologic study of 150 cases. Cancer 55: 1060-1073

Dunnick NR, Reaman GH, Head GL, Shawker TH, Ziegler JL (1979) Radiographic manifestations of Burkitt's lymphoma in American patients. AJR 132: 1-6

Dworkin B, Wormser GP, Rosenthal WS, Heier SK, Braumstein M, Weiss L, Jankowski R, Levy D, Weiselberg S (1985) Gastrointestinal manifestations of the acquired immunodeficiency syndrome: a review of 22 cases. Am J Gastroenterol 80: 774-778

Edwards RT (1969) Hodgkin's sarcoma of the small bowel. Va Med Mon 96: 521-525

Ehrlich AN, Stalder G, Geller W, Sherlock P (1968) Gastrointestinal manifestations of malignant lymphoma. Gastroenterology 54: 1115-1121

Federman J, Goldstein ME, Weingarten A (1963) Malignant lymphoma of over 15 years' duration masquerading as ulcerative colitis. AJR 89: 771-778

Fork FT, Haglund U, Hogstrom H, Wehlin L (1985) Primary gastric lymphoma versus gastric cancer: an endoscopic and radiographic study of differential diagnostic possibilities. Endoscopy 17: 5-7

Fox ER, Laufer I, Levine MS (1984) Response of gastric lymphoma to chemotherapy: radiographic appearance. AJR 142: 711-714

Frager DH, Frager JD, Brandt LJ, Wolf EL, Rand LG, Klein RS, Beneventano TC (1986) Gastrointestinal complications of AIDS: radiologic features. Radiology 158: 597-603

Freeman C, Berg JW, Cutler SJ (1972) Occurrence and prognosis of extranodal lymphomas. Cancer 29: 252-260

Fu YS, Perkin KH (1972) Lymphosarcoma of the small intestine. A clinicopathologic study. Cancer 29: 645-659

Goldthorn JF, Canizaro PC (1986) Gastrointestinal malignancies in infancy, childhood, and adolescence. Surg Clin North Am 66: 845-861

Greco A, Leung AWL, Swi LJ, Burdett-Smith P, Spencer J, Gibson RN, Allison DJ (1986) Ileocolic intussusception in large cell lymphoma of the terminal ileum. Report of a case. Acta Radiol [Diagn] (Stockh) 27: 687-690

Green JA, Dawson AA, Jones PF, Brunt PW (1979) The presentation of gastrointestinal lymphoma: study of a population. Br J Surg 66: 798-801

Hamza H, Ben Romdhane MH, Allegue M, Fodha M, Tlili-Graiess K, Kraiem C, Letaief R, Laarif M, Jedd M (1987) Les lésions tumorales cavitaires du grêle. Diagnostic radioéchographique. A propos de 4 observations. J Radiol 68: 537-543

Harris ARC, Herrmann RP, Carroll J (1976) Extensive primary lymphoma of the gastrointestinal tract. Aust NZ J Med 6: 571-575

Herrmann R, Panahon AM, Barcos MP, Walsh D, Stutzman L (1980) Gastrointestinal involvement in non-Hodgkin's lymphoma. Cancer 46: 215-222

Hoffken K, Hornung G, Becker G, Schmidt CG (1973) Die gastrointestinale Manifestation des Morbus Hodgkin. Med Welt 24: 731-732

Hricak H, Thoeni RF, Margulis AR, Eyler WR, Francis IR (1980) Extension of gastric lymphoma into the oesophagus and duodenum. Radiology: 135: 309-312

Isaacson P, Wright DH, Judd MA, Mepham BC (1979) Primary gastrointestinal lymphomas. A classification of 66 cases. Cancer 43: 1805-1819

Jones SE, Bull M, Kadin ME, Dorfman RF, Kaplan HS, Rosenberg SA, Kim H (1973) Non-Hodgkin's lymphomas. IV. Clinicopathologic correlation in 405 cases. Cancer 31: 806-823

Joseph JI, Lattes R (1966) Gastric lymphosarcoma. Clinicopathologic analysis of 71 cases and its relation to disseminated lymphosarcoma. Am J Clin Pathol 45: 653-669

Kahn LB, Selzer G, Kaschula ROC (1972) Primary gastrointestinal lymphoma. A clinicopathologic study of fifty-seven cases. Am J Dig Dis 17: 219-232

Kini SU, Pai PK, Rao PK, Kini AU (1986) Primary gastric lymphoma associated with Crohn's disease of the stomach. Am J Gastroenterol 81: 23-25

Kline TS, Goldstein F (1973) Malignant lymphoma involving the stomach. Cancer 32: 961-968

Krudy AG, Long JL, Magrath IT, Shawker TH, Paling M (1983) Gastric manifestations of North American Burkitt's lymphoma. Br J Radiol 56: 697-702

Kushelev AE (1975) Lymphogranulomatosis of the caecum. Vrach Delo 10: 99-100

Laurin S (1975) Cavography and lymphography in Hodgkin's disease. Acta Radiol [Diagn] (Stockh) 16: 98-106

Lecomte P, Bruneton JN, Eloit J, Bourry J, Aubanel D, Schneider M (1980a) Manifestations radiologiques des localisations digestives extragastriques ... lymphomes non-hodgkiniens. A propos de 25 observations. Ann Gastroenterol Hepatol 16: 463-471

Lecomte P, Bruneton JN, Rouison D (1980b) Lymphomes malins de l'estomac. J Can Assoc Radiol 31: 101-106

Lee KR, Levine E, Moffat RE, Bigongiari LR, Hermeck AS (1979) Computed tomographic staging of malignant gastric neoplasms. Radiology 133: 151-155

Lerman-Sagie T, Ziv Y, Rubin M, More C, Dintsman M (1985) Gastric lymphoma versus pseudolymphoma: the importance of immunological differentiation. Am J Gastroenterol 80: 763-766

Levine MS, Sunshine AG, Reynolds JC, Saul SH (1985) Diffuse nodularity in esophageal lymphoma. AJR 145: 1218-1220

Levine MS, Drooz AT, Herlinger H (1987) Annular malignancies of the small bowel. Gastrointest Radiol 12: 53-58

Lewin KJ, Ranchod M, Dorfman RF (1978) Lymphomas of the gastrointestinal tract. A study of 117 cases presenting with gastrointestinal disease. Cancer 42: 693-707

Libshitz HI, Lindell MM, Maor MH, Fuller LM (1985) Appearance of the intact lymphomatous stomach following radiotherapy and chemotherapy. Gastrointest Radiol 10: 25-29

Loehr WJ, Mujahed Z, Zahn FD, Gray GF, Thorbjarnarson B (1969) Primary lymphoma of the gastrointestinal tract: a review of 100 cases. Ann Surg 170: 232-238

Lorenz R, Zankowich R, Modder U, Beyer D (1987) Primares malignes Lymphom des Magens. MDP, Sonographie, Computer Tomographie. Fortschr Geb Roentgenstr 147: 156-160

Lozowski W, Hajdu SI (1984) Preoperative cytologic diagnosis of primary gastrointestinal malignant lymphoma. Acta Cytol (Baltimore) 28: 563-570

Lunderquist A, Lunderquist A, Holmdahl KH, Clemens F (1971) Selective superior mesenteric arteriography in reticular-cell sarcoma of the small bowel. Radiology 98: 113-115

Marshak RH, Lindner AE, Maklansky D (1976a): Lymphosarcoma of the stomach. Am J Gastroenterol 66: 176-184

Marshak RH, Lindner AE, Maklansky D (1976b) Immunoglobulin disorders of the small bowel. Radiol Clin North Am 14: 477-491

Matsura H, Saito R, Nakajima S, Yoshihara W, Enomoto T (1985) Non-Hodgkin's lymphoma of the esophagus. Am J Gastroenterol 80: 941-946

McNeer G, Berg JW (1959) The clinical behavior and management of primary malignant lymphoma of the stomach. Surgery 46: 829-840

Megibow AJ (1986) Gastrointestinal lymphoma: the role of CT in diagnosis and management. Semin Ultrasound CT MR 7: 43-57

Menuck LS (1976) Gastric lymphoma, a radiologic diagnosis. Gastrointest Radiol 1: 157-161

Meyers MA, Katzen B, Alonso DR (1975) Transpyloric extension to duodenal bulb in gastric lymphoma. Radiology 115: 575-580

Miller JH, Hindman BW, Lam AHK (1980) Ultrasound in the evaluation of small bowel lymphoma in children. Radiology 135: 409-414

Morrison FS, Critz F, Tatum WT, Stauss HK (1973) Hodgkin's disease of the esophagus: successful treatment of a rare complication. Cancer 31: 1244-1246

Musshoff K (1977) Klinische Stadieneinteilung der Nicht-Hodgkin-Lymphome. Strahlentherapie 153: 218-221

Nassar VH, Salem PA, Shadid MJ, Alami SY, Balikian JB, Salem AA, Nasrallah SM (1978) "Mediterranean abdominal lymphoma" or immunoproliferative small intestine disease. Part II. Pathological aspects. Cancer 41: 1340-1354

Nicoloff DM, Haynes LB, Wangensteen OH (1963) Primary lymphosarcoma of the gastrointestinal tract. Surg Gynecol Obstet 117: 433-437

Norfray J, Calenoff L, Zanon B (1973) Aneurysmal lymphoma of the small intestine. AJR 119: 335-341

Novak D, Probst P (1973) Morbus Hodgkin: Häufigkeit und Lokalisation der Lungen-, Knochen- und Magen-Darm-Manifestation. Strahlentherapie 146: 403-413

Novak S, Caraveo J, Trowbridge AA, Peterson RF, White RR (1979) Primary lymphomas of the gastrointestinal tract. South Med J 72: 1154-1158

O'Connell DJ, Thompson AJ (1978) Lymphoma of the colon: the spectrum of radiologic changes. Gastrointest Radiol 2: 377-385

Okamato M, Ushio Y, Kinoshita A (1973) Roentgenologic diagnosis of gastrointestinal malignant lymphomas. Stomach Intest (Tokyo) 8: 149-163

O'Rourke MGE, Lancashire RP, Vattoune JR (1986) Lymphoma of the small intestine. Aust NZ J Surg 56: 351-355

Peeples WJ, El Mahdi AM, Rosato FE (1979) Achalasia of the oesophagus associated with Hodgkin disease. J Surg Oncol 11: 213-216

Perfettini C, Cosnard G, Bassoulet J, Tardivel M, Lallemand D (1985) Localisation oesophagienne primitive de lymphome non hodgkinien. A propos d'un cas. J Radiol 66: 377-379

Petzel H, Mathea H (1972) Ausgedehnte lymphatische Hyperplasie im Magen-Darm-Trakt und Lymphosarkomatose. Fortschr Geb Roentgenstr 116: 523-529

Portmann UV, Dunne EF, Hazard JB (1954) Manifestations of Hodgkin's disease of the gastrointestinal tract. AJR 72: 772-787

Privett JTJ, Rhys Davies E, Roylance J (1977) The radiological features of gastric lymphoma. Clin Radiol 28: 457-463

Ramos L, Marcos J, Illanas M, Hernandez-Mora M, Perez-Paya F, Picouto JL, Santana P, Chantar C (1978) Radiologic characteristics of primary intestinal lymphoma of the "Mediterranean" type: observations on twelve cases. Radiology 126: 379-385

Remine SG, Braasch JW (1986) Gastric and small bowel lymphoma. Surg Clin North Am 66: 713-722

Richards MA (1986) Lymphoma of the colon and rectum. Postgrad Med J 62: 615-620

Rosenberg SA, Diamond HD, Jaslowitz B, Craver LF (1961) Lymphosarcoma: a review of 1269 cases. Medicine 40: 31-84

Salem S, Hiltz CW (1978) Ultrasonographic appearance of gastric lymphosarcoma. J Clin Ultrasound 6: 429-430

Salmela H, Kohler R (1969) Roentgenological characteristics of mesenchymal tumours of the stomach. Ann Clin Res 1: 57-63

Sandler RS (1984) Primary gastric lymphoma: a review. Am J Gastroenterol 79: 21-25

Sartoris DJ, Harell GS, Anderson MF, Zboralske FF (1984) Small-bowel lymphoma and regional enteritis: radiographic similarities. Radiology 152: 291-296

Sato T, Sakai Y, Ishiguro S, Furukawa H (1986) Radiologic manifestations of early gastric lymphoma. AJR 146: 513-517

Schmid U, Gloor F, Schildknecht O (1980) Das maligne nicht-Hodgkin-Lymphom des Magens. Dtsch Med Wochenschr 105: 1147-1152

Scoazec JY, Brousse N, Potet F, Jeulain JF (1986) Focal malignant lymphoma in gastric pseudolymphoma. Histologic and immunohistochemical study of a case. Cancer 57: 1330-1336

Sherrick DW, Hodgson JR, Dockerty MB (1965) The roentgenologic diagnosis of primary gastric lymphoma. Radiology 84: 925-932

Shukla HS, Misra MC (1979) Dysphagia in Hodgkin's disease. A case report. Clin Oncol 5: 371-381

Skinner JM (1985) Gastrointestinal lymphoma. Pathology 17: 193-203

Spinelli P, Lo Gullo C, Pizzetti P (1980) Endoscopic diagnosis of gastric lymphomas. Endoscopy 12: 211-214

Steinberg JJ, Bridges N, Feiner HD, Valensi Q (1985) Small intestinal lymphoma in three patients with acquired immune deficiency syndrome. Am J Gastroenterol 80: 21-26

Stetter G, Maydam K, Hering KG (1984) Computertomographische Untersuchungsmerkmale zwischen Adenokarzinom und malignen Lymphom des Magens. Röntgenblätter 37: 317-319

Taal BG, Den Hartog Jaeger FCA, Tytgat GNJ (1987) The endoscopic spectrum of primary non-Hodgkin's lymphoma of the stomach. Endoscopy 19: 190-192

Taleb N, Khouri K, Nassar W (1975) Les lymphomes à localisation digestive primitive. Considérations cliniques, radiologiques et thérapeutiques à propos de 42 observations. J Med Liban 28: 233-258

Thompson WM, Halvorsen RA (1987) Computed tomographic staging of gastrointestinal malignancies. Part II. The small bowel, colon, and rectum. Invest Radiol 22: 96-105

Thorling K (1984) Gastric lymphomas. Clinical features, treatment and prognosis. Acta Radiol [Oncol] 23: 193-197

Tio TL, Den Hartog Jaeger FCA, Tytgat GN (1986) Endoscopic ultrasonography in detection and staging of gastric non-Hodgkin lymphoma. Comparison with gastroscopy, barium meal, and computerized tomography scan. Scand J Gastroenterol 21 (Suppl 123): 52-58

Tokunaga O, Watanabe T, Morimatsu M (1987) Pseudolymphoma of the stomach. A clinicopathologic study of 15 cases. Cancer 59: 1320-1327

Trotman BW, Glick JH, Debarros SGS, Atkinson BF (1980) Dysphagia in a patient with Hodgkin's disease. JAMA 244: 2552-2553

Vessal K, Dutz W, Kohout E, Rezvani L (1980) Immunoproliferative small intestine disease with duodenojejunal lymphoma: radiologic changes. AJR 135: 491-497

Wall SD, Ominsky S, Altman DF, Perkins CL, Sollitto R, Goldberg HI, Margulis AR (1986) Multifocal abnormalities of the gastrointestinal tract in AIDS. AJR 146: 1-5

Wang CC, Petersen JA (1956) Malignant lymphoma of the gastrointestinal tract: roentgenographic consideration. Acta Radiol [Diagn] 46: 523-532

Wig JD, Kohli PK, Kaushik SP, Talwar BL, Bushwarmath SR, Dutta TK (1980) Unusual cause of massive rectal bleeding. Indian J Cancer 17: 276-278

Williams SM, Berk RN, Harned RK (1984) Radiologic features of multinodular lymphoma of the colon. AJR 143: 87-91

Wood NL, Coltman CA (1973) Localized primary extranodal Hodgkin's disease. Ann Intern Med 78: 113-118

Wychulis AR, Beahrs OH, Wollner LB (1966) Malignant lymphoma of the colon. A study of 69 cases. Arch Surg 93: 215-225

Yeh HC, Rabinowitz JG (1981) Ultrasonography and computed tomography of gastric wall lesions. Radiology 141: 147-155

Zeller C, Schmutz G, Giron JP, Kempf F (1983) Aspects radiologiques des localisations rectales et coliques des lymphomes non hodgkiniens. A propos de 30 cas. J Radiol 64: 233-239

Zeller C, Schmutz G, Pauline D, Giron JP, Kempf F (1983) Aspects radiologiques des localisations gastriques des lymphomes malins non hodgkiniens. A propos de 50 observations. J Radiol 64: 225-232

Zornoza J, Dodd GD (1980) Lymphoma of the gastrointestinal tract. Semin Roentgenol 15: 272-287

17 Metastases*

Gastrointestinal metastases of solid tumors are rare. In addition to the relatively common period of clinical latency, an interval of several years can separate diagnosis of the primary carcinoma from the appearance of metastatic disease. Radiographic identification of gastrointestinal metastases can be difficult because imaging features frequently suggest a primary carcinoma, radiation-induced lesions, or benign tumors. Diagnostic accuracy is essential, though, because the course of numerous malignancies such as lung cancer and melanoma, which cause the majority of gastrointestinal metastases, is rapidly unfavorable (Antler et al. 1982; Libshitz et al. 1982; McNeill et al. 1987; Mosimann et al. 1982; Reintgen et al. 1984; Telerman et al. 1985).
A review of the literature was conducted to define the general and radiologic features of these rare lesions. Apparently primary metastases associated with melanoma were excluded (Beirne 1955; De La Pava et al. 1963; Lund 1929; Oddson et al. 1978). The general and radiologic features of esophageal, gastric, intestinal, and colorectal metastases are discussed hereafter by anatomic site. The pathogenetic mechanisms are reviewed together with the radiologic patterns, because they clearly explain the features observed during imaging examinations. Gastrointestinal metastases have a wide variety of appearances. Barium studies are particularly valuable for investigation of intraluminal and ulcerating, nodular lesions while CT and ultrasonography are indicated for exploration of intramural and subserosal lesions (Coscina et al. 1986). In our experience, gastrointestinal metastases are multiple in nearly one-third of cases (Caramella et al. 1983). Radiologic studies of the entire gastrointestinal tract are mandatory complements to local barium examinations when suspicious images, possibly corresponding to a secondary disease site, are detected, especially in patients with melanoma.

17.1 Esophagus

In all, 179 cases of esophageal metastases were reviewed (Agha 1987; Anderson and Hareu 1980; Asch et al. 1968; Atkins 1966; Aubert et al. 1974; Badib et al. 1968; Biller et al. 1982; Butler et al. 1975; Caramella 1983; Chene et al. 1962; Das Gupta and Brasfield 1964a,b; Fisher 1976; Gale et al. 1984; Goldstein et al. 1977; Gouin et al. 1972; Holyoke et al. 1969; Joffe 1978; LeBreuil et al. 1971; Patel et al. 1978; Phadke et al. 1976; Polk et al. 1967; Steiner et al. 1984; Toreson 1944; Touraine et al. 1975; Wood and Wood 1975). The esophagus is the least frequent gastrointestinal site of metastases, accounting for only 0.6%-3.2% of autopsy findings in patients with malignant tumors (Fisher 1976; Toreson 1944).
Breast carcinoma (49.5%) and malignant melanoma (33%) are the most frequent primary etiologies. Lung, thyroid, and other gastrointestinal tract cancers can also metastasize to the esophagus (Agha 1987; Anderson and Harell 1980; Gale et al. 1984; Libshitz et al. 1982; Steiner et al. 1984). The esophagus is the most frequent gastrointestinal site for metastases of breast cancer, but the least common location for metastases of melanomas (Butler et al. 1975; Das Gupta and Brasfield 1964a,b).

---

* Written in collaboration with A. Geoffray.

17.1.1 Clinical Features

Reports of presenting symptoms were available for 56 cases (Table 17.1). Dysphagia, a prevalent feature, had several particularities: sudden onset, unpredictable course with occasional spontaneous improvement (Debaud 1961), indolent and often well-tolerated course (Chene et al. 1962). The incidence of latent esophageal metastases is undoubtedly higher than revealed by our literature review, because Atkins (1966) emphasized the frequency of asymptomatic forms discovered at autopsy.

After contiguous spread of pharyngeal or gastric cancers to the esophagus has been eliminated, and extension of primary mediastinal malignancies and recurrences have been ruled out, the pathogenesis of secondary esophageal involvement is limited to lymphatic spread and hematogenous dissemination. Lymphatic spread is responsible for neoplastic mediastinal fibrosis, histologically comparable to that encountered in the peritoneum with pelvic carcinomas (Lortat-Jacob et al. 1964). This explains metastatic sites in the middle third of the esophagus, especially with carcinoma of the breast, because of the lymphatic connections at this level. Tumor spread along the transdiaphragmatic pathways produces the circumferential stricture of the lower esophagus observed with certain bronchopulmonary tumors involving the lower lobes (Antler et al. 1982; Joffe 1978). Metastases in the cervical esophagus and lower esophagus are rare (Biller et al. 1982; Steiner et al. 1984). Hematogenous metastases are infrequent, and the primary malignancy is usually a melanoma (Fisher 1976).

17.1.2 Radiologic Features (Figs. 17.1–17.3)

The radiologic features identified by review of 92 cases in the literature are summarized in Table 17.2. In the 62 cases analyzed by Agha (1987), secondary esophageal involvement was accurately diagnosed radiologically in 89.3% of patients with direct tumoral extension, in 72.7% with mediastinal spread from the lymph nodes, and in 68.2% with hematogenous spread. Overall, the accurate diagnosis was suggested in 78% of patients. Lymphatic

Table 17.1. Clinical symptoms (associated or not) of gastrointestinal metastases reported in the literature (635 cases)

	Esophagus (56 cases)	Stomach (125 cases)	Small intestine (354 cases)	Colon/rectum (100 cases)
Dysphagia	80.3%	5.6%	–	–
Bleeding	3.6%	27.6%	36.7%	24%
Pain	5.4%	34.4%	15.8%	54%
Chronic obstruction	–	18.4%	6%	13%
Acute obstruction	–	8%	21.7%	7%
Weight loss	21.4%	29.6%	37.0%	10%
Mass	–	4%	3.1%	14%
Asymptomatic	7.5%	32.8%	9.9%	14%

Table 17.2. Radiologic features of gastrointestinal metastases reported in the literature (868 cases)

	Esophagus (92 cases)	Stomach (193 cases)	Small intestine (407 cases)	Colon/rectum (176 cases)
Intramural	14.1%	10.3%	8.3%	15.3%
Intraluminal	14.1%	56.5%	39.9%	19.9%
Subserosal	53.5%	7.3%	20.9%	13.1%
Infiltrating	18.5%	25.9%	30.9%	51.7%
Ulcerative	16.3%	47.6%	25.6%	11.9%

spread from breast carcinoma usually produces subserosal or infiltrating lesions causing stricture of the middle third of the esophagus. Intramural and intraluminal lesions are associated with hematogenous spread, and thus with melanoma. The differential diagnosis for concentric stenosis due to infiltrative disease is radiation damage, especially for breast cancer patients, who are often treated by radiotherapy. Less frequent differential diagnoses based on radiologic features include primary esophageal carcinoma and peptic esophagitis. The radiologic diagnosis for intramural lesions may be a benign tumor. Awareness of the pathophysiology and features of esophageal metastases can have a major influence on the endoscopic, histologic, and therapeutic results. Endoscopy can identify atresia and infiltration (Chene et al. 1962), but the usual diagnosis is stenosis due to scar tissue formation rather than a neoplasm; this is because the mucosa is merely only congestive or the folds are intact

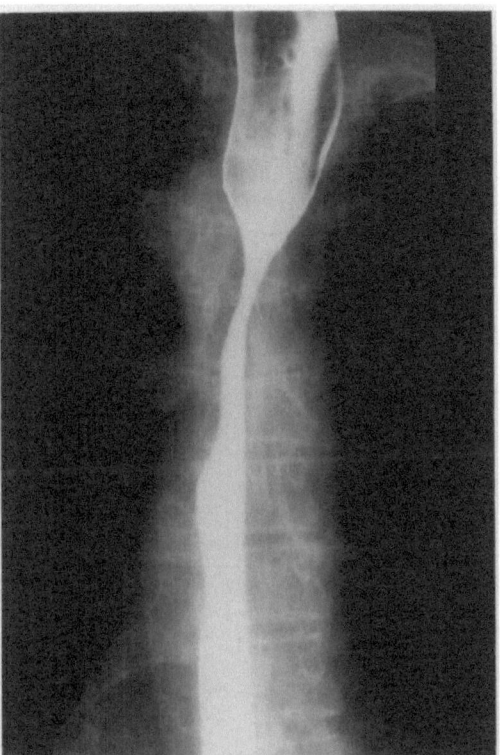 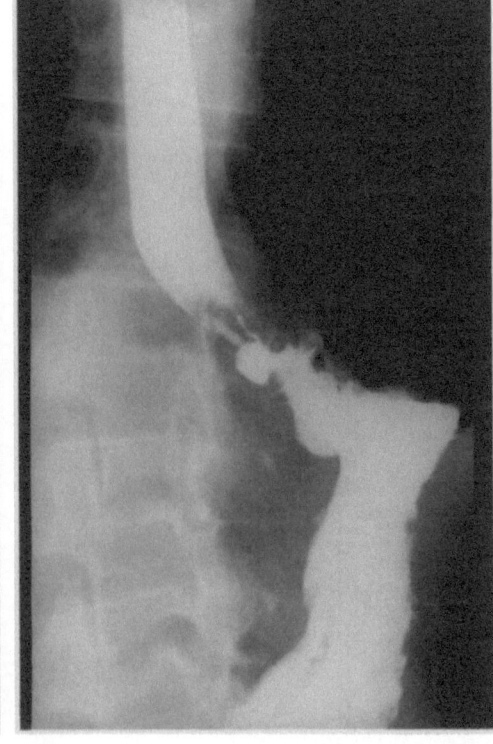

Fig. 17.1. Stenosis of the middle third of the esophagus caused by a metastasis of breast cancer

Fig. 17.2. Ulcerated lesion of the esogastric junction (lung cancer metastasis)

(Atkins 1966). Failure of biopsy to detect lesions can be explained by the exceptional, and often late occurrence of mucosal invasion. Deep biopsies are not advisable because of the risk of perforation of the weakened wall (Biller et al. 1982; Gouin et al. 1972), but comprehensive analysis of clinical, etiologic, radiologic, and endoscopic findings often allows appropriate therapy. Instrumental dilatation of the esophagus is contraindicated (Atkins 1966), but radiotherapy with or without adjuvant chemotherapy has proved effective (Holyoke et al. 1969; Polk et al. 1967). In conclusion, apparently extrinsic stricture of the middle third of the esophagus, with the presence of normal mucosa, should suggest the diagnosis of esophageal metastasis in patients with recognized breast cancer (Chene et al. 1962; Gouin et al. 1972).

17.2 Stomach

A total of 259 cases was reviewed in the literature (Asch et al. 1968; Auriol et al. 1958; Backman 1969; Badib et al. 1968; Beckly 1974; Choi et al. 1964; Das Gupta and Brasfield 1964a,b; Dick and Pattinson 1972; Doutre et al. 1972; Faguer et al. 1975; Fingerhut et al. 1977; Fraser-Moodie et al. 1976; Glick et al. 1985; Goldstein et al. 1977; Hartmann and Sherlock 1961; Higgins 1962; Hillemans et al. 1961; Joffe 1975; Klein and Sherlock 1972; Laval-Jeantet et al. 1975; Lebreuil et al. 1971; Lorriaux and Capron 1974; Menuck and Amberg 1975; Michalet et al. 1977; Morton and Tedesco 1974; Patel et al. 1978; Rodde et al. 1987; Rubin and Davis 1985; Scobie 1966; Shah et al. 1977; Simao 1963).

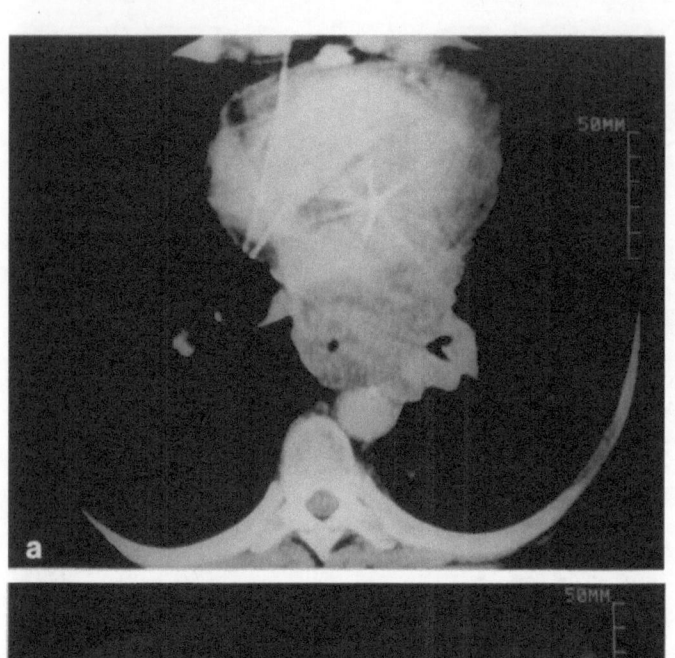

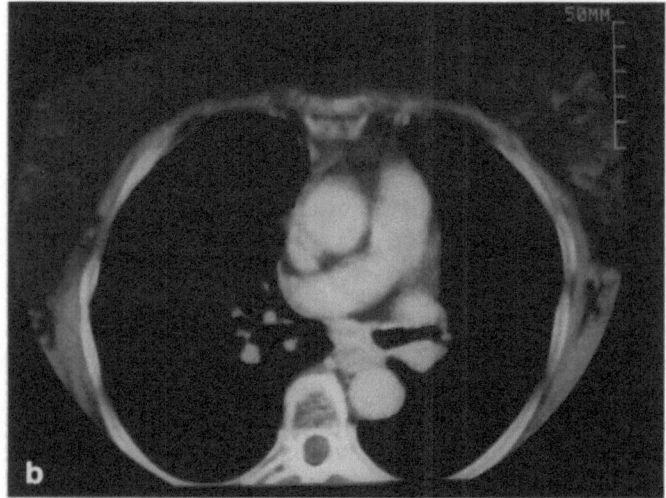

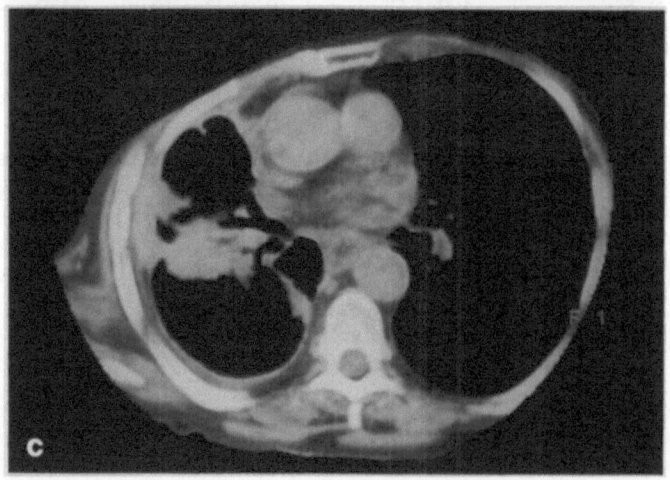

◄ **Fig. 17.3a–c.** CT study of esophageal metastases. **a** Lung cancer metastases. **b** Breast cancer metastases with infiltration of the subtracheal region. **c** Metastases of bilateral breast cancer; apparently intraparietal infiltration without peripheral extension. Note the right mediastinal and parenchymatous postirradiation fibrosis

17.2.1 Clinical Features

Metastases are rare in the stomach, representing only 0.36% of autopsy findings for cancer patients (Davis and Zollinger 1960; Menuck and Amberg 1975). In our literature review, gastric involvement was reported for 25% of the cases. The following primary etiologies accounted for nearly all of the literature cases: melanoma 44.8%, carcinoma of the breast 39%, bronchogenic carcinoma 5.1%.

Of all melanoma patients, 10%–20% develop gastric metastases, usually in the distal stomach (Das Gupta and Brasfield 1964b), and 2.1%–15.2% of all breast cancer patients develop at least histologic evidence of gastric involvement (Choi et al. 1964; Hartmann and Sherlock 1961). Small cell lung cancers are the main bronchogenic cause of gastric metastases (Antler et al. 1982). The incidence of metastases from bronchogenic carcinomas appears to be on the rise, as previously reported by Menuck and Amberg (1975). Most recent studies have mentioned considerable progression in the frequency of gastric involvement by lung cancer, and figures of up to 30% have been cited in autopsy series (Dick and Pattinson 1972; Morton and Tedesco 1974; Willis 1973). This is probably because the discrete improvement in the prognosis for lung cancer now allows time for such metastases to develop, at least on a histologic level. Only 125 cases for which presenting symptoms were reported could be analyzed. The most common clinical features were bleeding (often occult) and chronic obstruction accompanied by pain. Acute symptoms (occlusion 8%, hematemesis 6.2%) were less frequent, as was detection of a mass on physical examination (4%). Asymptomatic cases were fairly common (32.8%).

Metastatic neoplasms of the stomach have two main origins: hematogenous dissemination and spread along the mesenteric attachments. Blood-borne dissemination can create nodular lesions when metastatic deposits in the submucosal layer elicit a desmoblastic response. These intramural lesions can undergo local transformation, becoming intraluminal or subserosal, and ulcerate. Evolution of this type is encountered in patients with melanoma and bronchogenic carcinoma (Joffe 1978). Metastases can also acquire an infiltrating appearance while leaving the mucosal layer intact (Graham 1964; Menuck and Amberg 1975; Meyers 1976; Shah et al. 1977). So-called linitis plastica is common with breast cancer metastatic to the stomach (Choi et al. 1964).

Gastric metastases can also result from disease extension along the mesenteric attachments, especially in the region of the gastrocolic ligament, between the transverse colon and the greater curvature of the stomach. Carcinoma of the transverse colon can thus spread to the stomach along a centripetal trajectory, changing from a subserosal to an infiltrating lesion until it finally reaches the submucosa (Bachman 1954; Meyers 1976).

Direct invasion by a contiguous lesion, such as carcinoma of the pancreas (Chiat and Faegenburg 1960; Krestin et al. 1983), and lymphatic spread are two less frequent origins of gastric metastases. Lymphatic spread is responsible for metastases in the upper stomach from cancer of the lower lobe of the left lung (Joffe 1978) or esophageal carcinoma (Glick et al. 1985; Saito et al. 1985).

17.2.2 Radiologic Features (Figs. 17.4–17.7)

Radiologic features were reviewed for 193 cases in the literature. Several abnormalities have been described: metastasis is suggested by ulcerated, intraluminal, or intramural lesions, especially when multiple. These lesions are small, the diameter of the ulceration is large in comparison to the tumor filling defect, and the peripheral mucosa appears normal (Beckly 1974; Meyers 1976; Shah et al. 1977). Non-ulcerated, intramural, and intraluminal lesions are less frequent and generally multiple. The linitis plastica pattern observed in the distal stomach is similar to that seen with primary carcinoma (Rodde et al. 1987). Subserosal lesions (7.3% of the cases reviewed) appear associated with gastric extension of a carcino-

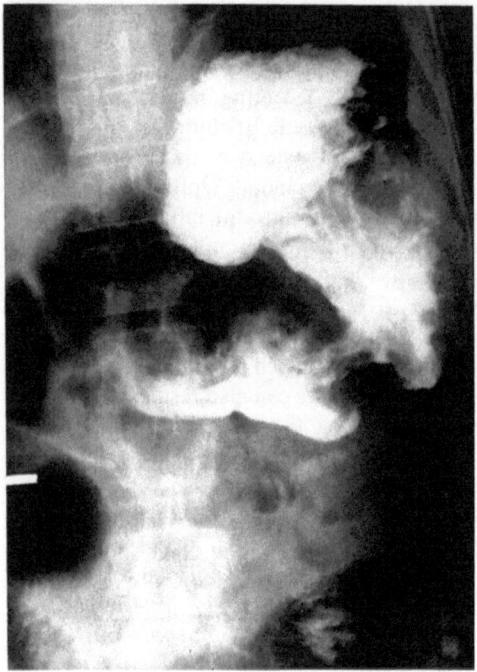

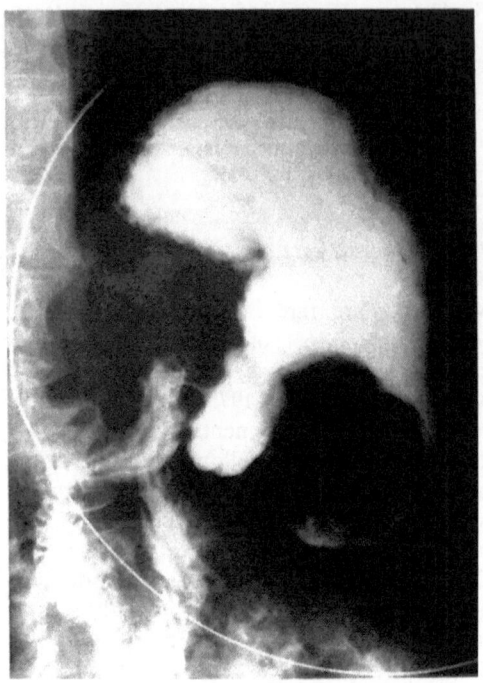

Fig. 17.4. Gastric metastasis of breast cancer (infiltrating pseudo-linitis lesion)

Fig. 17.5. Bulky gastric metastasis of a lung cancer

ma of the transverse colon along the gastrocolic ligament. The extent of involvement and subserosal character are best evaluated by ultrasonography and CT (Rodde et al. 1987; Yeh and Rabinowitz 1981).

Although there are no pathognomonic radiologic features that differentiate metastases of malignant melanomas from those of breast cancer, several somewhat distinctive patterns have been defined: multiple target or bull's eye images suggest metastases from melanoma, while linitis plastica, which should first suggest primary gastric cancer, may also be due to progressive breast cancer.

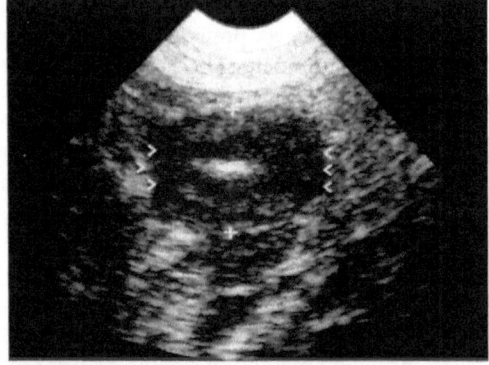

Fig. 17.6. Gastric metastasis of lung cancer: ultrasound revealed parietal infiltration of the gastric antrum. The examination was performed after the patient had fasted. The true lumen of the stomach is represented by the central echogenic area (*arrows;* 24 mm between the *two crosses*)

17.3 Small Intestine

This review covered 477 cases of intestinal metastases (Asch et al. 1968; Backman 1969; Badib et al. 1968; Beckly 1974; Beirne 1955; Benisch et al. 1972; Boquien et al. 1961; Boulez and Berard 1975; Chometowski et al. 1977; Dalmas et al. 1976; De Castro et al. 1957;

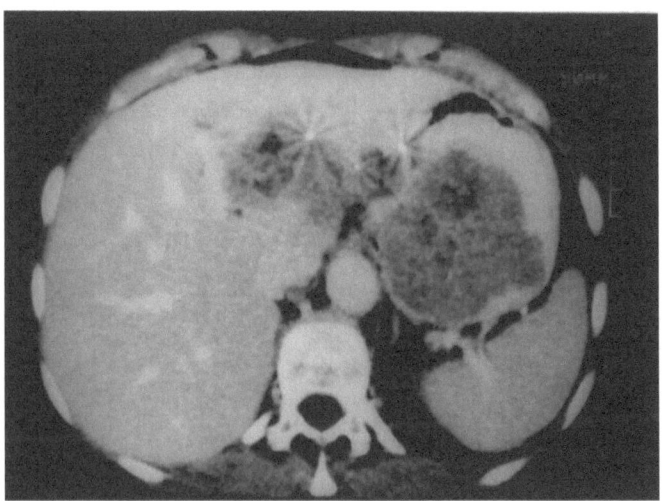

Fig. 17.7. Gastric metastasis of a pancreatic carcinoma

Estrade 1955; Farmer and Hawk 1964; Fingerhut et al. 1977; Fraser-Moodie et al. 1976; Frelot 1958; Goldstein et al. 1977; Grisoli et al. 1973; Hartmann and Sherlock 1961; Hery et al. 1978; Joffe 1978; Khilnani and Wolf 1960; Laval-Jeantet et al. 1975; Lebreuil et al. 1971; Legre et al. 1963; Levine et al. 1987; Mathieu 1973; Meyers 1975; Midell and Lochman 1972; Ngan 1970; Oddson et al. 1978; Patel et al. 1978; Poteshman 1967; Reeder and Cavanagh 1974; Rees at al. 1976; Roy 1979; Smith et al. 1977; Tongio et al. 1977; Treitel et al. 1970; Veen et al. 1976; Willbanks and Fogelman 1970; Zornoza and Goldstein 1977).

17.3.1 Clinical Features

The respective frequencies of primary cancers causing intestinal metastases are hard to define, but pelvic lesions are responsible for most intestinal metastases. It is often impossible to clinically distinguish generalized disease from direct invasion (De Castro et al. 1957; Farmer and Hawk 1964).
Melanomas are responsible for 25%–33% of intestinal metastases (Walther and Gilespie 1960; Willis 1973). Diffusion occurs by hematogenous spread. Breast, lung, colon, and kidney carcinomas metastasize less often to the small intestine (De Castro et al. 1957; Farmer and Hawk 1964; Walther and Gilespie 1960; Willis 1973).
Clinical features were reviewed for 354 cases (Table 17.1). Although presenting symptoms can be as obvious as hemorrhage or acute bowel obstruction, chronic signs that do not suggest metastases are more common. An abdominal mass was mentioned in only 3.1% of cases. Asymptomatic lesions were infrequent in the literature review (9.9%).
The histopathology of intestinal metastases was described by Meyers (1975). In addition to direct invasion by a contiguous primary tumor, dissemination may occur by direct extension from a non-contiguous primary carcinoma (along the fascia or the mesenteric attachments, or by lymphatic permeation), intraperitoneal malignant seeding, or hematogenous spread.

17.3.2 Radiologic Features (Figs. 17.8–17.14)

For the intestine and the colon, radiologic signs which are explained by the pathophysiology are discussed for each mode of dissemination. Direct invasion by a non-contiguous primary carcinoma generally takes place along the mesenteric attachments. This is particularly true for tumors with a high malignant potential which destroy the fascias that normally separate the intestine from these organs.

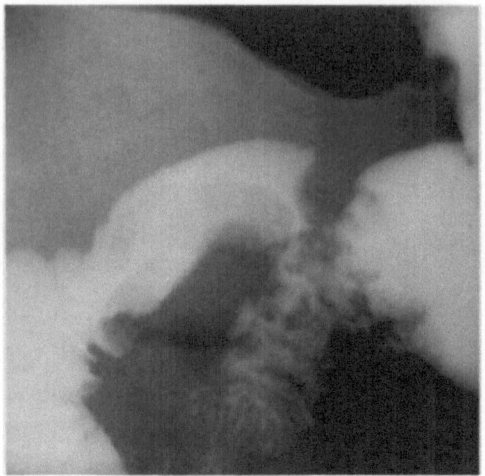

Fig. 17.8. Duodenal metastasis of a lung cancer

Fig. 17.9. Jejunal metastasis of a lung cancer   ▶

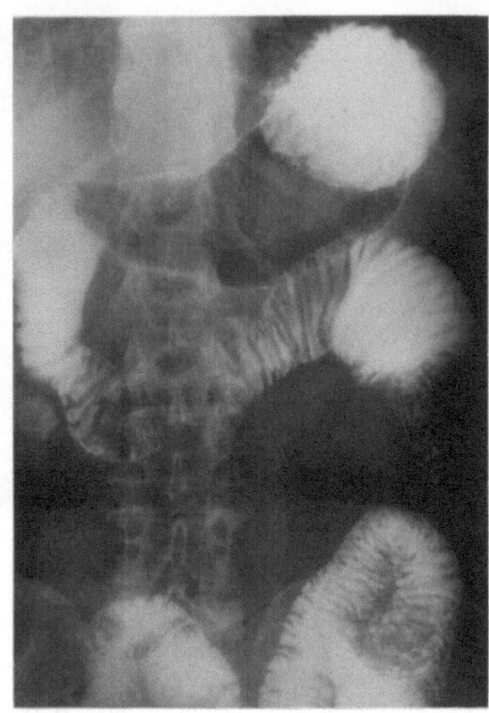

The usual cause is a pelvic carcinoma (ovary, uterus), and the degree of infiltration of the resultant tumor depends on the desmoblastic response.

Carcinoma of the kidney can also metastasize to the small intestine (Laval-Jeantet et al. 1975; Meyers and MacSweeney 1972). Carcinoma of the right kidney especially may displace, then progressively invade the second part of the duodenum. The desmoblastic reaction creates a nodular polypoid mass that projects into the lumen. Metastases of this type are hypervascularized, and hemorrhage is frequent (Tongio et al. 1977).

Carcinoma of the hepatic flexure of the colon can invade the duodenum through the first portion of the transverse mesocolon (Treitel et al. 1970). Direct abdominal spread to the subperitoneal space, as observed in neuroblastoma, is readily demonstrated by CT (Oliphant and Berne 1987).

Direct invasion by lymphatic permeation from a non-contiguous primary carcinoma is less frequent. Lymphatic stasis in the involved nodal chains can cause lymphatic reflux; subsequent retrograde passage along other lymphatic pathways can lead to paradoxal involvement by neoplastic emboli (Heller 1945). Radiographically, such lesions appear rigid, with angulation of the intestinal loops by mesenteric attachments; the mucosal folds appear thickened due to infiltration of the wall, associated or not with submucosal nodules, when the metastases have formed a tumoral mass. Occlusion is fairly rare. Even in cases of focal involvement, this feature may be helpful in distinguishing metastasis from a primary intestinal cancer (Farah et al. 1987; Zboralske and Bessolo 1967).

The notion of intraperitoneal seeding was first proposed by De Castro et al. (1957), and was later developed by Meyers (1975). After breaking through the peritoneal cavity, the primary cancer or its lymphatic metastases leaves metastatic implants along the intraperitoneal lymphatic pathways. Sites of predilection include the pouch of Douglas, the terminal portion of the mesentery, the sigmoid mesocolon, and the right paracolic gutter.

The radiologic features depend on the local fibroblastic reaction. If the reaction is weak, the tumor displaces the intestinal loops

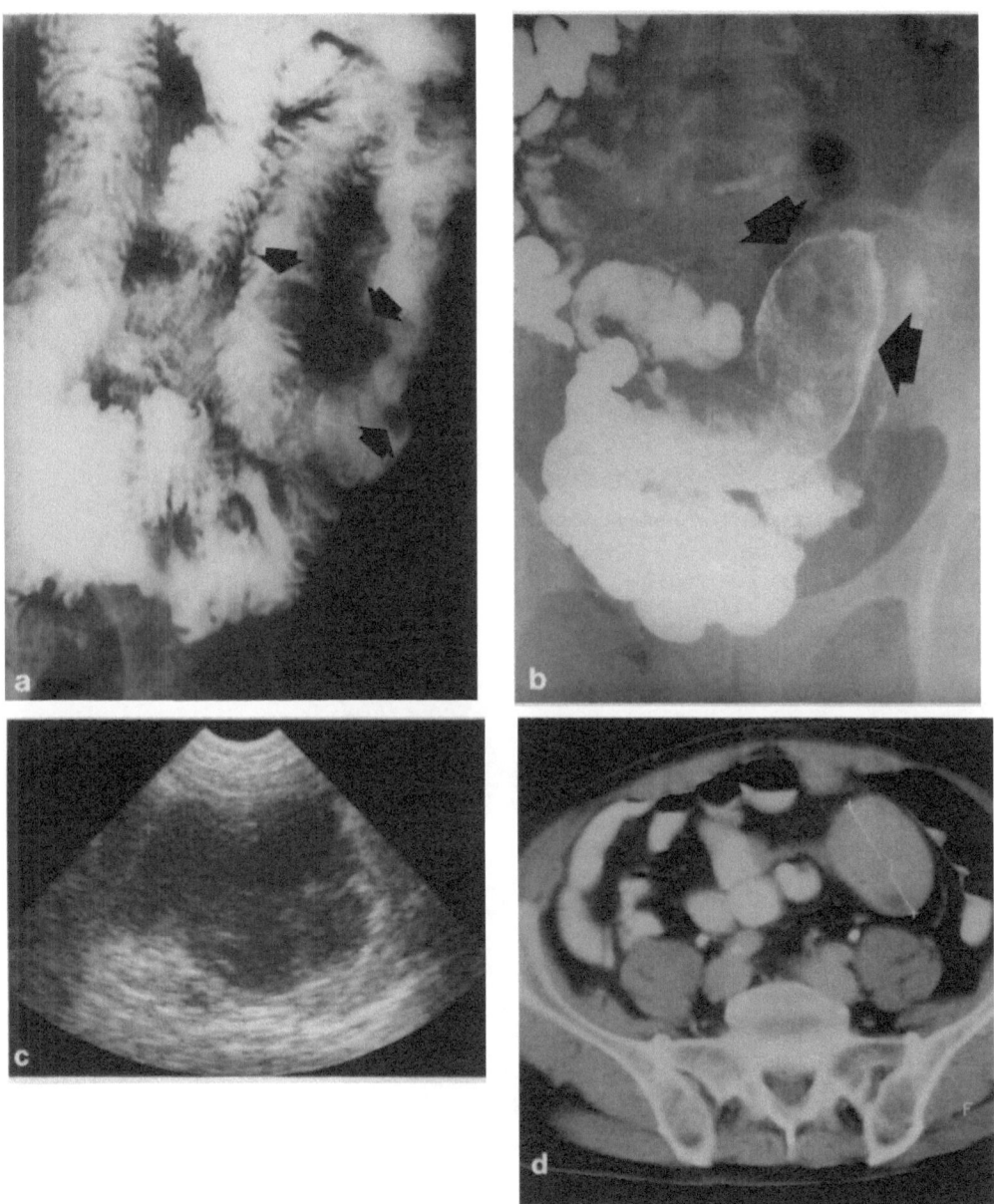

Fig. 17.10a–d. Intestinal metastases of melanoma. **a** Multinodular lesion *(arrow)*. **b** Tumoral lesion *(arrows; barium study)*. **c** Sonographically solid tumoral lesion (68 mm between the *two crosses*). **d** CT appearance of a tumoral lesion (6 cm; *line 1*)

downwards and inwards, and the mesenteric border appears stretched (Meyers 1976). A strong fibroblastic reaction will create an infiltrated, rigid, and angulated appearance of the intestinal loops, which is often most prevalent in the terminal ileum.

Blood-borne metastatic disease spread to the small intestine occurs with such primary tumors as melanoma, breast cancer, and bronchogenic carcinoma. McNeill et al. (1987) reported finding intestinal metastases at autopsy in 10.6% of primary lung cancer patients. Clin-

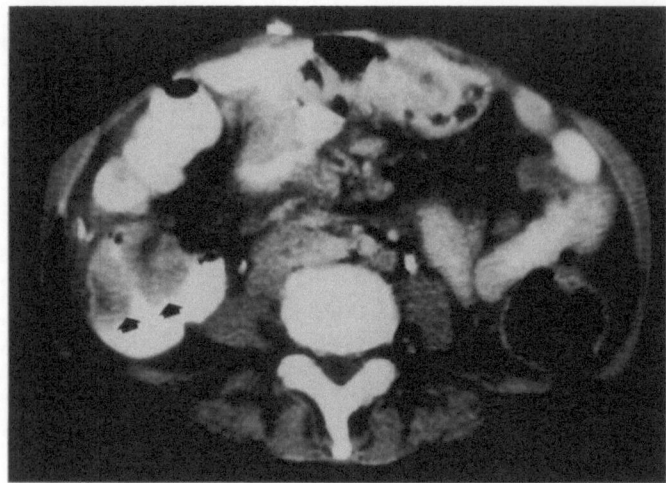

Fig. 17.11. Cecal metastasis of an ovarian carcinoma

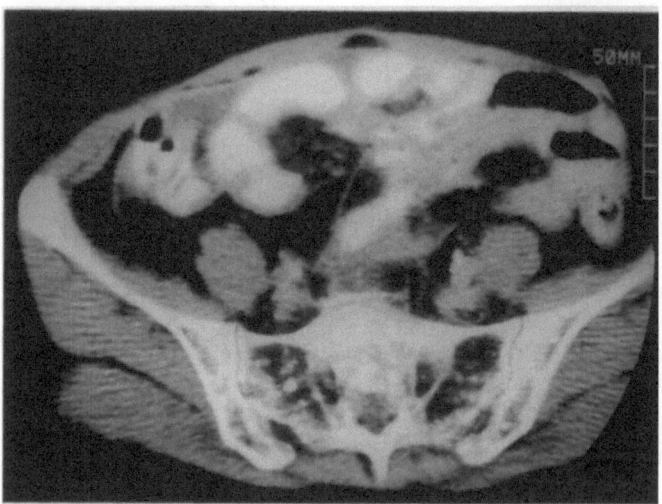

Fig. 17.12. Peritoneal carcinosis in a patient with breast cancer

ical discovery of hematogenous intestinal metastases is always correlated with a poor prognosis.

The small intestine is the most frequent site of metastases from melanoma, probably because this organ receives most of the mesenteric blood flow (Oddson et al. 1978). As in the stomach, metastases develop in the submucosa, creating intraluminal, often multiple polypoid masses (Reintgen et al. 1984). Ulceration is frequent, producing bull's eye images. Intraluminal growth probably explains the higher frequency of intestinal intussusception with melanoma (Backman 1969; Das Gupta and Brasfield 1964a,b). Infiltrating lesions, in which stenotic zones alternate with dilated areas, are more frequent with breast cancer than with other malignancies (Meyers 1976). Intestinal metastases of lung cancer frequently manifest as intramural or intraluminal lesions along the

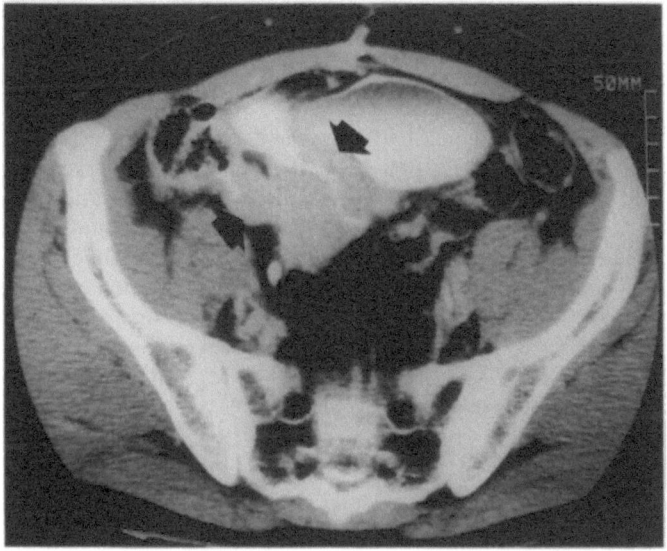

Fig. 17.13. Infiltration of the colon wall *(arrow)* causing extensive stenosis in a patient treated for ovarian cancer

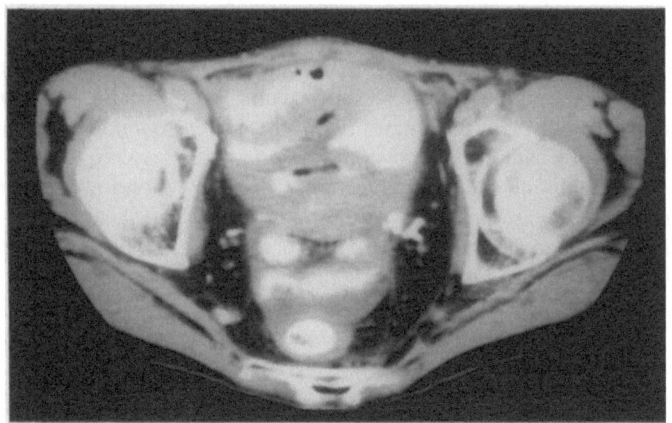

Fig. 17.14. Radiation-induced lesion after treatment of cervix uteri carcinoma. Note the symmetrical nature of the wall thickening, which contrasts with the appearance seen in carcinosis

antimesenteric border. As with melanoma, intussusception appears frequent, and the radiologic appearance is thus similar to secondary involvement by melanoma (Joffe 1978; Midell and Lochman 1972).

Whether ulcerated or not, a polypoid lesion may not be correctly diagnosed as metastasis, in particular if there are signs of intussusception. The focal nature of such lesions often leads to diagnosis of a benign tumor or even endometriosis (Marshak et al. 1965). In practice, radiation-induced lesions are the greatest diagnostic challenge, especially for pelvic cancer, since the radiologic features can be identical. The gross intraoperative features are insufficient for positive diagnosis, which requires histologic examination or analysis of the patient's clinical course.

17.4 Colon and Rectum

In all, 270 cases of metastases to the colon and rectum were reviewed (Asch et al. 1968; Badib et al. 1968; Baillet et al. 1977; Becker 1965; Boulez and Berard 1975; Bret 1976; Das Gupta and Brasfield 1964a,b; Fraser-Moodie et al. 1976; Goldstein et al. 1977; Joffe 1974; Klein and Sherlock 1972; Krestin et al. 1985; Lebreuil et al. 1971; L'Hermine et al. 1978; Marchal 1970; Mathieu 1973; Meyers et al. 1975; Patel et al. 1978; Rees et al.1976; Sacks et al. 1977; Smith and Vlasak 1978; Wigh and du V. Tapley 1958; Willbanks and Fogelman 1970).

17.4.1 Clinical Features

In the literature, the incidence of colonic metastases is similar to that of secondary gastric neoplasms. Pelvic tumors, and especially ovarian and prostate cancer, are the prime etiology. Estimates of secondary colonic involvement by malignant melanoma vary. For Fraser-Moodie et al. (1976), colonic metastases are less frequent than gastric or intestinal lesions because of the differences in vascularization. However, for Backman (1969), the incidence is the same as in the stomach, with the cecum being the site of predilection. Carcinoma of the breast was cited as the main cause of hematogenous metastasis to the colon by Asch et al. (1968). Other authors have reported a similar frequency of involvement (Graham 1964; Klein and Sherlock 1972). Metastatic invasion of the colon by bronchogenic carcinoma is rare, and less frequent than in the stomach (Joffe 1978).

The initial clinical features of secondary colonic involvement have rarely been reported, and such data was only available for 100 cases (Table 17.1). Acute symptoms are infrequent whereas asymptomatic cases are fairly common (14%). Physical examination may reveal a palpable mass (14% of patients) that often corresponds to stercoral stasis above a site of stenosis.

The histogenesis of colonic mestastases is similar to that for intestinal metastases. Direct invasion by a non-contiguous primary tumor along the fascia and the mesenteric attachments can occur with pelvic cancers. The sigmoid colon is the preferential site for metastases of ovarian carcinoma; prostate cancer can invade the rectum after rupturing through the fascia of Denonvilliers (Theander et al. 1963). Pelvic malignancies can metastasize to the transverse colon by spread along the greater omentum (Krestin et al. 1985).

In addition to pelvic cancers, carcinoma of the left kidney can spread towards the proximal portion of the descending colon. Gastric carcinoma may extend into the transverse colon along the gastrocolic ligament: the preferential site is above and along the row of sacculations between the taenia mesocolica and the taenia omentalis (Meyers 1976). Likewise, carcinoma of the pancreas can invade the lower border of the transverse colon through the transverse mesocolon.

17.4.2 Radiologic Features (Figs. 17.16, 17.17)

Radiologic features include infiltrating lesions, associated or not with subserosal formations which may or not be ulcerated. Lymphatic metastatic permeation in the colon is even less common than in the small intestine, but can explain tumoral recurrence after colonic resection for carcinoma (Grinnel 1966). Intraperitoneal seeding generally affects the pouch of Douglas (Meyers 1976); radiologic findings include both infiltration and a nodular mass. Involvement of the mesosigmoid and the right paracolic gutter is less frequent; the infiltrating, subserosal radiologic images are the result of a strong fibroblastic response. Metastasis by hematogenous spread occurs with malignant melanoma, breast cancer, and bronchogenic carcinoma. As in the small intestine, metastases from melanoma elicit a weak desmoblastic response; these often multiple, intramural or intraluminal lesions can ulcerate, creating a bull's eye image (Sacks et al. 1977). Colonic metastases of breast cancer may be nodular or stenosing, depending on the fibroblastic reaction; they are often associated with involvement of the terminal ileum (Meyers and McSweeney 1972). Secondary involvement by bronchogenic carcinoma, which can resemble breast cancer metastases, also depends on the fibroblastic reaction.

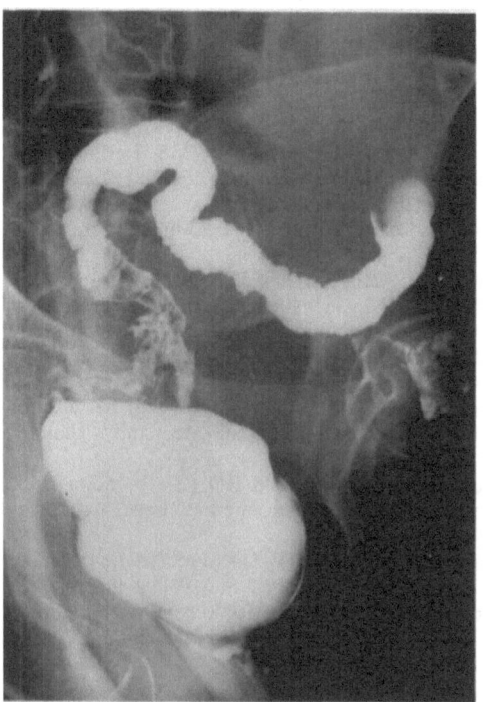

Fig. 17.15. Sigmoid metastasis of an ovarian cancer (infiltrating lesion)

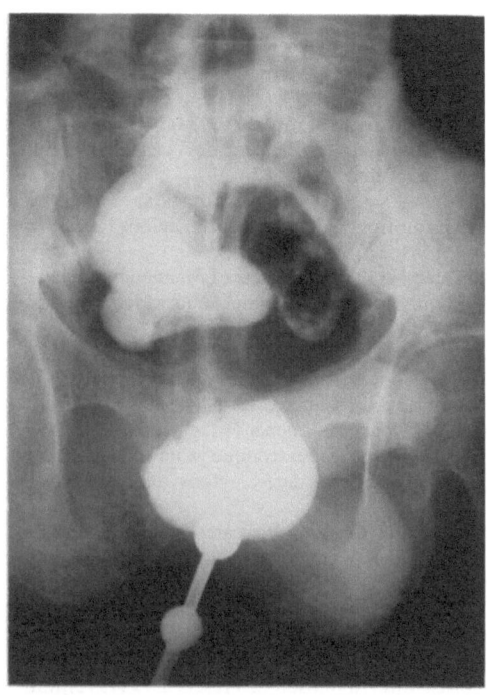

Fig. 17.16. Rectal metastasis of lung cancer

Intraluminal and intramural lesions can be confused radiographically with a benign tumor. Focal infiltrating lesions may resemble primary colon carcinoma or even inflammatory colitis (Meyers et al. 1975). As for the small intestine, the most difficult diagnostic problem is radiation-induced lesions. However, intestinal and colonic radiation lesions are more frequently associated than metastatic involvement of the small intestine and colon. Detection of more or less stenosing, infiltrating images in both the colon and small intestine is in favor of radiation damage (Goldstein 1979).

17.5 Conclusion

Gastrointestinal metastases involve two basic situations: (1) for patients with a predominantly gastrointestinal localization (the least frequent case), awareness of the pathogenesis of gastrointestinal metastases can orient the search for detection of the primary cancer. (2) in patients with a known malignancy (the most common situation), familiarity with the mode of dissemination of the primary cancer can prevent a secondary gastrointestinal site from being overlooked, even if clinical signs are minimal.

17.6 References

Agha FP (1987) Secondary neoplasms of the oesophagus. Gastrointest Radiol 12: 187–193

Anderson MF, Harell GS (1980) Secondary esophageal tumors. AJR 135: 1243–1246

Antler AS, Ough Y, Pitchumoni CS, Davidian M, Thelmo W (1982) Gastrointestinal metastases from malignant tumors of the lung. Cancer 49: 170–172

Asch MJ, Wiedel PD, Habif DV (1968) Gastrointestinal metastases from carcinoma of the breast. Autopsy study and 18 cases requiring operative intervention. Arch Surg 96: 840–843

Atkins JP (1966) Metastatic carcinoma to the esophagus. Endoscopic considerations with special reference to carcinoma of the breast. Ann Otol Rhinol Laryngol 75: 356–367

Aubert P, Lainee J, Duron JJ, Bisson A, Guilleausseau PJ (1974) Dysphagie révélatrice d'un cancer du sein. Ann Med Interne (Paris) 125: 927–931

Auriol M, Cesari J, Prade M (1958) Métastases gastrointestinales des cancers de l'oesophage. Bull Cancer (Paris) 45: 77–82

Bachman AL (1954) Roentgen appearance of gastric invasion from carcinoma of the colon. Radiology 63: 814–822

Backman H (1969) Metastases of malignant melanoma in the gastrointestinal tract. Geriatrics 24: 112–120

Badib AO, Kurohara SS, Webster JH, Pickren JW (1968) Metastasis to organs in carcinoma of the uterine cervix. Cancer 21: 434–439

Baillet P, Nouel P, Rouanet P, Lichtenstein H, Bloch P (1977) Métastase colique d'un cystadénocarcinome ovarien calcifié. Nouv Presse Med 6: 2977

Becker JA (1965) Prostatic carcinoma involving the rectum and sigmoid colon. AJR 94: 421–428

Beckly DE (1974) Alimentary tract metastases from malignant melanoma. Clin Radiol 25: 385–389

Beirne MF (1955) Malignant melanoma of the small intestine. Radiology 65: 749–752

Benisch BM, Abramson S, Present DH (1972) Malabsorption and metastatic melanoma. Mt Sinai J Med 39: 474–477

Biller HF, Diktaban T, Fink W, Lawson W (1982) Breast carcinoma metastasizing to the cervical esophagus. Laryngoscope 92: 999–1000

Boquien Y, Kerneis JP, Alliot G, Delumeau G (1961) Epithéliomas secondaires de l'intestin grêle (à propos de 5 cas). Presse Med 59: 879–882

Boulez J, Berard P (1975) Les métastases intestinales multiples dans les cancers du sein. A propos d'une forme rare simulant la maladie de Crohn. Lyon Med 233: 627–631

Bret P (1976) Etude radiologique en double contraste des lésions coliques par métastases ou propagation d'un cancer du voisinage. Ann Radiol 19: 289–293

Butler ML, Van Heertum RL, Teplick SK (1975) Metastatic malignant melanoma of the esophagus: a case report. Gastroenterology 69: 1334–1337

Caramella E, Bruneton JN, Roux P, Aubanel D, Lecomte P (1983) Metastases of the digestive tract. Report of 77 cases and review of the literature. Eur J Radiol 3: 331–338

Chene P, Markovits A, Debaud B (1962) Le cancer métastatique de l'oesophage. Gaz Med Fr 69: 371–389

Chiat H, Faegenburg DH (1960) Illusory neoplasms of the stomach and duodenum as a manifestation of carcinoma of the pancreas. Radiology 74: 771–777

Choi SH, Shehan FR, Pickren JW (1964) Metastatic involvement of the stomach by breast cancer. Cancer 17: 791–797

Chometowski S, Nguyen Cat R, Assadourian R, Bourdes J, Lamy J (1977) Métastases iléales tardives d'un mélanome cutané périphérique. Manifestation hémorragique prédominante (1 cas). J Chir (Paris) 113: 537–542

Coscina WF, Arger PH, Levine MS, Herlinger H, Cohen S, Coleman BG, Mintz MC (1986) Gastrointestinal tract focal mass lesions: role of CT and barium evaluations. Radiology 158: 581–587

Dalmas H, Anfossi G, Dor JF, Basbous D, Guidicelli C (1976) Invaginations jéjuno et iléo-iléales révélatrices de multiples métastases mélaniques de l'intestin grêle. Présentation d'une observation. J Chir (Paris) 111: 341–346

Das Gupta TK, Brasfield RD (1964a) Metastatic melanoma: a clinicopathological study. Cancer 17: 1323–1339

Das Gupta TK, Brasfield RD (1964b) Metastatic melanoma of the gastrointestinal tract. Arch Surg 88: 969–973

Davis GH, Zollinger RW (1960) Metastatic melanoma of the stomach. Am J Surg 99: 94–96

De Castro CA, Dockerty MB, Mayo CW (1957) Metastatic tumors of the small intestine. Surg Gynecol Obstet 105: 159–165

De La Plava S, Nigogosyan G, Pickren JW, Cabrera A (1963) Melanosis of the esophagus. Cancer 16: 48–50

Dick R, Pattinson JW (1972) Metastasis of the stomach presenting as single polyps. Br J Radiol 45: 761–764

Doutre LP, Leger H, Perissat J, Paccalin J, Beaulieu JC, Valentin F (1972) Les cancers secondaires de l'estomac. Bordeaux Med 5: 269–275

Engelman RE, MacNamara ML (1954) Bronchiogenic carcinoma. A statistical review of two hundred and thirty-four autopsies. J Thorac Cardiovasc Surg 27: 227–237

Estrade J (1955) Deux tumeurs secondaires sténosantes du grêle. Bull Cancer (Paris) 42: 498–502

Faguer P, Tomasson N, Lambert R (1975) Les métastases gastriques du mélanome malin. Présentation d'un cas. Arch Fr Mal Appar Dig 64: 139–144

Farah MC, Jafri SZH, Schwab RE, Mezwa DG, Francis IR, Noujaim S, Kim C (1987) Duodenal neoplasms: role of CT. Radiology 162: 839–843

Farmer RG, Hawk WA (1964) Metastatic tumors of the small bowel. Gastroenterology 57: 496–504

Fingerhut A, Eugene C, Pourcher J, Bergue A, Ronat R (1977) Mélanomes malins de l'estomac et du grêle révélés par une occlusion fébrile. Sem Hop 53: 1719–1721

Fisher MS (1976) Metastasis to the esophagus. Gastrointest Radiol 1: 245–251

Fraser-Moodie A, Hughes G, Jones SM, Shorey BA, Snape L (1976) Malignant melanoma metastases to the alimentary tract. Gut 17: 206–209

Frelot C (1958) Cancer secondaire de l'intestin grêle. Medical thesis, University of Paris

Gale ME, Birnbaum SB, Gale DR, Vincent ME (1984) Esophageal invasion by lung cancer: CT diagnosis. J Comput Assist Tomogr 8: 694-698

Glick SN, Teplick SK, Levine MS (1985) Squamous cell metastases to the gastric cardia. Gastrointest Radiol 10: 339-344

Glick SN, Teplick SK, Levine MS, Caroline DF (1986) Gastric cardia metastasis in esophageal carcinoma. Radiology 160: 627-630

Goldstein HM (1979) Small bowel and colon. In: Libshitz HI (ed) Diagnostic roentgenology of radiotherapy change. Williams and Wilkins, Baltimore, pp 85-100

Goldstein HM, Bemdoun MT, Dodd GD (1977) Radiologic spectrum of melanoma metastatic to the gastrointestinal tract. AJR 129: 605-612

Gouin B, Couturier D, Hardouin JP, Debray C (1972) Les médiastinites néoplasiques. Complications tardives des cancers du sein. A propos de 3 observations. Nouv Presse Med 1: 1563-1568

Graham WP (1964) Gastrointestinal metastases from carcinoma of the breast. Ann Surg 159: 477-480

Grinnel RS (1966) Lymphatic block with atypical and retrograde lymphatic metastasis and spread in carcinoma of the colon and rectum. Ann Surg 163: 272-280

Grisoli J, Farisse J, Argene M, Delmont JP, Lebreuil G (1973) Métastase entéromésentérique tardive d'une tumeur de la granulosa. Sem Hop 49: 640-655

Hartmann WH, Sherlock P (1961) Gastroduodenal metastases from carcinoma of the breast: an adrenal steroid-induced phenomenon. Cancer 14: 426-431

Heller EL (1945) Carcinoma of the stomach with multiple annular metastatic intestinal infiltrations. Arch Pathol 40: 392-394

Hery MD, Aubanel D, Monticelli J, Occelli JP, Galli J, Lecomte P (1978) Localisations secondaires des mélanomes malins au niveau du grêle. A propos de 4 observations. J Radiol 59

Higgins PM (1962) Pyloric obstruction due to a metastatic deposit from carcinoma of the bronchus. Can J Surg 5: 438-441

Hillemans P, Maillard JN, Conte A (1961) Les cancers malpighiens de l'estomac. Arch Fr Mal Appar Dig 50: 1001-1009

Holyoke ED, Nemoto T, Dao TL (1969) Esophageal metastases and dysphagia in patients with carcinoma of the breast. J Surg Oncol 1: 97-107

Joffe N (1974) Medical cecal defect associated with metastatic pancreatic carcinoma. Radiology 111: 297-300

Joffe N (1975) Metastatic involvement of the stomach secondary to breast carcinoma. AJR 123: 297-300

Joffe N (1978) Symptomatic gastrointestinal metastases secondary to bronchogenic carcinoma. Clin Radiol 29: 217-225

Khilnani MT, Wolf BS (1960) Late involvement of the alimentary tract by carcinoma of the kidney. Am J Dig Dis 5: 529-540

Klein MS, Sherlock P (1972) Gastric and colonic metastases from breast cancer. Am J Dig Dis 17: 881-886

Krestin GP, Beyer D, Lorenz R, Thul H (1983) Kolonbeteiligung bei Magen- und Pankreasprozessen. Fortschr Geb Roentgenstr 138: 276-282

Krestin GP, Beyer D, Lorenz R (1985) Secondary involvement of the transverse colon by tumors of the pelvis: spread of malignancies along the greater omentum. Gastrointest Radiol 10: 283-288

Laval-Jeantet M, Plainfosse MC, Tristant H, Chelloul N (1975) Les cancers du rein et de la loge rénale à expression digestive. Ann Radiol (Paris) 18: 733-737

Lebreuil G, Payan H, Varette I, Cornil J, Duchassin M (1971) Les métastases digestive. Arch Anat Pathol 19: 195-202

Legre J, Padovani J, Salamon G, Clement JP (1963) Tumeurs métastatiques du grêle. J Radiol 44: 126-127

Levine MS, Drooz AT, Herlinger H (1987) Annular malignancies of the small bowel. Gastrointest Radiol 12: 53-58

L'Hermine C, Froment T, Lescut J, Roger J, Lemaitre G (1978) Extension au côlon transverse des cancers infiltrants de l'estomac. J Radiol 59: 261-266

Libshitz HI, Lindell MM, Dodd GD (1982) Metastases to the hollow viscera. Radiol Clin North Am 20: 487-499

Lorriaux A, Capron JP (1974) Métastases gastriques d'un cancer épidermoïde de l'oesophage. Sem Hop 50: 2507-2509

Lortat-Jacob JL, Fekete F, Garcia-Moran M (1964) Dysphagie et cancer du sein. Ann Chir 18: 975-985

Lund FB (1929) Melanotic sarcoma of the small intestine. New Engl J Med 201: 1133-1136

Marchal G (1970) Cancer colo-rectal révélé par une greffe métastatique dans une fistule anale (3 cas). Arch Fr Mal Appar Dig 59: 815-816

Marshak RH, Khilnani MT, Eliasoph J, Wolf BS (1965) Metastatic carcinoma of the small bowel. AJR 94: 385-394

Mathieu I (1973) Cancer métastatique du grêle et du côlon (1 cas). J Belge Radiol 56: 149-150

Mc Neill PM, Wagman LD, Neifeld JP (1987) Small bowel metastases from primary carcinoma of the lung. Cancer 59: 1486-1489

Menuck LS, Amberg JR (1975) Metastatic disease involving the stomach. Am J Dig Dis 20: 903-913

Meyers MA (1975) Metastatic seeding along the small bowel mesentery. AJR 123: 67-73

Meyers MA (1976) Dynamic radiology of the abdomen. Normal and pathologic anatomy. Springer, Berlin Heidelberg New York, pp 37-80

Meyers MA, McSweeney J (1972) Secondary neoplasm of the bowel. Radiology 105: 1–11

Meyers MA, Oliphant M, Teixidor H, Weiser P (1975) Metastatic carcinoma simulating inflammatory colitis. AJR 123: 74–83

Michalet JP, Faivre J, Klepping C (1977) Métastase gastrique: manifestation révélatrice très inhabituelle d'un cancer bronchique. J Med Lyon 58: 647–650

Midell AI, Lochman DJ (1972) An unusual metastatic manifestation of a primary bronchogenic carcinoma. Cancer 30: 806–809

Morton WJ, Tedesco FJ (1974) Metastatic bronchogenic carcinoma seen as a gastric ulcer. Am J Dig Dis 19: 766–770

Mosimann F, Fontolliet C, Genton A, Gertsch P, Pettavel J (1982) Resection of metastases to the alimentary tract from malignant melanoma. Int ᴜurg 67: 257–260

Ngan H (1970) Involvement of the duodenum by metastases from tumours of the genital tract. Br J Radiol 43: 701–705

Oddson TA, Rice RP, Seigler HF, Thompson WM, Kelvin FM, Clark WM (1978) The spectrum of small bowel melanoma. Gastrointest Radiol 3: 419–423

Oliphant M, Berne AS (1987) Mechanism of direct spread of abdominal neuroblastoma: CT demonstration and clinical implications. Gastrointest Radiol 12: 59–66

Patel JK, Didolkar MS, Pickren JW, Moore RH (1978) Metastatic pattern of malignant melanoma. A study of 216 autopsy cases. Am J Surg 135: 807–810

Phadke M, Rao U, Takita H (1976) Metastatic tumors of esophagus. NY State J Med 76: 963–965

Polk HC, Camp FA, Walker AW (1967) Dysphagia and esophageal stenosis. Manifestation of metastatic mammary cancer. Cancer 20: 2002–2004

Poteshman NL (1967) Metastatic tumor to the small bowel; three cases simulating primary malignant tumour. AJR 99: 122–126

Reeder AM, Cavanagh RC (1974) "Bull's eye" lesions: solitary or multiple nodules in the gastrointestinal tract with large central ulceration. JAMA 229: 825–826

Rees BI, Okwonga W, Jenkins IL (1976) Intestinal metastases from carcinoma of the breast. Clin Oncol 2: 113–119

Reintgen DS, Thompson W, Garbutt J, Seigler HF (1984) Radiologic, endoscopic, and surgical consideration of melanoma metastatic to the gastrointestinal tract. Surgery 95: 635–639

Rodde A, Stines J, Regent D, Becker S, Conroy T, Weber M, Delgoffe C, Bour C (1987) Les pseudolinites gastriques d'origine mammaire. J Radiol 68: 269–274

Roy G (1979) Les métastases jéjuno-iléales du mélanome malin. Medical thesis, University of Amiens

Rubin SA, Davis M (1985) "Bull's eye" or "target" lesions of the stomach secondary to carcinoma of the lung. Am J Gastroenterol 80: 67–69

Sacks BA, Joffe N, Antonioli DA (1977) Metastatic melanoma presenting clinically as multiple colonic polyps. AJR 129: 511–513

Saito T, Iizuka T, Kato H, Watanabe H (1985) Esophageal carcinoma metastatic to the stomach. A clinicopathologic study of 35 cases. Cancer 56: 2235–2241

Scatarige JC, Allen HA, Fishman EK (1987) Computed tomography of the small bowel. Semin Ultrasound CT MR 8: 403–423

Scobie BA (1966) Malignant gastric ulcer due to metastasis. Aust Radiol 10: 119–123

Shah SM, Smart DF, Texter EC, Morris WD (1977) Metastatic melanoma of the stomach: the endoscopic and roentgenographic findings and review of the literature. South Med J 70: 379–381

Simao A (1963) Metastatic carcinoma of the stomach: Med Radiogr Photogr 39: 15–18

Smith HJ, Vlasak MG (1978) Metastasis to the colon from bronchogenic carcinoma. Gastrointest Radiol 2: 393–396

Smith MJ, Carlson HC, Gisvold JJ (1977) Secondary neoplasm of the small bowel. Radiology 125: 29–33

Steiner H, Lammer J, Hackl A (1984) Lymphatic metastases to the esophagus. Gastrointest Radiol 9: 1–4

Telerman A, Gerard B, Van den Heule B, Bleiberg H (1985) Gastrointestinal metastases from extra-abdominal tumors. Endoscopy 17: 99–101

Theander G, Wehlin L, Langeland P (1963) Deformation of the rectosigmoid junction in peritoneal carcinomatosis. Acta Radiol [Diagn] (Stockh) 1: 1071–1076

Tongio J, Peruta O, Wenger JJ, Warter P (1977) Métastases duodénales et pancréatiques du néphro-épithéliome. A propos de 4 observations. Ann Radiol (Paris) 20: 641–647

Toreson WE (1944) Secondary carcinoma of the esophagus as a cause of dysphagia. Arch Pathol 38: 82–84

Touraine R, Onagnier C, Braillon G (1975) Les sténoses oesophagiennes par métastase tardive du cancer du sein. Lyon Chir 71: 394–398

Treitel H, Meyers MA, Maza V (1970) Changes in the duodenal loop secondary to carcinoma of the hepatic flexure of the colon. Br J Radiol 43: 209–213

Veen HF, Oscarson JEA, Malt RA (1976) Alien cancers of the duodenum. Surg Gynecol Obstet 143: 39–42

Wade BN (1945) Jejunal intussusception of melanoma of the small intestine. Northwest Med 44: 388–390

Walther CW, Gilepsie DR (1960) Metastatic hypernephroma of fifty years duration. Minn Med 43: 126–129

Wigh R, Tapley N du V (1958) Metastatic lesions to large intestine. Radiology 70: 222–229

Willbanks OL, Fogelman MJ (1970) Gastrointestinal melanosarcoma. Am J Surg 120: 602–606

Willis RA (1973) The spread of tumours in the human body 3rd edn. Butterworths, London, pp 209–213

Wood CB, Wood RAB (1975) Metastatic malignant melanoma of the esophagus. Am J Dig Dis 20: 786–789

Yeh HC, Rabinowitz HG (1981) Ultrasonography and computed tomography of gastric wall lesions. Radiology 141: 147–155

Zboralske FF, Bessolo RJ (1967) Metastatic carcinoma to the mesentery and gut. Radiology 88: 302–310

Zornoza J, Goldstein HM (1977) Cavitating metastases of the small intestine. AJR 129: 613–615

18 Kaposi's Sarcoma*

In parallel with the appearance of acquired immune deficiency syndrome (AIDS), a marked increase was noted in the incidence of Kaposi's sarcoma. This epidemic-type sarcoma differs in several ways from the classic form of Kaposi's sarcoma (Rothman 1962; Safai 1987).

18.1 General Features

AIDS-related Kaposi's sarcoma has the same histogenesis as the classic form and the endemic African variant. The essential difference is that it is currently an epidemic affection with a very marked aggressivity (Gottlieb et al. 1983).

Kaposi's sarcoma is a multiple, pigmented cutaneous sarcoma associated with visceral manifestations. The classic form involves primarily cutaneous lesions of the lower limbs in men; it is only slightly lymphophilic, and gastrointestinal manifestations are of late onset. The natural course usually extends over some 15 years. By contrast, the AIDS-related disease is remarkable because of the virulence of visceral, gastrointestinal and nodal manifestations. Associated opportunistic infections are frequent, and survival is currently less than 20% at 2 years (Mitsuyasu 1987; Safai 1984). During AIDS, Kaposi's sarcoma causes gastrointestinal manifestations which may or may not be the most common visceral lesions (Marche et al.1986; Rose et al. 1982). Gastric and intestinal lesions predominate; colic lesions are less common. The esophagus is the least common site of gastrointestinal Kaposi's sarcoma. There have been several rare reports of purely gastrointestinal Kaposi's sarcoma, where

---

* Written in collaboration with G. Schmutz.

physical examination failed to detect any cutaneous or nodal involvement (Hanno et al. 1979). While Kaposi's sarcoma is often asymptomatic in AIDS patients, clinical symptoms may include bleeding. Acute signs such as intestinal obstruction, intussusception, and perforation are rare.

Malignant hematologic diseases such as lymphoma are also common in patients with Kaposi's sarcoma. The frequency of this association was approximately 10% in a review of the literature (Safai 1987).

Along with Kaposi's sarcoma, AIDS can be complicated by infections with a predilection for the gastrointestinal tract, such as candidal esophagitis and *Cryptosporidium, Mycobacterium avium-intracellulare,* cytomegalovirus, and herpes simplex infections of the intestine. Development of a Kaposi's sarcoma, associated or not with a gastrointestinal tract infection, is currently synonymous with a rapidly fatal outcome.

18.2 Imaging (Figs. 18.1–18.4)

Barium studies and CT are less sensitive than endoscopy for detection of early disease. The small macular mucosal lesions are generally asymptomatic (Friedman et al. 1985) and have no specific features (Albin et al. 1987). Wall et al. (1986) described the following radiographic abnormalities: thickened folds (87%), nodules (66%), aphthous lesions (58%), and irregular mucosa (47%). A mass effect (26%) and stenosis (21%) are less frequent. These images can be grouped together in three forms:

- Tumoral lesions with a polypoid appearance, encountered in the esophagus (Rose et al. 1982).
- Multifocal nodular pattern, seen essentially in the stomach and the colon. In the colon,

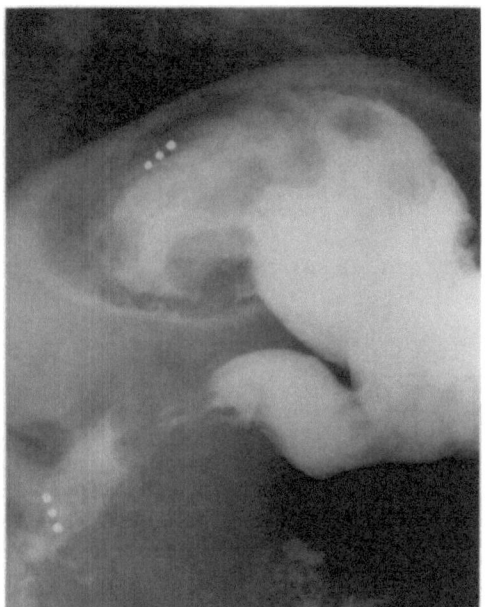

Fig. 18.1. Multinodular gastric lesion

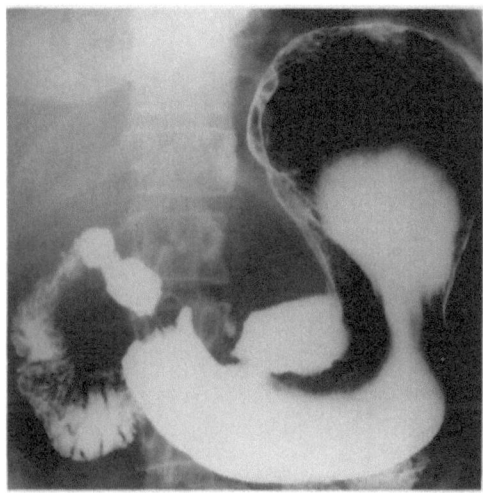

Fig. 18.2. Ulcerated bulky lesion of the body of the stomach

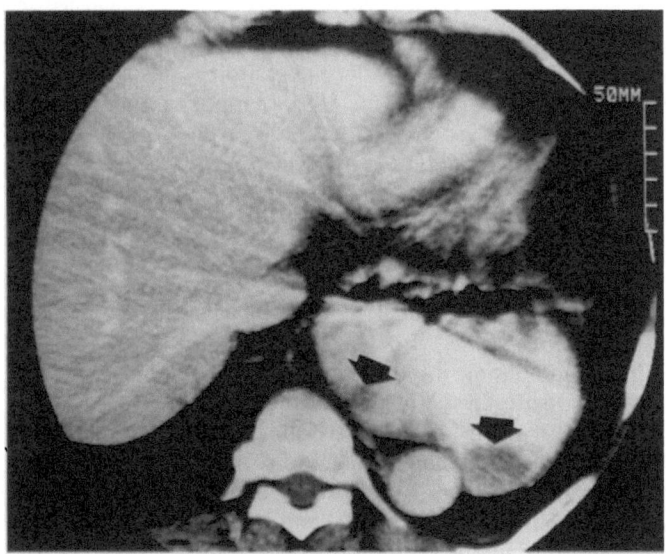

Fig. 18.3. Multinodular Kaposi's sarcoma lesion *(arrows)* (CT study)

an increase in the number of nodules and their coalescence may ultimately cause stenosis. Diffuse intestinal nodules are sometimes ulcerated.

- Disseminated micropolyposis, a pattern similar to that seen in familial polyposis.

Depending on the pattern, the differential diagnosis is lymphoma, hematogenous metastases, polyposis, infiltrating cancer, or Crohn's disease (Bryk et al. 1978; Calenoff 1972).

CT may visualize associated signs; involvement of the retroperitoneal and mesenteric

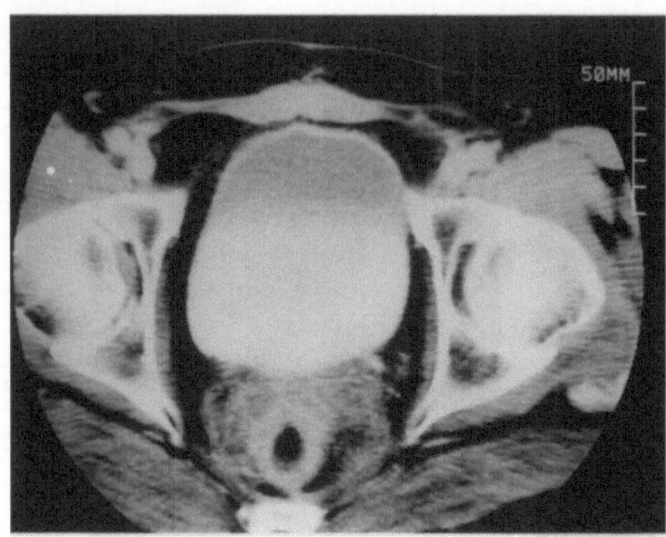

Fig. 18.4. Rectal wall thickening and perirectal infiltration by Kaposi's sarcoma

nodes is quite common. Hepatic, pancreatic, and bile duct involvement are less frequent. Lesions may decrease or even disappear radiologically in response to chemotherapy.

Infectious associations are possible in the abdominal cavity, and in particular the gastrointestinal tract (Balthazar et al. 1985; Frager et al. 1986; Jeffrey et al. 1986; Nyberg et al. 1985). Except for tumoral lesions, which may suggest the diagnosis of Kaposi's sarcoma, submucosal involvement, ulcerations, edema, and thickened folds are seen not only as a complication of AIDS, but also with certain parasites especially frequent in homosexuals *(Giardia, Strongyloides)*.

Furthermore, during Kaposi's sarcoma, other sites may exist, in particular in the lungs (McCauley et al. 1982). The most valuable information when searching for Kaposi's sarcoma in an AIDS patient is provided by barium studies (for micronodular disease) and CT (for tumoral forms and detection of extragastrointestinal subdiaphragmatic involvement). Gallium-67 scans are useful for detecting infection, but are of no benefit for detection of Kaposi's sarcoma (Woolfenden et al. 1987).

18.3 References

Albin J, Lewis E, Eftekhari F, Shirkhoda A (1987) Computed tomography of rectal and perirectal disease of AIDS patients. Gastrointest Radiol 12: 67-70

Balthazar EJ, Megibow AW, Fazzini E, Opulencia JF, Engel I (1985) Cytomegalovirus colitis in AIDS: radiographic findings in 11 patients. Radiology 155: 585-590

Bryk D, Farman J, Dallimond S, Meyers M, Wecksell A (1978) Kaposi's sarcoma of the intestinal tract: roentgen manifestations. Gastrointest Radiol 3: 425-430

Calenoff L (1972) Gastrointestinal Kaposi's sarcoma: roentgen manifestations. AJR 114: 525-528

Frager DH, Frager JD, Brandt LJ, Wolf EL, Rand LG, Klein RS, Beneventano TC (1986) Gastrointestinal complications of AIDS: radiologic features. Radiology 158: 597-603

Friedman SL, Wright T, Altman DF (1985) Gastrointestinal Kaposi's sarcoma in patients with acquired immunodeficiency syndrome. Endoscopic and autopsy findings. Gastroenterology 89: 102-108

Gottlieb MS, Groopman JE, Weinstein WM, Fahey JL, Detels R (1983) Acquired immunodeficiency syndrome. Ann Intern Med 99: 208-220

Hanno R, Owen L, Callen J (1979) Kaposi's sarcoma with extensive silent internal involvement. Int J Dermatol 9: 718-721

Jeffrey RB, Nyberg Da, Bottles K, Abrams DI, Federle MP, Wall SD, Wing VW, Laing FC (1986) Abdominal CT in acquired immunodeficiency syndrome. AJR 146: 7-13

Marche C, Zoubi D, Rene E, Girard PM (1986) Les lésions digestives en relation avec le SIDA. Valeur diagnostique. Ann Pathol 6: 282-286

McCauley DI, Naidich DP, Leitman BS, Reede DL, Laubenstein L (1982) Radiographic patterns of opportunistic lung infections and Kaposi sarcoma in homosexual men. AJR 139: 653-658

Mitsuyasu RT (1987) Clinical variants and staging of Kaposi's sarcoma. Semin Oncol 14 (Suppl 3): 13-18

Nyberg DA, Federle MP, Jeffrey RB, Bottles K, Wofsy CB (1985) Abdominal CT findings of disseminated mycobacterium avium intracellulare infection in AIDS. AJR 145. 297-299

Rose HS, Balthazar EJ, Megibow AJ, Horowitz L, Laubenstein LJ (1982) Alimentary tract involvement in Kaposi sarcoma: radiographic and endoscopic findings in 25 homosexual men. AJR 139: 661 566

Rothman S (1962) Remarks on sex, age and racial distribution of Kaposi's sarcoma and on possible pathogenetic factors. Acta Un Int Cancer 18: 326-329

Safai B (1984) Kaposi's sarcoma: a review of classical and epidemic forms. Ann NY Acad Sci 437: 373-381

Safai B (1987) Pathophysiology and epidemiology of epidemic Kaposi's sarcoma. Semin Oncol 14 (Suppl 3): 7-12

Wall SD, Ominsky S, Altman DF, Perkins CL, Sollitto R, Goldberg HI, Margulis AR (1986) Multifocal abnormalities of the gastrointestinal tract in AIDS. AJR 146: 1-5

Woolfenden JM, Carrasquillo JA, Larson SM, Simmons JT, Masur H, Smith PD, Shelhamer JH, Ognibene FP (1987) Acquired immunodeficiency syndrome: Ga-67 citrate imaging. Radiology 162: 383-387

19 Malignant Neurogenic Tumors*

Malignant neurogenic tumors are very rare entities often seen in patients with von Recklinghausen's disease. Neurofibrosarcomas are more common than schwannosarcomas. The tumor, which originates from the Schwann cell develops on a normal nerve or on a neurofibroma (Mouchet et al. 1969). For Fouet et al. (1962), the frequency of malignant degeneration is less than 10%. The prognosis for solitary malignant neurogenic tumors is better than for neoplasms occurring within the context of von Recklinghausen's disease (Sordillo et al. 1981). As for benign neurogenic tumors, the only gastrointestinal sites warranting mention are the stomach and the small intestine. Malignant neurogenic tumors in these two sites are dealt with in succession, before the description of these tumors in von Recklinghausen's disease.

19.1 Stomach
(Excluding von Recklinghausen's Disease)

19.1.1 General Features

Thirty-six cases were reviewed in the literature (Bruneton et al. 1983; De Oliviera et al. 1986; Fouet et al. 1962; Galea et al. 1984; Lescut et al. 1968; Mouchet et al. 1969; Nielsen and Eiken 1961; Pape and Hackensellner 1952; Peycelon and Replumaz 1958; Piattelli et al. 1978; Rautureau et al. 1971; Roux and Delavierre 1972; Rutten 1965; Schirmer et al.1975; Schwesinger and Teichmann 1977; Van der Hoeden et al. 1972; Yovanovitch and Yovanovitch 1962).
Malignant schwannomas account for 0.3%–0.8% of all malignant gastric tumors

---

* Written in collaboration with G. Schmutz.

(Belikian et al. 1980; Delannoy 1965). Compared to all benign neurogenic tumors, malignant tumors represent around one-quarter of all cases (Hill and Schmitt-Koppler 1972; Leroy et al. 1962). This high percentage emphasizes the importance of histologic examination and surgical treatment of neurogenic tumors. The site of predilection is the body of the stomach (58.1% of the cases reviewed); antral sites are rare (10.9%). Lesions are often bulky at diagnosis: 71.4% of the review cases measured over 10 cm (Table 19.1). This feature differentiates malignant tumors from benign tu-

Table 19.1. Schwannosarcomas of the stomach and small intestine

	Stomach	Small intestine
Clinical symptom	(36 cases)	(39 cases)
Pain	55.5%	33.3%
Upper gastrointestinal bleeding	72.2%	48.7%
Vomiting	11.1%	7.7%
Weight loss	36.7%	7.7%
Obstruction	–	25.6%
Palpable mass	30.5%	43.6%
Radiologic pattern	(28 cases)	(22 cases)
Intraluminal	14.3%	13.6%
Intramural	28.6%	13.6%
Subserosal	42.8%	63.6%
Dumbbell	14.3%	9.2%
Ulceration	60.7%	41.9%
Radiologic diagnosis	(28 cases)	(27 cases)
Benign	21.4%	7.4%
Malignant	25%	40.7%
Unknown	53.6%	51.9%
False-negative	–	–
Diameter	(28 cases)	(23 cases)
<5 cm	–	21.7%
5–10 cm	28.6%	43.5%
>10 cm	71.4%	34.8%

mors, which are usually under 5 cm in diameter at diagnosis. More than 75% of all solitary malignant neurogenic tumors occur in males; average patient age is 54 years. All of the cases reviewed were symptomatic; as for benign neurogenic tumors, bleeding and pain are the most frequent clinical symptoms. Less than one-third of patients present with a palpable mass. Surgery is the usual therapy. However, the prognosis is not as good as for carcinoma (Flabeau et al. 1962).

19.1.2 Imaging (Figs. 19.1, 19.2)

Review of the literature failed to disclose any false-negative errors for detection of gastric schwannosarcomas, undoubtedly because these lesions are usually bulky, despite the frequency of subserosal forms (42.8% of review cases). Ulceration is just as frequent as for benign neurogenic tumors. In 21.4% of cases, the appearance suggests a benign lesion; this is particularly true for intraluminal lesions (De Oliveira et al. 1986). The frequency of subserosal lesions reduces the value of barium studies for these tumors in the stomach. Ultrasonography and especially CT can suggest the origin of the tumor with better accuracy. Leiomyosarcoma is the most common presumptive diagnosis because of the greater frequency of this pathology.

19.2 Small Intestine (Excluding von Recklinghausen's Disease)

19.2.1 General Features

Thirty-nine cases of solitary malignant neurogenic tumors of the small intestine were reviewed in the literature (Cedermak 1949; Cherigie et al. 1954; Delorme et al. 1971; Dubourg et al. 1963; Fraisse and Etaix 1963; Leroy et al. 1962; Innocenti et al. 1978; Juan et al. 1980; Klepping et al. 1965; Lemaitre et al. 1976; Nillson and Jonsson 1957; Pape and Hackensellner 1952; Poulat and Grandmottet 1963; Viandier et al. 1982). Malignant schwannomas account for 0.2%–0.6% of all intestinal malignancies (Ostermiller et al. 1966;

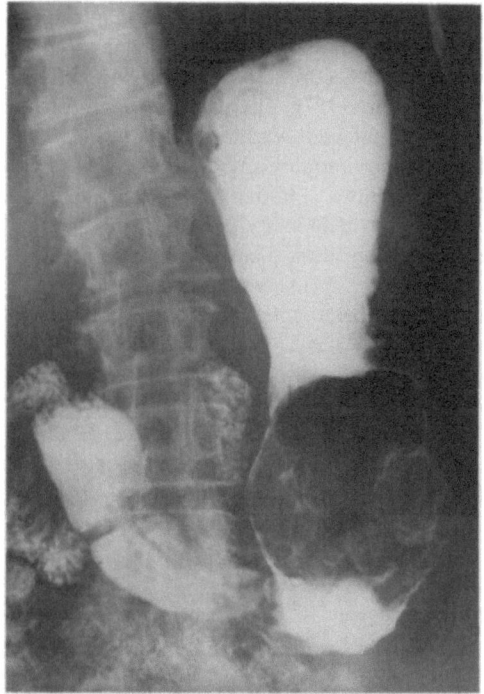

Fig. 19.1. Bulky tumoral lesion in the middle third of the stomach

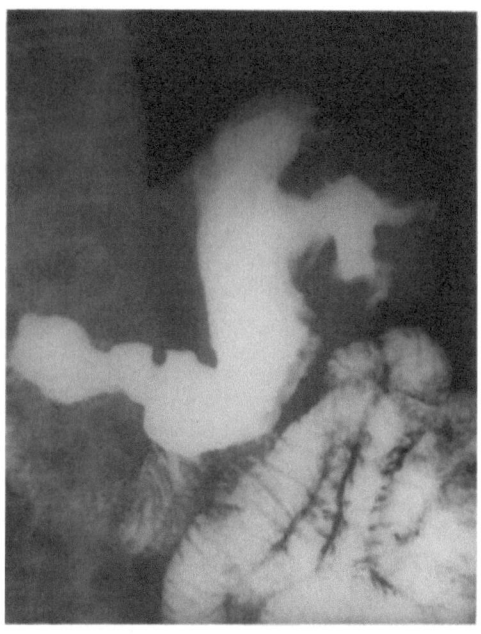

Fig. 19.2. Large ulcerated subserosal lesion

Sivak et al. 1975). Compared to all intestinal neurogenic tumors, malignant lesions represent 15%–40% (Bruneton et al. 1984; Nillson and Jonsson 1957). There are apparently no sites of predilection within the gastrointestinal tract. In the literature review, the distribution was as follows: duodenum 41.7%, jejunum 41.7%, ileum 16.6%. At diagnosis, lesions often measure more than 5 cm along their greatest axis (Table 19.1). Discrete masculine predominance has been noted (60.5%) and average age at diagnosis is 51 years. The clinical symptoms are nonspecific (bleeding and pain) but obstruction (25.6% of review cases) and a palpable mass (43.6% of review cases) are fairly common. Other acute clinical pictures such as intraperitoneal bleeding or perforation are rare (Poulat and Grandmottet 1963).

19.2.2 Imaging

In the literature review, there were no reports of false-negative errors for diagnosis of solitary malignant neurogenic tumors of the small intestine; this is probably due to the large size of these lesions. Despite the frequency of subserosal lesions (63.6%), barium studies are often positive; when they are negative, angiography can demonstrate the tumor. The tumoral

calcifications sometimes observed on plain films are not seen with benign lesions, and may thus be considered an element in favor of malignancy (Cedermak 1949; Lemaitre et al. 1976). Angiography constantly demonstrates hypervascularity; the heterogeneous nature of increased vascularization appears essentially related to the large size of the tumor and possible necrotic reorganization (Delorme et al. 1971; Lagache et al. 1974; Lemaitre et al. 1976). Too few cases have been investigated with angiography to define patterns suggestive of malignancy, but venous thrombosis appears to be correlated with a neoplastic etiology. No reports have been published on CT or ultrasound studies of these lesions, but the radiologic features demonstrated by barium examination and angiography are such that their appearance is probably similar to that of other connective tissue tumors, and in particular leiomyosarcoma. Conventional imaging studies correctly diagnose malignancy in over one-half of cases.

19.3 Malignant Neurogenic Tumors in von Recklinghausen's Disease

The estimated frequency of malignant degeneration of neurofibromas in patients with von

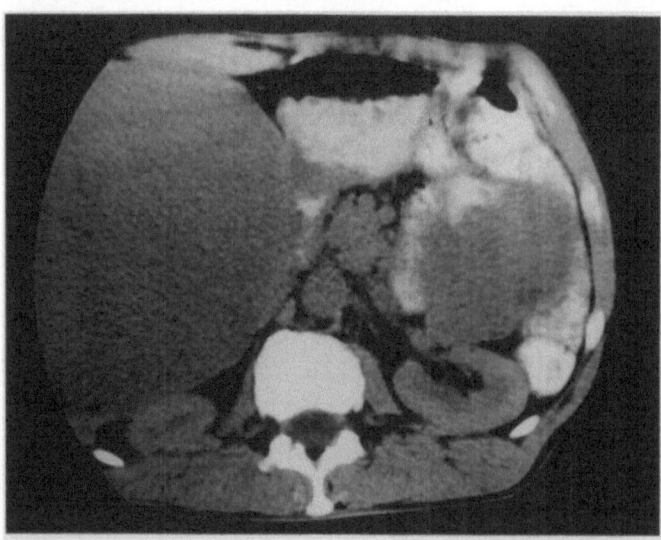

Fig. 19.3. Solid tumor infiltrating the jejunum (jejunal schwannosarcoma)

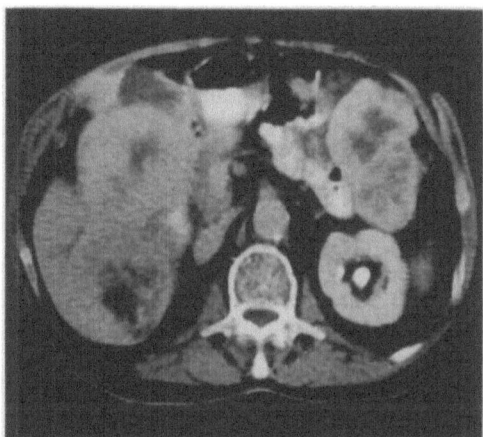

Fig. 19.4 Multifocal degeneration of intestinal lesions in a patient with von Recklinghausen's disease

Recklinghausen's disease is comparable to that of solitary neurogenic tumors: 3%–16% (Baldi et al. 1979; Croker and Greenstein 1979; Hochberg et al. 1974). Degenerated forms are usually associated with lesions elsewhere in the gastrointestinal tract, and especially in the stomach and small intestine (Figure 19.4). The generally small size of neurofibromas in von Recklinghausen's disease should be kept in mind when a lesion at least 10 cm in greatest axis is detected during examinations prompted by bleeding. Such large lesions may actually be a malignancy. Appearance of a malignant neurogenic tumor and degeneration of a neurofibroma are associated with a rapidly fatal outcome in patients with von Recklinghausen's disease.

19.4 References

Baldi A, Azzario G, Merli G (1979) Le localizzazioni digestive della neurofibromatosi di Recklinghausen. Minerva Chir 34: 365–374

Bedikian AY, Khankhanian N, Heilburn LK, Valdivieso M (1980) Primary lymphomas and sarcomas of the stomach. South Med J 73: 21–24

Bruneton JN, Drouillard J, Roux P, Ettore F, Lecomte P (1983) Neurogenic tumors of the stomach. Report of 18 cases and review of the literature. Fortschr Geb Roentgenstr 139: 192–198

Bruneton JN, Drouillard J, Roux P, Ettore F, Aubanel D (1984) Les tumeurs nerveuses de l'intestin grêle. Revue de la littérature à propos de 6 cas personnels. Ann Gastroenterol Hepatol (Paris) 20: 79–84

Cedermak J (1949) Neurinomas of the gastrointestinal tract. J Int Coll Surg 12: 5–11

Cherigie J, Tavernier C, Verspyck R, Raynal M (1954) Tumeurs bénignes du cadre duodénal. Difficulté du diagnostic. J Radiol 45: 788–789

Croker JR, Greenstein RJ (1979) Malignant schwannosarcoma of the stomach in a patient with von Recklinghausen's disease. Histopathology 3: 79–85

Delannoy E (1965) Les tumeurs bénignes de l'estomac. Lyon Chir 61: 161–175

Delorme G, Tavernier J, Labat JP, Grelet P, Lafitte JJ, Fagola M, Diard F (1971) Apport de l'angiographie dans le diagnostic des tumeurs du grêle. Ann Radiol 52: 673–680

De Oliveira FJ, Cabral Silveira JM, Martins MI, Marthinho F, Soares F, De Oliveira F (1986) Schwannomas gastricos. A proposito de cinco casos siendo tres malignos. Rev Esp Enferm Ap Digest 69: 124–128

Dubourg G, Fontan F, Gourdon A (1963) Hémorragie digestive massive par schwannome pseudo-diverticulaire du duodénum. Arch Fr Mal Appar Dig 52: 552–556

Flabeau F, Terquem J, Henry JG (1962) A propos de l'évolution et du traitement chirurgical des schwannomes gastriques. Presse Med 70: 1519–1520

Fouet A, Lescut J, Dauchy J (1962) Schwannome dégénéré. Arch Fr Mal Appar Dig 51: 223–234

Fraisse H, Etaix JP (1963) Tumeur maligne primitive du duodénum: à propos de deux nouveaux cas. Arch Fr Mal Appar Dig 52: 1058–1061

Galea S, Garieri R, Fodero G, Bertucci A (1984) Un raro caso di schwannoma maligno dello stomaco. Minerva Chir 70: 416–417

Hill K, Schmitt-Koppler A (1972) Zur Klinik und Histogenese der neurogenen Tumoren des oberen gastrointestinal Trakts. Dtsch Med Wochenschr 97: 899–902

Hochberg FH, Dasilva AB, Galdabini J, Richardson EP (1974) Gastrointestinal involvement in von Recklinghausen's neurofibromatosis. Neurology 24: 1144–1151

Innocenti P, Caizzi N, Ucchino S, Angelone A (1978) Il neurosarcoma della papilla di Vater. A proposito di un caso. Minerva Chir 33: 51–56

Juan IK, Sono F, Okada T, Muto M, Furuki A (1980) Neurogenic tumor of small intestine. Report of a case with review of literature. Gastroenterol Jpn 15: 112–119

Klepping C, Cortet P, Michiels R, Dusserre P, Jacquot B, Gaudet M, Michelot M (1965) Les schwannomes de l'intestin grêle (revue de la littérature à propos de deux observations personnelles). J Med Lyon 46: 1607–1632

Lagache G, Proye C, Laurent JC (1974) Schwannome sous-séreux du deuxième duodénum à symptomatologie tumorale et anémique. Sem Hop 50: 1208-1210

Lemaitre G, L'Hermine C, Proye C, Marache P, Ribet M (1976) Aspect radiologique des schwannomes du 2ème duodénum à développement extrinsèque (à propos de 3 observations). Lille Med 21: 827-832

Leroy A, Blanc P, Henry J (1962) Etude analytique des schwannomes digestifs. A propos d'une statistique de 72 cas de schwannomes. J Chir (Paris) 83: 683-708

Lescut J, Hamon G, Triquet O (1968) Schwannome exogastrique calcifiè. Presse Med 76: 984

Mouchet A, Marquand J, Guivarc'h M, Benoist JP, Saglier G (1969) A propos de 45 cas de tumeurs dites bénignes de l'estomac. Ann Chir 23: 1297-1308

Nielsen R, Eiken M (1961) Gastric tumours of neuᵒ:genic origin. Dan Med Bull 8: 121-125

Nillson B, Jonsson I (1957) Malignant neurinoma of the duodenum. Report of a case and review of the literature. Acta Chir Scand 113: 357-363

Ostermiller W, Joergenson EJ, Weibel L (1966) A clinical review of tumors of the small bowel. Am J Surg 111: 403-409

Pape R, Hackensellner HA (1952) Das röntgenologische Erscheinungsbild der neurogenen Tumoren des Verdauungstrakts. Fortschr Geb Roentgenstr 76: 691-711

Peycelon R, Replumaz P (1958) A propos des schwannomes gastriques. Arch Fr Mal Appar Dig 47: 465-479

Piattelli A, Innocenti P, Baiocchi A, Mancini G (1978) Il neurinosarcoma delle stomaco. Ann Ital Chir 50: 27-32

Poulat R, Grandmottet P (1963) Hémorragie intra-péritonéale par rupture d'un schwannome dégén-

éré de l'iléon. Résection-guérison. Arch Fr Mal Appar Dig 52: 359-361

Rautureau J, Gross G, Clot JP, Chomette G (1971) Schwannome kystique géant exogastrique. Ses difficultés diagnostiques. A propos d'une observation. Arch Fr Mal Appar Dig 60: 542-552

Roux M, Delavierre P (1972) Schwannome malin du moignon gastrique chez un ancien gastrectomisé. Sem Hop 48: 1260-1264

Rutten APM (1965) Neurogenic tumours of the stomach. Br J Surg 52: 920-925

Schirmer G, Kozuschek W, Helpap B (1975) Neurogene Magentumoren: solitare Schwannome und Neurofibrome. Fortschr Geb Roentgenstr 122: 534-541

Schwesinger G, Teichmann W (1977) Monstroses malignes Magenneurinom. Z Gesamte Inn Med Ihre Grenzgeb 32: 233-235

Sivak MV, Sullivan BH, Farmer RG (1975) Neurogenic tumor of the small intestine. Review of the literature and report of a case with endoscopic removal. Gastroenterology 68: 374-380

Sordillo PP, Helson L, Hajdu SI, Magill GB, Kosloff C, Golbey RB, Beattie EJ (1981) Malignant schwannoma. Clinical characteristics, survival, and response to therapy. Cancer 47: 2503-2509

Van der Hoeden R, Bremien A, Hins C, Parmentier R, Tala H (1972) Schwannome malin de l'estomac à développement exogastrique. Sem Hop 48: 1255-1259

Viandier A, Clot P, Gayet B, Douard MC (1982) Schwannomes et schwannosarcomes duodénaux et de l'angle duodénojéjunal. A propos de 3 cas. Ann Chir 36: 368-370

Yovanovitch BY, Yovanovitch DM (1962) Les tumeurs bénignes de l'estomac. Etude à propos de 13 observations personnelles. Bull Soc Chir Paris 52: 77-86

20 Primary Malignant Melanoma of the Gastrointestinal Tract*

Primary malignant melanoma of the digestive mucosa is very rare, accounting for only 0.05%–0.5% of all malignant tumors of the gastrointestinal tract. Furthermore, the histogenesis of these lesions within segments of the gastrointestinal tract is controversial, because secondary gastrointestinal involvement is common during the course of melanomas.

20.1 Pathology

Gastrointestinal melanomas are identical to melanomas in other anatomic sites (Go and Zirkin 1982). The tumoral tissue is composed of varying forms of melanocytes (Arnaud et al. 1978), ranging from an epithelial structure with round cells to a pseudosarcomatous structure with independent spindle-shaped cells. Fontana's stain reveals melanin in the tumoral cells as well as in the cytoplasm of cells of the stroma and the submucosa (Chalkiadakis et al. 1985). In certain cases, no pigment is visualized (achromic malignant melanoma). On electron microscopy, the cytoplasm of the tumoral cells contains a variable number of premelanomas and denser and more developed melanosomes (Go and Zirkin 1982). The primary nature of malignant gastrointestinal tract melanomas is debated because melanoblasts, the origin of these tumors, do not exist in the stomach, duodenum, small bowel, colon, or rectum (Masson 1951; Saby et al. 1978). Nevertheless, islands of heterotopic cells, while a very exceptional possibility, could give rise to such primary tumors. Esophageal and anorectal lesions are less controversial because 4% of normal subjects have melanic cells in the esophagus, and melanocytes

are present in the normal transitional mucosa of the anorectal junction (Phade and Lawrence 1981). Malignant melanomas of the anal margin are classed as cutaneous malignant melanomas (Schmutz et al. 1988).

20.2 General Features

Differentiation of a primary melanoma from secondary involvement requires demonstration of junctional activity at the periphery of the tumor, i.e., solitary theques or nevus cells within the malpighian layer (Vayre et al. 1978).

The frequencies of secondary anorectal and esophageal melanomas (respectively, 5% and 4%) are markedly lower than secondary involvement in other gastrointestinal sites: small intestine 58%, stomach 26%, colon 22%, duodenum 12% (De La Pava et al. 1963).

20.3 Gastrointestinal Sites

A number of cases were reviewed in the literature (Cattan et al. 1957; Delavierre et al. 1973; Fingerhut et al. 1979; Milton et al. 1967; Robertson 1954). Even though their primary origin is debated, several dozen cases had features highly suggestive of a primary lesion (Banzet et al. 1953; Reed et al. 1962; Saby et al. 1978; Vachon et al. 1967). These lesions are usually discovered in patients presenting with acute intestinal obstruction secondary to intussusception (Dalmas et al. 1976; Fingerhut et al. 1979) or following massive gastrointestinal hemorrhage of sudden onset in an elderly individual (Chometowski et al. 1977; Harris 1964). The tumor is often large, ulcerated, and very invasive, with a distinctive blackish color at surgery. The recent history often includes

---

* Written in collaboration with G. Schmutz.

acute disease, progressive deterioration in general condition, diarrhea and obstruction, or vague abdominal pain.

Complementary examinations are rarely performed because of the emergency situation at discovery of the lesion. *Barium studies* may reveal a malignant-appearing lesion as an asymmetrical, irregular stenosing tumor or a large endoluminal nodular lesion with central ulcerations, sometimes creating a bull's eye or target image (Reeder and Cavanagh 1974). This nodular lesion may be partially masked by intussusception (Arnauud et al. 1978; Dalmas et al. 1976). *Angiography* can evidence anarchic malignant-type tumoral hypervascularity (Arnaud et al. 1978). No reports of *CT* studies of primary malignant gastrointestinal melanomas were found in a review of the literature. However, CT would probably demonstrate a solid density tumoral mass enhancing strongly after contrast medium injection.

20.4 Primary Melanoma of the Esophagus

Reports on the subject by numerous authors were reviewed (Baur 1906, Chaput et al. 1974; Chalkiadakis et al. 1985; De La Pava et al. 1963; Go and Zirkin 1982; Jaleski and Waldo 1910; Ludwig et al. 1981; Robertson 1954; Schmutz et al. 1988; Vayre et al. 1978; Witonsky 1968). Primary melanoma of the esophagus accounts for only 0.1% of all primary esophageal malignancies (Chalkiadakis et al. 1985; Lagache et al. 1977). Baur described the first case in 1906; 52 additional cases have been reported since then (Chalkiadakis et al. 1985; Lagache et al. 1977). Males are affected twice as often as women, and mean age at diagnosis is 59 years (Chalkiadakis et al. 1985; Lagache et al. 1977).

There are no specific clinical manifestations, but dysphagia is nearly always present, and one-half of patients complain of pain (epigastric or retrosternal, continuous or intermittent). Pain may appear before dysphagia and suggest a gastroduodenal lesion. Less often, regurgitation, hypersialorrhea, or even deterioration in general condition are noted. The physical examination is normal (Schmutz et al. 1988).

Barium studies may demonstrate an obviously malignant lesion in the form of an asymmetrical, eccentric, irregular, ulcerated nodule associated with rigidity and parietal infiltration; the esophagogram may also show a regular,

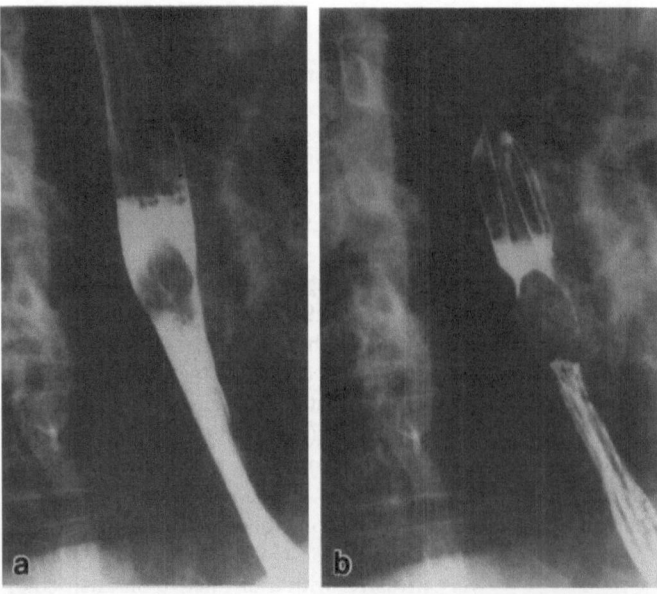

Fig. 20.1 a, b. Primary melanoma of the esophagus (intraluminal lesion < 3 cm)

rounded, 2-3-cm diameter endoluminal nodule with or without a pedicle. The esophageal walls remain pliable and mould to the lesion; over half of these lesions occur in the lower third of the esophagus (Go and Zirkin 1982). This second appearance is suggestive of a benign submucosal tumor such as leiomyoma, fibroma, or Abrikosof's tumor; a fibrovascular polyp is less probable, but an extrinsic lesion is sometimes described. A benign-appearing submucosal tumor was mentioned in 24% of the cases reviewed (Chalkiadakis et al. 1985) (Figure 20.1).

Endoscopy may allow immediate diagnosis if the tumor has the typical black coloration, but often it is gray or blue or even unpigmented (achromic forms). Gross diagnosis at endoscopy is thus possible in only a quarter of cases (Chaput et al. 1974). These ulcerated, friable, exophytic tumors tend to bleed easily. Bulky tumors may have a hard, slightly elastic consistency, with soft zones (Vayre et al. 1978). Biopsy is indispensable yet is diagnostic only half of the time. Besides the negative nature of certain biopsy specimens, interpretation is difficult because of the cellular polymorphism. Differential diagnoses include anaplastic carcinoma, undifferentiated or poorly differentiated adenocarcinoma, and fibroblastic sarcoma (Arnaud et al. 1978; Dalmas et al. 1976). Diagnosis by examination of surgical specimens is easier: spread to the muscle wall is rare, as is invasion of the peripheral tissues; by contrast, 50% of patients have nodal involvement (Vayre et al. 1978) and metastatic spread through the bloodstream is rapid.

20.5 Anorectal Melanoma

Several reports were reviewed in the literature (Guivarc'h et al. 1973; Huguier and Luboinski 1973; Ludwig et al. 1981; Phade and Lawrence 1981). Anorectal melanomas account for 0.25%-0.5% of all anal cancers (Vayre et al. 1978); they are the most frequent gastrointestinal localization, and the third site of primary malignant melanomas after the skin (67%) and the eye (8%), before the vulva (4%) and the bucco-sinusal mucosa (Guivarc'h et al. 1973; Phade and Lawrence 1981).

The first case was reported in 1857 by Moore (Chalkiadakis et al. 1985); over 200 cases had been published by 1981. Primary malignant melanomas have a predilection for the anus; only 14 cases concern the rectum (Schmutz et al. 1988). There is no sex predominance; average age at diagnosis is 64 years.

Rectal bleeding is the predominant clinical symptom; melena (blood containing melamine) has also been reported (Schmutz et al. 1988). Because these lesions often lie near the anal margin, patients may complain of tenesmus, false sensations of defecation, a sensation of prolapse, etc. The patient's general condition is unaffected. Digital rectal examination will detect a smooth, well-limited polypoid lesion of variable size.

Rectoscopy allows visualization of the tumor, which sometimes has a distinctive black coloration. It is often ulcerated, bleeds easily, and feels hard on palpation. Biopsies are often diagnostic, provided the sample fragments are large enough.

Barium enema may be negative if the lesion is small (under 5 mm); lesions in the lower part of the rectum may be masked by the intrarectal canula (Figure 20.2). These usually nodular lesions with sharp margins can vary in size from several millimeters to several centimeters. Sessile lesions predominate, but a stalk occurs occasionally. The mucosa is smooth or only slightly irregular. When the dimensions are larger than 2 cm, the nodular appearance suggests a submucosal tumor with sharp limits;

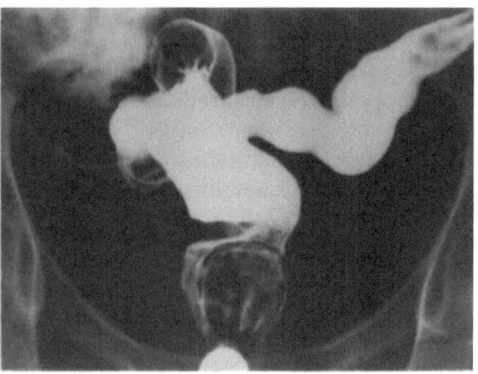

Fig. 20.2. Primary melanoma of the rectum (polypoid lesion <5 cm)

lesions under 2 cm correspond to common polyps.

Histologically, the lesion originates in the submucosa (melanocytes) but rapidly spreads to the entire rectal wall, then to the ischiorectal space. The pelvic and inguinal lymph nodes are often invaded; hepatic and lung metastases are possible (Vayre et al. 1978).

Regardless of the location of the lesion, surgical resection remains the treatment of choice, especially since preoperative histologic diagnosis is inconclusive. Chemotherapy (actinomycin) (Fingerhut et al. 1979) or immunotherapy are often offered. Despite the radioresistance of these tumors, postoperative external beam or interstitial implant irradiation is sometimes used, especially for recurrent disease (Lagache et al. 1977). Regardless of the therapeutic attitude and the disease stage at the time of surgery, the prognosis is very poor: average survival is only 7 months for esophageal lesions (Lagache et al. 1977) and less than 12 months for anorectal lesions (Schmutz et al. 1988).

20.6 Conclusion

Primary malignant melanomas of the digestive tract are very exceptional compared to other primary tumors and especially to secondary involvement by melanoma. Whereas secondary gastrointestinal sites of malignant melanoma essentially occur in the small intestine and the stomach, primary lesions are found almost exclusively in the esophagus and the anorectal region. The gross appearance may be very suggestive of the diagnosis. Radiologically, these tumors may be either obviously malignant, or benign-appearing submucosal nodules. Contrary to secondary localizations, there is no large central ulceration. Surgery often provides the diagnosis but improves survival only slightly (less than 12 months).

20.7 References

Arnaud JP, Miclo S, Aprahamiam M, Weill-Bousson M, Adloff M (1978) Métastases intestinales et vésiculaires d'un naevo épithélioma. A propos d'une observation révélée par une hémorrhagie occulte. J Chir (Paris) 115: 29–34

Banzet P, Delarue J, Chappelart S, Santagostini F, Civatte J (1953) Un cas de mélanome à localisations gastro-intestinales multiples apparemment primitives. Presse Med 61: 1732–1734

Baur E (1906) Ein Fall von primaren Melanoma des Ösophagus. Arch Anal Inst Tübingen 5: 343–354

Chaput JC, Gourdier S, Martin E, Carrieu H, Etienne JP (1974) Naevocarcinome primitif de l'oesophage. Sem Hop 2: 151–157

Cattan R, Champeau M, Frumusan P, Cerf M, Nivet P, Habib L (1957) Tumeur mélanique gastro-duodénale. Arch Fr Mal Appar Dig 46: 1125–1132

Chalkiadakis G, Wihlm JM, Morand G, Weill-Bousson M, Witz JP (1985) Primary malignant melanoma of the esophagus. Ann Thorac Surg 39: 5–7

Chometowski S, Nguyen Cat R, Assadourian R, Bourde J, Lamy J (1977) Métastases iléales tardives d'un mélanome cutané périphérique. Manifestations hémorragiques prédominantes. J Chir (Paris) 113: 537–542

Dalmas H, Anfossi G, Dor JF, Basbous D, Guidicelli C (1976) Invaginations jéjuno et iléo-iléales révélatrices de multiples métastases mélaniques de l'intestin grêle. J Chir (Paris) 111: 341–346

De la Pava S, Nigo Gosyan G, Pickren J, Cabrera A (1963) Melanosis of the esophagus. Cancer 16: 48–50

Delavierre P, Vayre P, Hureau J, Martignon C, Bourdais JP, Roux M, Justin-Besancon L (1973) Tumeurs gastriques non carcinomateuses. A propos de 35 observations. Sem Hop 47: 3119–3127

Fingerhut A, Eugene C, Pourcher J, Bergue A, Ronat R (1979) Mélanomes malins de l'estomac et du grêle révélés par une occlusion fébrile. Sem Hop 53: 1719–1721

Go ATS, Zirkin RM (1982) Primary malignant melanoma of the esophagus: a case report with endoscopic and electron microscopic studies. Am J Gastroenterol 77: 840–843

Guivarch M, Nathan G, Mouchet A, Saglier G (1973) Un cas de mélanome malin primitif de l'ampoule du rectum. Arch Fr Mal Appar Dig 62: 613–624

Harris MN (1964) Massive gastro-intestinal hemorrhage due to metastatic malignant melanoma of small intestine. Arch Surg 88: 1049–1051

Huguier M, Luboinski J (1973) Les mélanomes malins ano-rectaux. Arch Fr Mal Appar Dig 62: 579–590

Jaleski TC, Waldo PV (1910) Primary melanotic sarcoma of the esophagus: report of a case. Am J Anat 24: 340–344

Lagache G, Heraud M, Leduc M (1977) A propos d'un cas de mélanome rectal. Lille Med 22: 2–3

Ludwig MC, Shaw R, De Suto-Nagy C (1981) Primary malignant melanoma of the esophagus. Cancer 48: 2528–2534

Masson P (1951) My conception of cellular nevi. Cancer 4: 9

Milton GW, Lanebrown M, Gilder M (1967) Malignant melanoma with an occult primary lesion. Br J Surg 54: 651-658

Phade VR, Lawrence WR (1981) Anorectal melanoma. Br J Surg 68: 667-668

Reed PL, Raskin HF, Graff PW (1962) Malignant melanoma of stomach. JAMA 182: 298-299

Reeder HM, Cavanagh RC (1974) "Bull's eye" lesions. Solitary or multiple nodules in the gastrointestinal tract with large center ulcerations. JAMA 825-826

Robertson JW (1954) Malignant melanoma of the esophagus, as one of multiple malignant tumors. Gastroenterology 27: 121-126

Saby R, Chate M, Hypousteguy D, Baste JC (1978) Mélanome malin du grêle, point de départ cutané régressif, survie à 4 ans. Chir Paris 104: 916-918

Schmutz G, Drape JL, Weill-Bousson M, Wihlm JM, Adloff M, Bockel R (1988) Les mélanomes malins primitifs du tractus digestif: oesophage et rectum. J Radiol 69: 285-289

Vachon A, Tete R, Gauthier J, Abry M (1967) Les tumeurs mélaniques de l'estomac. Rev Lyon Med 16: 437-443

Vayre P, Hureau J, Jost JL, Delavierre P, Lambert D, Benit C, Bourdais JP, Jost B, Letailleur M, Germain M (1978) Les mélanomes malins primitifs du tube digestif. Chirurgie 104: 968-972

Witonsky O (1968) Primares Melanoblastum malignum des Ösophagus. Krebsarzt 23: 94-96

21 Malignant Fibrous Histiocytoma*

Malignant fibrous histiocytoma (MFH) is the most common sarcoma in adults, with a frequency of 15%–20% (Suit et al. 1975; Weiss and Enzinger 1978). Soft tissue lesions of the extremities predominate. Only 16% of published cases concern the abdominal cavity, where the retroperitoneum represents the most frequent site (Weiss and Enzinger 1978). If secondary abdominal lesions are excluded, in particular after retroperitoneal involvement (Goldman et al. 1986), primary digestive tract MFH is very rare.

21.1 General Features

MFH involved a diagnostic problem in publications prior to 1970, because this tumor was poorly recognized and often classified under other designations (Enzinger et al. 1969). Macroscopically, these essentially subserosal lesions may spread to the digestive tract lumen (Shibuya et al. 1985; Wawman et al. 1983) or contiguous viscera (Balpe et al. 1981). Stenosing forms (Lin et al. 1983) and endoluminal pedunculated tumors that can cause intussusception (Sewell et al. 1980) are less common. Multiple lesions have been described only rarely (Shibuya et al. 1985; Adams 1984; Levinson and Tsang 1982). These bulky, often necrotic tumors generally do not invade the adjacent lymph nodes, and hepatic metastases are a late occurrence (Balpe et al. 1981; Sewell et al. 1980).

The pleomorphic histologic appearance of MFH associates fibrogenic areas with spindle cells arranged in storiform pattern, clusters or sheets of histiocyte-like cells, benign and malignant giant cells, foam cells, inflammatory cells, scattered mitotic figures, and anaplasia of stromal cells (Weiss and Enzinger 1978).

Four histologic subtypes of MFH have been identified (fibrous, giant cell, myxoid, and inflammatory), but they have no prognostic significance (Kearney et al. 1980). Fibrous MFH is the most common type. MFH generally affects the limbs (68% of all cases for Weiss and Enzinger 1978). Intra-abdominal involvement, which is very rare, occurs essentially in the retroperitoneum (Goldman et al. 1986; Ros et al. 1984).

A review of the literature revealed very few reports of gastrointestinal MFH. Published cases included sites in the stomach (Adams et al. 1983; Balpe et al. 1981; O'Brien and Stout 1964; Radner et al. 1985; Shibuya et al. 1985), small intestine (Lin et al. 1983; Ros et al. 1984; Shibuya et al. 1985; Singh et al. 1985; Suster 1986), colon and rectum (Adams 1984; Baratz et al. 1986; Levinson and Tsang 1982; Rubbini et al. 1983; Sewell et al. 1980; Verma et al. 1979; Wawman et al. 1983), and appendix (Zazzaro et al. 1980). MFH generally affects individuals aged 50–60 years (Ros et al. 1983); there is no sex predominance. Owing to the deep-seated nature of these lesions, diagnosis is often not made until an advanced stage. All types of gastrointestinal symptoms have been described; a mass syndrome is frequent (Levinson and Tsang 1982; Lin et al. 1983). Endoluminal lesions can cause intussusception (Sewell et al. 1980; Shibuya et al. 1985) while tumors exerting pressure on adjacent viscera may be responsible for chronic obstruction (Lin et al. 1983; Suster 1986).

Although the histologic subtype has no prognostic value, the following elements are all associated with a favorable prognosis: small diameter tumor, superficial location, inflammatory form (Rydholm and Syk 1986; Weiss and Enzinger 1978). By contrast, a diameter greater

---

* Written in collaboration with G. Schmutz.

than 5 cm, the possibility of only partial resection, and early relapse (less than 1 year after surgery) are all factors pointing to a poor outcome (Bertoni et al. 1985).

Both early relapses (before 12 months) and prolonged, relapse-free survival lasting several years (Adams 1984) have been reported in patients with gastrointestinal MFH (Adams et al. 1983; Wawman et al. 1983). Generally speaking, MFH recurs in 37.5%–51% of cases (Bertoni et al. 1985; Kearney et al. 1980; Weiss and Enzinger 1978). For Weiss and Enzinger (1978), 42% of patients develop metastases, essentially in the lungs and lymph nodes. Hepatic metastases account for only 15% of relapses. Overall survival is 60% at 2 years and 14%–36% at 5 years (Bertoni et al. 1985; Kearney et al. 1980; Weiss and Enzinger 1978).

21.2 Imaging

Ultrasonography and *CT* are the two most valuable imaging techniques; barium examinations, angiography, and gallium scanning are of less interest. Goldman et al. (1986) defined three sonographic patterns: a hypoechoic pattern (the most frequent), a mixed pattern that may include extensive necrotic areas, and a predominantly anechoic pattern with thick septa. Other authors have emphasized the frequency of the mixed pattern with necrotic zones (Ros et al. 1984; Rubbini et al. 1983). Despite the few literature reports on abdominal MFH, no particular pattern appears associated with a given organ, whether it be the liver or a segment of the digestive tract.

CT images MFH as a solid lesion (Ros et al. 1984); the frequent areas of necrosis may contain calcifications (Levinson and Tsang 1982; Ros et al. 1984). Tumoral spread to adjacent viscera is correctly identified by CT (Balpe et al. 1981). Few authors have mentioned tumor enhancement following bolus injection of contrast medium.

Neither ultrasound nor CT findings are specific for MFH. Differential diagnoses for gastrointestinal tract sites include leiomyosarcoma, fibrosarcoma, liposarcoma, and malignant mesothelioma. Liposarcoma cannot be ruled out because not all liposarcomas exhibit areas of fat density. In general, abdominal MFH is diagnosed preoperatively as a malignant tumor of probably sarcomatous origin (Figs. 20.1, 20.2).

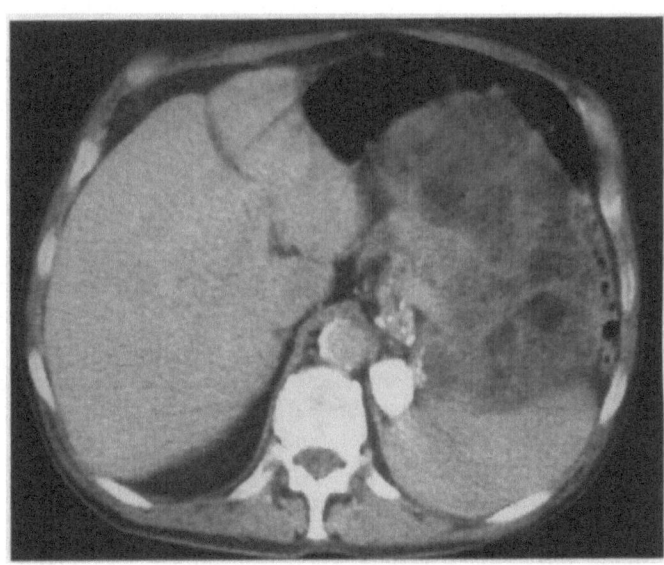

Fig. 21.1. Bulky lesion involving the left mesocolon. The posterior portion of this tumoral mass is calcified and there are extensive areas of necrosis

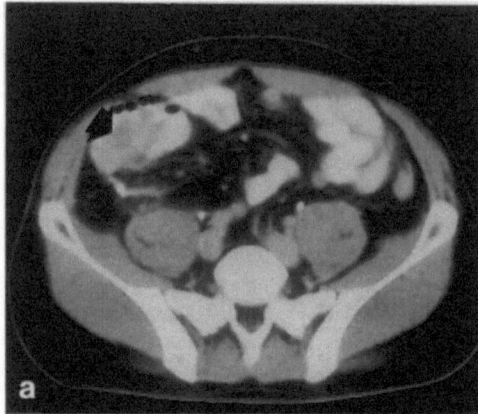

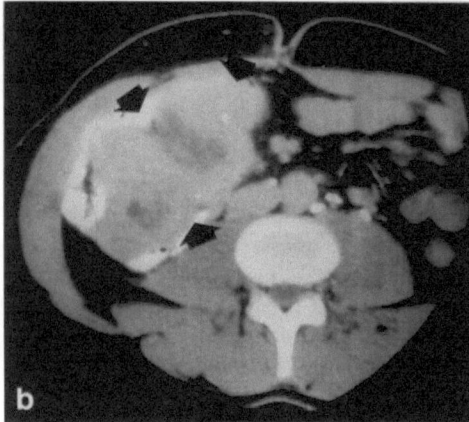

Fig. 21.2 a, b. Malignant fibrous histiocytoma of the right mesocolon. The initial examination **(a)** revealed parietal infiltration of the right colon *(arrow)*. Resection was performed, but a recurrence developed less than one year later in the form of extensive subserosal infiltration *(arrow)* which did not affect bowel function **(b)**

The other radiologic techniques have a complementary interest, but are performed only after CT and ultrasonography. Tumoral calcifications throughout the gastrointestinal tract can be visualized on *plain films* taken prior to barium studies (Levinson and Tsang 1982) Parietal involvement with intraluminal invasion is seen as filling defects or polypoid growths on *barium films* (Rubbini et al. 1983; Shibuya et al. 1985), although purely subserosal forms may be overlooked (Baratz et al. 1986). The variable *angiographic features* reported in the literature include both hypervascularity, as in osseous MFH, and hypovascularity, as with

cerebral and renal lesions (Burgener and Landman 1976; Goldman et al. 1986). *Gallium scanning* has no real interest for pretherapy workups but can be helpful for detection of recurrent disease (Verma et al. 1979).

21.3 Conclusion

MFH is a frequent sarcomatous tumor in adults but rarely affects the digestive tract. These deep, bulky, and extensively necrotic lesions are correctly analyzed by both ultrasonography and CT, but there are no specific imaging patterns suggestive of the diagnosis prior to surgery. CT and ultrasonography are useful for topographic workups aimed at detecting tumoral spread to contiguous organs. Owing to the risk of recurrence and the deep nature of MFH lesions, follow-up by imaging studies is particularly indicated.

21.4 References

Adams HW (1984) Malignant fibrous histiocytoma associated with diverticulitis of the colon. J Miss State Med Assoc 25: 205–206

Adams HW, Adkins JR, Rehak EM (1983) Malignant fibrous histiocytoma presenting as a bleeding gastric ulcer. Am J Gastroenterol 78: 212–213

Balpe DM, Koehler RE, Kartstaedt N, Stanley RJ, Sagel SS (1981) Computed tomography of gastric neoplasms. Radiology 140: 431–436

Baratz M, Ostrzega N, Michowitz M, Messer G (1986) Primary inflammatory malignant fibrous histiocytoma of the colon. Dis Colon Rectum 29: 462–465

Bertoni F, Capanna R, Biagini R, Bacchini P, Guerra A, Ruggieri P, Present D, Campanacci M (1985) Malignant fibrous histiocytoma of soft tissue. An analysis of 78 cases located and deeply seated in the extremities. Cancer 56: 356–367

Burgener FA, Landman S (1976) Angiographic features of malignant fibrous histiocytomas. Radiology 121: 581–583

Enzinger TM, Lattes R, Torloni M (1969) Histological typing of soft tumors. International histological classification of tumors. No 3. World Health Organization, Geneva

Goldman SM, Hartman DS, Weiss SW (1986) The varied radiographic manifestations of retroperitoneal malignant fibrous histiocytoma revealed through 27 cases. J Urol 135: 33–38

Kearny MM, Soule EH, Iving JC (1980) Malignant fibrous histiocytoma. A retrospective study of 167 cases. Cancer 45: 167–178

Levinson MM, Tsang D (1982) Multicentric malignant fibrous histiocytomas of the colon: report of a case and review of the subject. Dis Colon Rectum 25: 327-331

Lin JI, Kim CK, Tsung SH, Peoples JB (1983) Malignant fibrous histiocytoma of the ileum. Dis Colon Rectum 26: 335-338

O'Brien JE, Stout AR (1964) Malignant fibrous xanthomas. Cancer 17: 1445-1455

Radner H, Beham A, Weybora W (1985) Malignes fibröses Histiozytom des Magens. Ein Fallbericht mit Literaturübersicht. Pathologe 6: 313-318

Ros PR, Viamonte M, Rywlin AM (1984) Malignant fibrous histiocytoma: mesenchymal tumor of ubiquitous origin. AJR 142: 753-759

Rubbini M, Marzola A, Spaneda R, Scalco GB, Zamboni P, Guerrera C, Donini I (1983) Primary malignant fibrous histiocytoma of the sigmoid colon: a case report. Ital J Surg Sci 13: 299-302

Rydholm A, Syk I (1986) Malignant fibrous histiocytoma of soft tissue. Correlation between clinical variables and histologic malignancy grade. Cancer 57: 2323-2324

Sewell R, Levine BA, Harrison GK, Tio F, Schwesinger WH (1980) Primary malignant fibrous histiocytoma of the intestine. Intussusception of a rare neoplasm. Dis Colon Rectum 23: 198-201

Shibuya H, Azumi N, Onda Y, Abe F (1985) Multiple primary malignant fibrous histiocytoma of the stomach and small intestine. Acta Pathol Jpn 35: 157-164

Singh G, Gupta S, Gupta S (1985) Malignant fibrous histiocytoma of solitary jejunal diverticulum. J Surg Oncol 28: 273-276

Suit HD, Russell WO, Martin RG (1975) Sarcoma of soft tissue: clinical and histopathologic parameters and response to treatment. Cancer 35: 1478-1483

Suster S (1986) Transformation of Hodgkin's disease into malignant fibrous histiocytoma. Cancer 57: 264-268

Verma P, Chandra U, Bhatia PS (1979) Malignant histiocytoma of the rectum: report of a case. Dis Colon Rectum 22: 179-182

Wawman M, Faegenburg D, Waxman JS, Janelli DE (1983) Malignant fibrous histiocytoma of the colon associated with diverticulitis. Dis Colon Rectum 26: 339-343

Weiss SW, Enzinger FM (1978) Malignant fibrous histiocytoma. An analysis of 200 cases. Cancer 41: 2250-2266

Zazzaro PF, Bosworth JE, Schneider V, Zelenak JJ (1980) Gallium scanning in malignant fibrous histiocytoma. AJR 135: 775-779

Tumors with
an Indeterminate Prognosis

22 Carcinoid Tumors*

Rare lesions that represent 1.5% of all gastrointestinal tumors (Kowlessar 1973), carcinoids are unusual in several ways:

- Their malignant predisposition varies as a function of their anatomic site.
- They are classified as amine precursor uptake and decarboxylation (APUD) neoplasms.
- A relationship exists between the clinical carcinoid syndrome and the presence of hepatic metastases.
- Laboratory tests are important for diagnosis [serotoninemia, increased urinary excretion of 5-hydroxy-indolacetic acid (5-HIAA)].
- A malignant carcinoid does not invariably have a poor prognosis.

22.1 General Features

22.1.1 Gross Features

Gastrointestinal carcinoids are a heterogeneous group of neoplasms of the enterochromaffin cells of the gastrointestinal tract. Derived from the ectoderm, these APUD cells are believed to be programed for a neuroendocrine function (Pearse 1980). Carcinoids are divided into foregut, midgut, and hindgut tumors depending on their location in the tissues derived, respectively, from the anterior primitive intestine (bronchus, esophagus, stomach, duodenum, pancreas, bile ducts), the middle intestine (small intestine, appendix, right colon), and the posterior intestine (left colon and rectum); 90% of all carcinoid tumors occur in the intestinal tract. The main extragastrointestinal site (10%–14%) is the bronchus (Godwin 1975; Okike et al. 1976).

The gastrointestinal site incidence is as follows: appendix (35.5%–47%), small intestine (18.9%–30.3%), rectum (12.2%–17%), colon (2%–6.7%), stomach (2%–2.5%) (Godwin 1975; Orloff 1971). The marked proclivity for the appendix is further reflected by the fact that carcinoids are found in 0.5%–0.6% of appendectomies (Collins 1955; Glasser and Bhargavan 1980). Most tumors associated with the clinical carcinoid syndrome occur in the small intestine (Warner et al. 1979).

The frequently small (< 15 mm) primary tumor originates in the submucosa and propagates through the muscularis towards the mesentery. Five histologic types have been defined: insular, trabecular, glandular, undifferentiated, and mixed (Johnson et al. 1983). These histologic growth patterns have a prognostic significance, with undifferentiated lesions having a very poor prognosis (Hajdu et al. 1974).

The incidence of metastatic spread is a function of the gastrointestinal site. Metastases are extremely frequent with colonic tumors (55%–63%) but much less so for appendiceal lesions (6%) (Sanders 1973). Gastrointestinal carcinoids metastasize to the lymph nodes and liver. The clinical carcinoid syndrome is accompanied by liver metastases; solitary nodal metastases are less frequent (Feldman and Jones 1982). Metastatic spread is also correlated with invasion of the muscularis and the size of the primary tumor (Orloff 1971), although this last parameter is inconstant. Even ileal tumors smaller than 1 cm, for example, may be associated with metastatic spread (Thompson et al. 1985).

The frequency of multiple carcinoids varies according to the site, from 1%–4.2% in the appendix to 29%–37% in the ileum (Beaton et al. 1981; Moertel et al. 1961; Orloff 1971).

---

* Written in collaboration with J. Drouillard.

22.1.2 Clinical Features

Carcinoids occur with equal frequency in men and in women. They are rare in children, and mean age at the time of diagnosis is 50 years (Goldthorn and Canizaro 1986). Schematically, diagnosis of these tumors is made in three situations:

- As an incidental finding at laparotomy (non-secretory carcinoid, appendiceal carcinoid).
- Atypical carcinoid syndrome.
- Nonspecific, isolated clinical manifestations: intestinal hypermotility, vasomotor paroxysms, Koenig's syndrome, gastrointestinal bleeding, or tumoral hepatomegaly.

Many carcinoid tumors are discovered during surgery or at autopsy (60% for Thompson et al. 1985).
The initial manifestations are often nonspecific: abdominal pain, chronic diarrhea, intermittent obstruction. Hemorrhage is rare (Zeitels et al. 1982). The carcinoid syndrome, which does not become clear until the appearance of liver metastases, occurs in only 1.12%–5% of patients (McDonald 1956; Sanders 1973); 75% of such cases concern metastatic ileal tumors (Thompson et al. 1985). The carcinoid syndrome is responsible for cutaneous flushing, diarrhea, and cardiac involvement (Graham-Smith 1968). Four types of flushing have been described; the causative factor remains unclear, but bradykinin, histamine, and serotonin have all been implicated (Delcourt and Robberecht 1981). After flushing, diarrhea is the most common symptom of carcinoid syndrome, occurring in 70% of cases (Graham-Smith 1968); the intestinal hypermotility often develops over several years and is independent of flushing. Cardiac involvement manifests as right-sided heart failure, pulmonary stenosis, and tricuspid valve insufficiency. Bronchoconstriction and chronic telangiectasia are less common.

22.1.3 Diagnosis by Techniques Other than Imaging

Diagnosis is based on laboratory tests and fiberoptic endoscopy. Assays of 5-HIAA in 24-hr urine samples and serum and urinary serotonin remain the basic diagnostic tests for carcinoid tumors (Dreux 1977).
Endoscopy can diagnose gastric, colonic, and rectal carcinoid tumors. However, endoscopic biopsies are not always diagnostic because of the firm consistency and submucosal location of these tumors (Gutman et al. 1986; Lemozy 1973).

22.1.4 Evolution and Prognosis

Carcinoids are slowly-growing tumors, and 80% of patients survive longer than 5 years (Godwin 1975). Prognostic factors include the existence of metastases, the histologic type (with undifferentiated forms being particularly severe), tumor size at the time of diagnosis, and the location of the primary tumor in the gastrointestinal tract. Whereas appendiceal and rectal lesions have a good prognosis (83% and 99% survival at 5 years), gastric, intestinal and colonic lesions are less favorable (52%–54% at 5 years) (Godwin 1975).
Owing to their frequency, intestinal, rectal, colonic, and gastric carcinoids are dealt with first. Other sites, because of their rarity or the absence of interest of imaging studies (appendiceal sites) are discussed afterwards.

22.2 Imaging

22.2.1 Small Intestine (Figs. 22.1–22.9)

Carcinoids are the most frequent malignant tumor of the small bowel: 20%–45% (Good 1962; Barclay and Schapira 1983; Godwin 1975). The ileum is the most common site, accounting for over 90% of cases (Bruneton et al. 1980); jejunal (Balthazar 1978; Bancks et al. 1975) and duodenal carcinoids (Clements and Roche 1984; Lasson et al. 1983; Seymour et al. 1982) are rare. The incidence of these tumors appears to increase with proximity to the cecum. Two particularities of intestinal carcinoids warrant mention: the frequency of multiple forms and the high incidence (8%–47%) of concurrent neoplasms (Barclay and Schapira 1983; Godwin 1975; Peck et al. 1983; Warner et al. 1979a). Male predominance has been

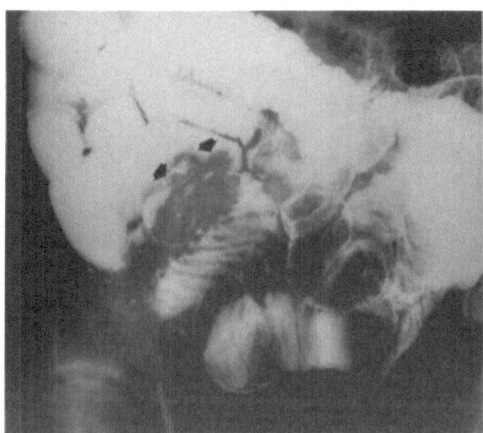

Fig. 22.1. Ileal carcinoid *(arrows)*: barium examination

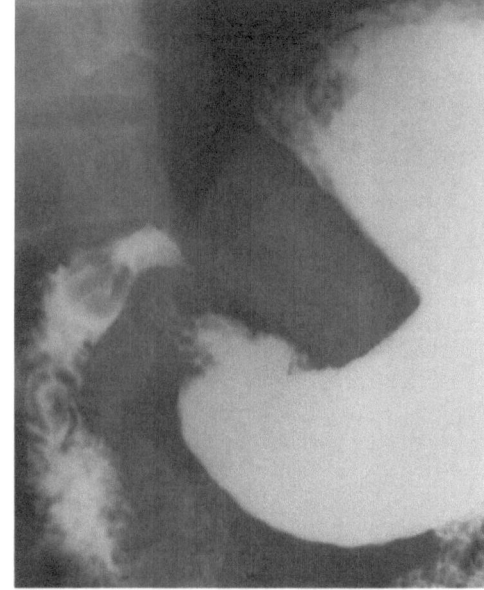

Fig. 22.3. Small polypoid lesion in the duodenum; surgery revealed a solitary carcinoid tumor

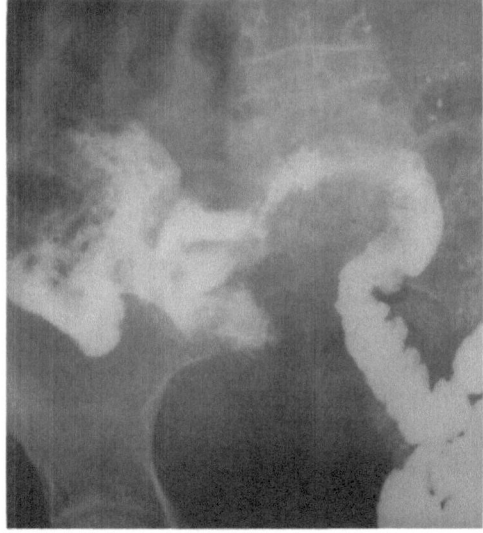

Fig. 22.2. Bulky ileocecal carcinoid extensively infiltrating the terminal ileum; this lesion caused hepatic metastases from the outset

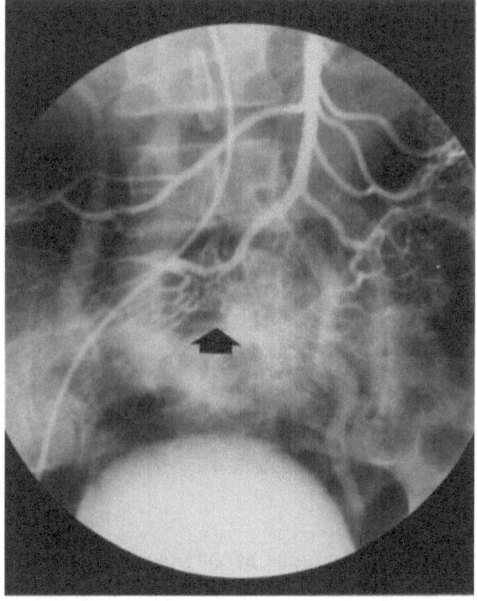

Fig. 22.4. Angiographic study of an ileal carcinoid: note the stellate appearance of the vasa recta *(arrow)*

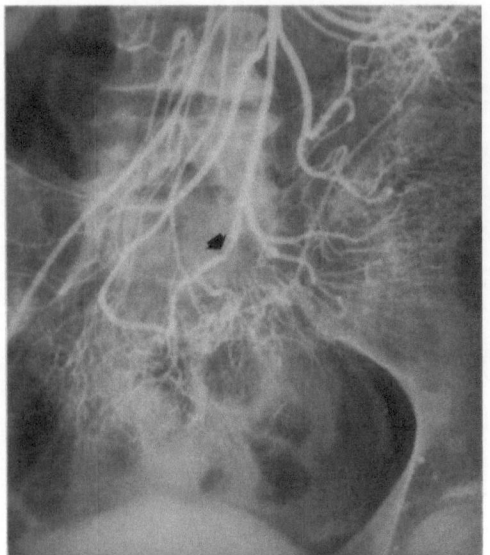

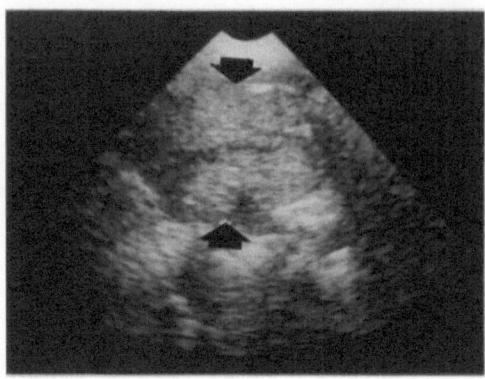

Fig. 22.5. Angiographic study of an ileal carcinoid: stellate appearance of the vasa recta and proximal arterial infiltration *(arrow)*

Fig. 22.6. Recurrence of an intestinal carcinoid: ultrasonography demonstrated a solid lesion (55 mm between the *two arrows*)

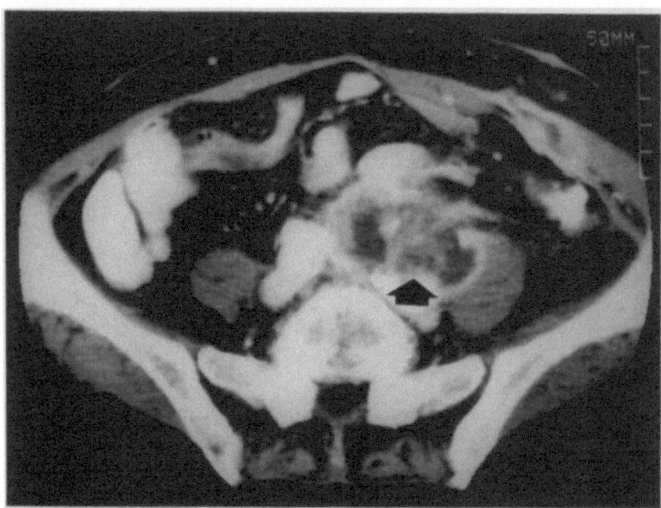

Fig. 22.7. Recurrence of a small bowel carcinoid: mesenteric involvement displacing and invading the adjacent digestive tract organs *(arrow)*

noted, and mean age at diagnosis is 60 years. The carcinoid syndrome, corresponding to the presence of hepatic metastases, occurs in 26%-29% of patients (Bruneton et al. 1980; Peck et al. 1983). Atypical or incomplete carcinoid syndromes are possible, but the most common clinical symptoms are pain, an abdominal mass, and weight loss. Upper or lower gastrointestinal bleeding (Gencsi et al. 1986;

Rees and Bancewicz 1984), acute occlusion (Faust et al. 1976), and intestinal infarction secondary to mesenteric angiopathy (Eckhauser et al. 1981) are other rare possibilities.

Various imaging techniques have been used for intestinal workups: barium, ultrasonography, CT and angiography.

Curvilinear calcifications less than 15 mm in diameter may be visible on *abdominal plain*

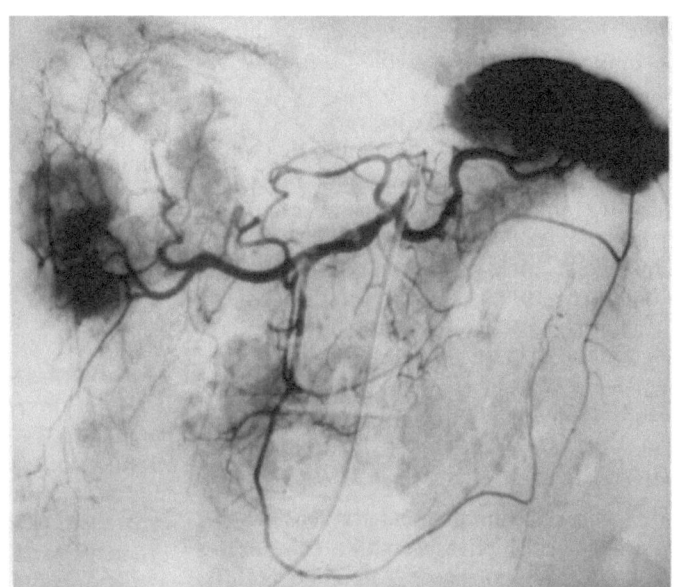

Fig. 22.8. Hepatic angiography demonstrating hypervascular liver metastases

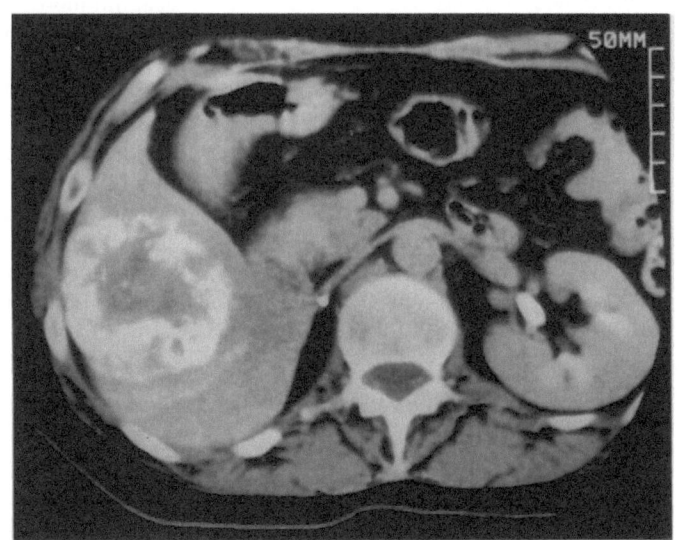

Fig. 22.9. CT scans after intra-arterial lipiodol injection: hypervascular right liver metastasis of an intestinal carcinoid

films (Boijsen et al. 1974). *Barium* examinations of the small intestine are positive in only 58% of cases (Bruneton et al. 1980). Radiologic features seen alone or in combination (Bancks et al. 1975; Jeffree et al. 1984) include a possibly eccentric intraluminal filling defect, with or without suprajacent dilatation, narrowing of ileal loops, and extrinsic compression with separation of intestinal loops by adenopathies. Intussusception and a radiologic pattern suggesting Crohn's disease are less frequent findings (Jeffree et al. 1984; Verma 1972). Acceleration of transit is less common, as is annular stenosis, which tends to suggest intestinal adenocarcinoma (Levine et al. 1987). Solitary or multiple polypoid lesions may be seen in the duodenum (Clements and Roche 1984; Lasson et al. 1983; Seymour et al. 1982).

Ultrasonography rarely succeeds in visualizing the tumor, although favorable cases may be evidenced as a solid, only slightly echoic mass (Skaane 1987). Extensive retraction of the mesentery can create a sonographically visible solid mass syndrome. Ultrasound is indicated primarily for examination of the liver and detection of hepatic metastases, which have a variable but often hyperechoic echostructure (Adolph et al. 1987).

CT allows better analysis of the mesentery, but carcinoids are rarely visible because of their small size (Adolph et al. 1987; Cockey et al. 1985; Gould and Johnson 1986; Scatarige et al. 1987; Seigel et al. 1980; Thompson and Halvoren 1987). CT patterns include:

- Small nodular intramesenteric densities associated with perivascular thickening. This pattern may correspond to adenopathies and initial infiltration of the mesentery.
- Rarely, focal thickening of the intestinal wall (Cockey et al. 1985).
- More often, presence of a mesenteric mass anterior to the spine, discretely enhanced by the injection of contrast medium, and displacing the small intestine anteriorly. This pattern corresponds to massive infiltration of the mesentery.
- Hepatic metastases of variable appearance: well defined, round and hypodense; poorly delimited, or exhibiting extensive hypervascularity after injection (Smevik et al. 1983).
- More rarely, presence of retroperitoneal adenopathies.

The CT patterns of mesenteric carcinoids resemble those of lymphoma, metastases, mesothelioma, and especially Crohn's disease. Improvement of CT units has increased the diagnostic accuracy of this technique, which was previously judged inferior to that of arteriography (Hemmingsson et al. 1981). The widely recognized angiographic features described by numerous authors (Bruneton et al. 1978; Gold and Redman 1972; Goldstein and Miller 1975; Kinkhabwala and Balthazar 1978; Reuter and Boijsen 1966) include:

- Nearly constant tumor hypovascularity, and failure to visualize venous return.
- Stellate appearance of the vasa recta, with or without stenosis of the proximal arteries, venous obstruction, or opacification of adenopathies.

- Possibility of hepatic metastases, which tend to be hypervascularized.

The stellate configuration of the vasa recta, a constant feature of positive angiograms, is not pathognomonic for carcinoid tumor, but is very suggestive of the diagnosis. This abnormality is also encountered in several fibrotic etiologies, including plastic peritonitis or idiopathic retractile mesenteritis, intestinal tuberculosis, and segmental enteritis (Gold and Redman 1972). Along with providing diagnostic and topographic information, angiography is also of therapeutic benefit for patients with carcinoid syndrome, because embolization produces at least temporary disappearance of clinical and biologic manifestations (Carrasco et al. 1986; Odurny and Birch 1985).

When diagnosis remains problematic, recourse is occasionally made to mesenteric phlebography by transparietal puncture of the portal vein. Selective venous opacification may reveal thrombosis. Above all, blood samples can be obtained at different levels for serotonin assays (Bigot and Roche 1981; Reichardt et al. 1979).

Despite the information they provide, these various imaging techniques are negative in half of all cases because of the small size and submucosal location of intestinal carcinoids (Peck et al. 1983). Moreover, nearly one-third of patients with an ileal carcinoid also have another lesion (Beaton et al. 1981).

22.2.2 *Rectum* (Fig. 22.10)

Rectal carcinoids are much less common than intestinal lesions, and they are account for only 0.04% of all lower endoscopic findings (Quan et al. 1964). Carcinoids represent 1.3% of rectal tumors (Godwin 1975), and 30% of cases are asymptomatic (Delcourt and Robberecht 1981). Proctoscopy is the most sensitive examination because these rectal tumors are often small (Pronay et al. 1982). The carcinoid syndrome is infrequent because these tumors are almost always smaller than 2 cm and rarely metastasize to the liver (Audebert et al. 1987). Aggressive therapy is indicated for lesions larger than 2 cm and whenever the muscularis propria has been invaded (Naunheim

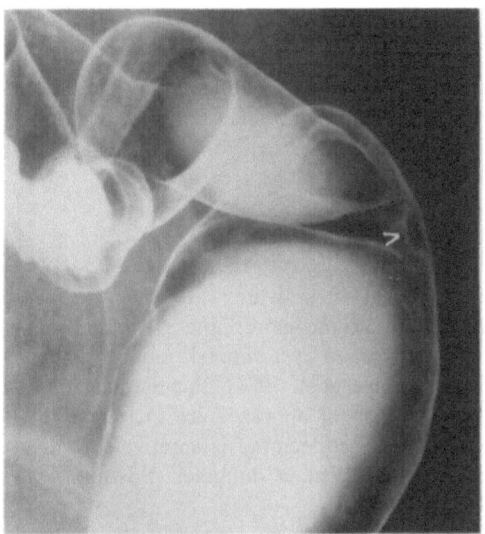

Fig. 22.10. Small polypoid lesion in the posterior rectum related to a carcinoid without any signs of degeneration

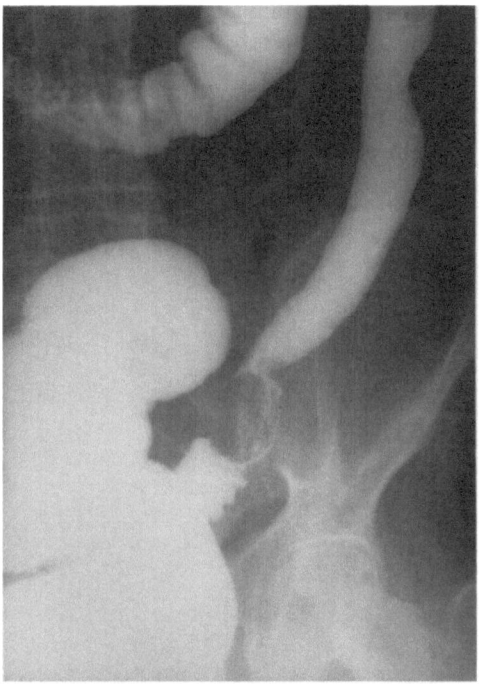

Fig. 22.11. Tumoral lesion in the left colon: surgery demonstrated a carcinoid

et al. 1983). Endoscopy and barium enemas usually demonstrate a sessile or pedunculated intraluminal mass (Hudson and Margulis 1964; Sato et al. 1984).

22.2.3 *Colon* (Fig. 22.11, 22.12)

Carcinoids account for 0.3% of all colon tumors (Godwin 1975); the site of predilection is the cecum, which is involved in more than one-half of all cases (Rosenberg and Welch 1985). Rectal carcinoids are associated with another colonic malignancy in 3%–10% of cases (Godwin 1975). There is female predominance. The carcinoid syndrome corresponding to the presence of hepatic metastases is very rare. Pain is the most common complaint, and one-third of patients present with an abdominal mass (Rosenberg and Welch 1985). Gastrointestinal bleeding or an obstructive syndrome may prompt colonic exploration. Barium enema examination is often positive, but findings (severe annular stenosis, polypoid filling defect, less often extrinsic impression by adenopathies) tend to be interpreted as adenocarcinoma. Multiple carcinoids are generally not detected radiologically (Bruneton et al.

1980). Angiography is rarely performed, but patterns are comparable to those observed in the small intestine (Kinkhabwala and Balthazar 1978).

22.2.4 *Stomach* (Fig. 22.12, 22.13)

Carcinoids, which represent only 0.5% of all gastric tumors (Godwin 1975), are often diagnosed by endoscopic biopsy (Pao-Huei et al. 1980). As in the colon, the carcinoid syndrome, corresponding to the presence of hepatic metastases, is rare. The major clinical manifestations are pain and a mass syndrome.

For Balthazar et al. (1982), gastric carcinoid tumors may be imaged as a solitary intramural filling defect, often multiple gastric polyps (Goldfarb et al. 1983), large gastric ulcerations, or an intraluminal polypoid tumor. More rarely, an infiltrative appearance suggests adenocarcinoma (Caletti et al. 1986; Okeon and Bieber 1968).

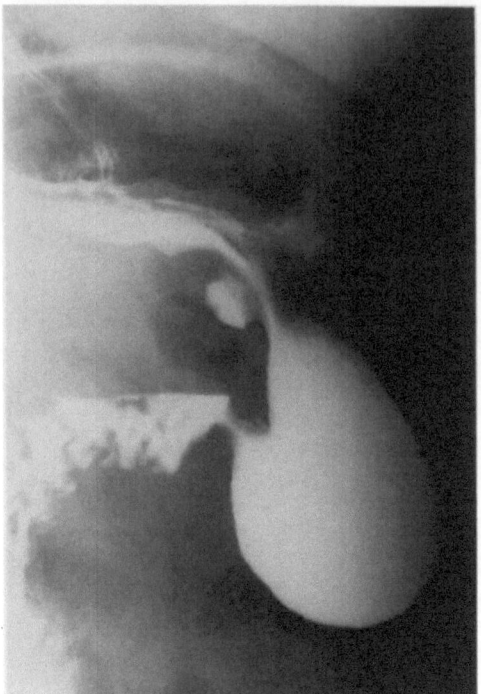

Fig. 22.12. Ulcerated bulky gastric lesion (carcinoid); adenopathies and liver metastases were found at surgery

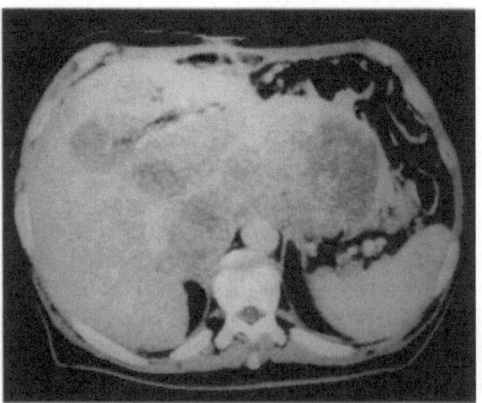

Fig. 22.13. Gastric carcinoid with diffuse hepatic metastases

Few reports concerning use of angiography for gastric carcinoid tumors exist in the literature; angiographic features may resemble those of connective tissue tumors, with tumoral hypervascularity.

22.2.5 Other Anatomic Sites

Appendiceal sites, which are very frequent from an anatomic standpoint, are actually exceptional causes of a clinical tumoral process (De Fresnoye et al. 1984). For Syracuse et al. (1979), 90.2% of all cases are incidental discoveries. Appendectomy is curative for carcinoids under 1 cm in diameter (Bowman and Rosenthal 1983).

Esophageal sites are exceptional. Brenner et al. (1969) reported a case that manifested clinically as dysphagia; barium esophagography disclosed an extramucosal filling defect in the lower esophagus. In their review of 50 cases affecting Meckel's diverticulum, Singhabhandhu et al. (1973) reported detection of a filling defect in the diverticulum on barium enema examination.

22.3 Conclusion

Overall, carcinoids are unusual lesions whose course (and thus the frequency of clinical manifestations) depends on their location. Imaging studies cannot always visualize the tumor, especially small lesions and those in the ileum. The main indications for CT and angiography are diagnosis of disease extension to the mesentery.

22.4 References

Adolph JMG, Kimmig BN, Georgi P, Winkel KZ (1987) Carcinoid tumors: CT and I-131 Meta-iodo-benzylguanidine scintigraphy. Radiology 164: 199–203

Audebert M, Huguier M, Valade S, Roland J (1987) Tumeurs carcinoïdes du rectum. A propos de deux cas avec métastases. Ann Gastroenterol Hepatol (Paris) 23: 229–231

Balthazar EJ (1978) Carcinoid tumors of the alimentary tract. I. Radiographic diagnosis. Gastrointest Radiol 3: 47–56

Balthazar EJ, Megibow A, Bryk D, Cohen T (1982) Gastric carcinoid tumors: radiographic features in eight cases. AJR 139: 1123-1127

Bancks NH, Goldstein HM, Dodd GD (1975) The roentgenologic spectrum of small intestinal carcinoid tumors. AJR 123: 274-280

Barclay THC, Schapira DV (1983) Malignant tumors of the small intestine. Cancer 51: 878-881

Beaton H, Homan W, Dineen P (1981) Gastrointestinal carcinoids and the malignant carcinoid syndrome. Surg Gynecol Obstet 152: 268-272

Bigot JM, Roche A (1981) Possibilités diagnostiques et thérapeutiques de l'angiographie dans les tumeurs carcinoïdes du tube digestif. Acta Gastroenterol Belg 64: 120-143

Boijsen E, Kaude J, Tylen U (1974) Radiologic diagnosis of ileal carcinoid tumours. Acta Radiol [Diagn] (Stockh) 15: 65-82

Bowman GA, Rosenthal D (1983) Carcinoid tumors of the appendix. Am J Surg 146: 700-703

Brenner S, Heimlich H, Widman M (1969) Carcinoid of esophagus. NY State J Med 69: 1337-1339

Bruneton JN, Sabatier JC, Drouillard J, Elie G, Amouretti M, Tavernier J (1978) Apport de l'angiographie dans le diagnostic radiologique des carcinoïdes du grêle. A propos de 2 observations. Med Chir Dig 7: 507-513

Bruneton JN, Roux P, Drouillard J, Elie G, Tavernier J (1980) Etude radiologique des tumeurs carcinoïdes du tube digestif. Revue de 150 cas de la littérature. Bordeaux Med 13: 881-888

Caletti GC, Guizzardi G, Brocchi E, Grigioni WF, D'Errico A, Labo G (1986) Gastric carcinoid: a clinical and endoscopic assessment of four cases. Endoscopy 18: 101-104

Carrasco CH, Charnsangavej C, Ajani J, Samaan NA, Richli W, Wallace S (1986) The carcinoid syndrome: palliation by hepatic artery embolization. AJR 147: 149-154

Clements JL, Roche RR (1984) Carcinoid of the duodenum: a report of six cases. Gastrointest Radiol 9: 17-21

Cockey BM, Fishman EK, Jones B, Siegelman SS (1985) Computed tomography of abdominal carcinoid tumor. J Comput Assist Tomogr 9: 38-42

Collins DC (1955) A study of 50000 specimens of the human vermiform appendix. Surg Gynecol Obstet 101: 437-445

De Fresnoye H, Brunel A, Delepierre A, Birembaut P, Loygue J (1984) Syndrome carcinoïde d'une tumeur isolée de l'appendice. Ann Chir 38: 633-636

Delcourt A, Robberecht P (1981) Tumeurs et syndrome carcinoïdes. Acta Gastroenterol Belg 64: 112-119

Dreux C (1977) Biochimie des tumeurs carcinoïdes du tube digestif. Méthode de dépistage précoce de ces tumeurs. Ann Gastroenterol Hepatol (Paris) 13: 367-377

Eckhauser FE, Argenta LC, Strodel WE, Wheeler RH, Bul FE, Appelman HD, Thompson NW (1981) Mesenteric angiopathy, intestinal gangrene, and midgut carcinoids. Surgery 90: 720-728

Faust H, Hehne HJ, Mueller W (1976) Karzinoide des Dunndarms. Retrospektive Studie der radiologischen Befunde von 15 Patienten. Radiol Clin (Basel) 45: 402-411

Feldman JM, Jones RS (1982) Carcinoid syndrome from gastrointestinal carcinoids without liver metastasis. Ann Surg 196: 33-37

Gencsi E, Lux E, Kaduk B, Roedl W, Schmidt H, Gebhardt C, Lux G (1986) Upper gastrointestinal bleeding as an unusual presentation of a duodenal carcinoid. Endoscopy 18: 105-107

Glasser CM, Bhargavan BS (1980) Carcinoid tumors of the appendix. Arch Pathol Lab Med 104: 272-275

Godwin JD (1975) Carcinoid tumors. An analysis of 2837 cases. Cancer 36: 560-569

Gold RE, Redman HC (1972) Mesenteric fibrosis simulating the angiographic appearance of ileal carcinoid tumor. Radiology 103: 85-86

Goldfarb JP, Gross F, Maxfield R, Rubin M, Janis R (1983) Gastric carcinoid: two unusual presentations. Am J Gastroenterol 78: 332-334

Goldstein HM, Miller M (1975) Angiographic evaluation of carcinoid tumors of the small intestine: the value of epinephrine. Radiology 114: 23-28

Goldthorn JF, Canizaro PC (1986) Gastrointestinal malignancies in infancy, childhood, and adolescence. Surg Clin North Am 66: 845-861

Good CA (1962) Tumors of the small intestine. Caldwell lecture. AJR 89: 685-705

Gould M, Johnson RJ (1986) Computed tomography of abdominal carcinoid tumour. Br J Radiol 59: 881-885

Graham-Smith DG (1968) The carcinoid syndrome. Am J Cardiol 21: 376-387

Gutman H, Deutsch AA, Leiser A, Reiss R (1986) Primary duodenal carcinoid with malignant carcinoid syndrome: a case report. Am J Gastroenterol 81: 112-114

Hajdu SI, Winawer SJ, Laird Myers WP (1974) Carcinoid tumors. A study of 204 cases. Am J Pathol 61: 521-528

Hemmingsson A, Lindgren PG, Lorelius LE, Oberg K (1981) Diagnosis of endocrine gastrointestinal tumours. Acta Radiol [Diagn] (Stockh) 22: 657-662

Hudson HL, Margulis AR (1964) The roentgen findings of carcinoid tumors of the gastrointestinal tract. A report of 12 recent cases. AJR 91: 835-839

Jeffree MA, Nolan DJ (1987) Multiple ileal carcinoid tumours. Br J Radiol 60: 402-403

Jeffree MA, Barter SJ, Hemingway AP, Nolan DJ (1984) Primary carcinoid tumours of the ileum: the radiological appearances. Clin Radiol 35: 451-455

Johnson LA, Lavin P, Moertel CG, Weiland L, Dayal Y, Doos WG, Geller SA, Cooper HS,

Nime F, Masse S, Simson IW, Sumner H, Folsch E, Engstrom P (1983) Carcinoids: the association of histologic growth pattern and survival. Cancer 51: 882-889

Kinkhabwala M, Balthazar EJ (1978) Carcinoid tumors of the alimentary tract. II. Angiographic diagnosis of small intestine and colonic lesions. Gastrointest Radiol 3: 57-61

Kowlessar OD (1973) The carcinoid syndrome. In: Sleizenger MH, Fortran JS (eds) Gastrointestinal disease. Saunders, Philadelphia, pp 1190-1201

Lasson A, Alwmark A, Nobin A, Sundler F (1983) Endocrine tumors of the duodenum. Ann Surg 197: 393-398

Lemozy J (1973) Les tumeurs carcinoïdes du rectum. Arch Fr Mal Appar Dig 62: 537-568

Levine MS, Drooz AT, Herlinger H (1987) Annular malignancies of the small bowel. Gastrointest Radiol 12: 53-58

McDonald RA (1956) Study of 356 carcinoids of the gastrointestinal tract. Report of four new cases of the carcinoid syndrome. Am J Med 21: 867-878

Moertel CG, Saver WG, Dockerty MB, Baggenstoss AH (1961) Life history of the carcinoid tumor of the small intestine. Cancer 14: 901-912

Naunheim KS, Zeitels J, Kaplan EL, Sugimoto J, Shen KL, Lee CH, Straus FH (1983) Rectal carcinoid tumors. Treatment and prognosis. Surgery 94: 670-676

Odurny A, Birch SJ (1985) Hepatic arterial embolisation in patients with metastatic carcinoid tumours. Clin Radiol 36: 597-602

Okeon MM, Bieber WP (1968) Carcinoid tumor of the stomach resembling carcinoma. Report of a case. AJR 103: 314-316

Okike N, Bernatz PE, Woolner LB (1976) Carcinoid tumors of the lung. Ann Thorac Surg 22: 270-277

Orloff MJ (1971) Carcinoid tumors of the rectum. Cancer 28: 175-180

Pao-Huei C, Chuan-Pau S, Kuang-Yang L, Gonq-Chin H, Jean-Dean L, Hsian-Chong K, Ting-Yao C (1980) Carcinoids of the gastrointestinal tract. Endoscopy 12: 299-305

Pearse AGE (1980) The APUD concept and hormone production. Clin Endocrinol Metab 9: 211-222

Peck JJ, Shields AB, Boyden AM, Dworkin LA, Nadal JW (1983) Carcinoid tumors of the ileum. Am J Surg 146: 124-132

Pronay G, Nagy G, Ujszaszy L, Minik K (1982) Carcinoid tumors of the rectum. Ann Gastroenterol Hepatol (Paris) 18: 313-315

Quan SHQ, Bader E, Berg JW (1964) Carcinoid tumors of the rectum. Dis Colon Rectum 7: 197-206

Rees WDW, Bancewicz J (1984) Endoscopic diagnosis of a bleeding ileal carcinoid tumour. Gut 25: 211-212

Reichardt W, Ingemanson S, Lunderquist A, Nobin A (1979) Selective mesenteric phlebography in patients with carcinoid tumors. Gastrointest Radiol 4: 179-189

Reuter SR, Boijsen E (1966) Angiographic findings in two ileal carcinoid tumors. Radiology 87: 836-840

Rosenberg JM, Welch JP (1985) Carcinoid tumors of the colon. A study of 72 patients. Am J Surg 149: 775-779

Sanders RJ (1973) Carcinoids of the gastrointestinal tract. Thomas, Springfield

Sato T, Sakai Y, Sonoyama A, Kawamoto S, Okawa M, Kajita A, Tanaka H, Nakanishi K, Fujino Y, Fujita M (1984) Radiologic spectrum of rectal carcinoid tumors. Gastrointest Radiol 9: 23-26

Scatarige JC, Allen HA, Fishman EK (1987) Computed tomography of the small bowel. Semin Ultrasound CT MR 8: 403-423

Scoma JA (1978) Carcinoid tumors of the rectum. Am J Surg 135: 708-709

Seigel RS, Kuhns LR, Borlaza GS, Mc Cormick TL, Simmons JL (1980) Computed tomography and angiography in ileal carcinoid tumor and retractile mesenteritis. Radiology 134: 437-440

Seymour EQ, Griffin CN, Kurtz SM (1982) Carcinoid tumors of the duodenal cap presenting as multiple polypoid defects. Gastrointest Radiol 7: 19-21

Singhabhandhu B, Gray SW, Krieger H (1973) Carcinoid tumor of Meckel's diverticulum: report of a case and review of literature. J Med Assoc Ga 62: 84-89

Skaane P (1987) The ultrasonic demonstration of carcinoid tumor of the ileocecal valve. Am J Gastroenterol 82: 168-170

Smevik B, Kolmannsko G, Aakhus T (1983) Computed tomography and angiography in carcinoid liver metastases. Acta Radiol [Diagn] (Stockh) 24: 189-193

Syracuse DC, Perzin KH, Price JB, Wichel PD, Mesatejada R (1979) Carcinoid tumors in the appendix. Ann Surg 190: 58-63

Thompson GB, Van Heerden JA, Martin JK, Schutt AJ, Ilstrup DM, Carney JA (1985) Carcinoid tumors of the gastrointestinal tract: presentation, management, and prognosis. Surgery 98: 1056-1063

Thompson WM, Halvorsen RA (1987) Computed tomographic staging of gastrointestinal malignancies. Part II. The small bowel, colon, and rectum. Invest Radiol 22: 96-105

Verma VK (1972) Multiple carcinoid tumour mimicking Crohn's disease. J Irish Med Ass 65: 413-414

Warner TF, O'Reilly G, Mc Lee GA (1979a) Mesenteric occlusive lesion and ileal carcinoids. Cancer 44: 758-762

Warner TF, O'Reilly G, Power LH (1979b) Carcinoid diathesis of the ileum. Cancer 43: 1900-1905

Zeitels J, Naunheim K, Kaplan EL, Strauss F (1982) Carcinoid tumors. A 37 year experience. Arch Surg 117: 732-737

23 Leiomyoblastoma*

Leiomyoblastomas of the gastrointestinal tract are very rare pathologic entities which differ from leiomyomas and leiomyosarcomas histologically. Stout (1962) described 69 gastric tumors with the same gross appearance and proposed the term leiomyoblastoma for these "bizarre smooth muscle tumors of the stomach". In France, Martin et al. (1960) referred to them as "myoid tumors".

Leiomyoblastomas are infrequent submucosal tumors that are much less common than leiomyomas and leiomyosarcomas (only one leiomyoblastoma for eight leiomyomatous lesions in our experience). They resemble smooth muscle macroscopically, and sheets of polygonal or rounded cells without smooth muscle fibers are evident on microscope examination (Hadju et al. 1982; Kay and Still 1969). Although an artefact of formalin fixation may surround the nucleus during electron microscopy (Salazar and Totten 1970), these tumors definitely appear to be of smooth muscle origin (Gupta and Chandler 1965). Most leiomyoblastomas occur in the stomach, but similar tumors have been described elsewhere in the intestinal tract and adnexa (Maaouni et al. 1980; Mouroux et al. 1986), in the uterus, and in the retroperitoneum (Lavin et al. 1972; Stout 1962).

23.1 Stomach

The stomach is by far the most prevalent site of gastrointestinal leiomyoblastomas. A total of 307 cases described in the literature since 1960 were reviewed by Lecomte et al. (1981).

23.1.1 General Features

The preferential gastric sites of leiomyoblastoma are the body and the antrum (over 90% of cases). Benign and malignant tumors tend to differ in size: 41.7% of benign lesions were under 5 cm whereas over 72.1% of the malignant cases reviewed were over 5 cm. Although size is not a specific criterion, leiomyoblastomas smaller than 5 cm are apt to be benign whereas those over 10 cm are more likely to be malignant.

Leiomyoblastomas are usually solitary lesions. Multiple tumors, reported in 2.3% of cases, were not correlated with the benign or malignant nature of the disease (2% of 244 benign leiomyoblastomas and 3.2% of 63 malignant leiomyoblastomas presented as multiple lesions).

Mean patient age was 58 years (range 8–88). Males were affected in 63.6% of cases. There was no predominance by race. Presenting symptoms are listed in Table 23.1. As for other muscle tumors of the gastrointestinal tract, hemorrhage was frequent. Both massive hemorrhage and bleeding confined to the peritoneum are possible (subserosal leiomyoblastoma) (Kelsey 1966). Reports on atypical clinical symptoms include jaundice (Salazar and Totten 1970), diarrhea (1.3%), and obstruction (0.6%) (Lenne and Delumeau 1973). Asymptomatic lesions are frequent.

Table 23.1. Clinical symptoms of gastric leiomyoblastoma

Hemorrhage or anemia	51.8%
Pain	30.9%
Palpable mass	20.8%
Muscle weakness	17.3%
Asymptomatic	21.2%

---

* Written in collaboration with M.Y. Mourou.

In addition to cases of fortuitous association with a gastric carcinoma (Viard et al. 1977), leiomyoblastoma has been described in conjunction with two other rare neoplasms, pulmonary chondroma and functioning extralienal paraganglioma. This synchronous combination may not be fortuitous (Carney 1979; De Castro et al. 1972; Graham et al. 1987).

As for other leiomyomatous lesions, most leiomyoblastomas are benign (79.5%) rather than malignant. Malignant forms accounted for 63 of the 307 cases (20.5%) reviewed by Lecomte et al. (1981) whereas the literature review by Graham et al. (1987) cited a malignancy rate of only 10%. These lesions were either malignant from the outset (87.3%) or degenerated after recurrence of what was considered a benign leiomyoblastoma at previous surgery (12.7%). The features of these lesions were specified for 31 of the 55 cases where malignancy was diagnosed at the outset: 41.9% of these 31 cases involved liver metastases, and nodal involvement was discovered at surgery in 38.7% of cases. Average survival after diagnosis was only 1 year. The disease-free interval for the eight recurrences of what had been considered benign lesions ranged from 2 years (Rachman et al. 1968) to 12 years (Martin et al. 1960). Some of these local recurrences were associated with liver metastases. Malignant recurrence of this type differentiates the course of leiomyoblastomas from gastric leiomyomas, which never recur.

The endoscopic pattern is often a submucosal and frequently intramural, ulcerated tumor (Bose and Candy 1970; Mann et al. 1975).

Histologic diagnosis of malignancy can be difficult for leiomyoblastomas. Stout (1962) suggested that their malignant potential could be evaluated by counting the number of mitoses in 50 high-power fields. Biologically benign tumors appear to have a low mitotic rate (less than 6 per 50 high-power fields) even though there are rare reports of benign courses despite mitotic rates over 20 (Sehgal et al. 1966; Stout 1962). Furthermore, certain malignant lesions have mitotic rates of 5 to 20 per high-power field (Rachman et al. 1968; Stout 1962). In the majority of cases, however, biologic behavior can be adequately predicted by evaluating mitotic activity (Ranchod and Kempson 1977).

Small tumors may be amenable to surgical resection (Viard et al. 1975). Because it is often difficult to predict their malignant potential, tumors of 5 cm or more are best managed by partial gastrectomy (Tallqvist et al. 1967).

23.1.2 Imaging

Radiologically, gastric leiomyoblastomas are similar to leiomyomas and leiomyosarcomas. Lecomte et al. (1981) reviewed 143 cases for which barium examination was performed; 15 of these studies were negative (10.5%). This technique was never used when there was a high risk of hemorrhage. The radiologic features of gastric leiomyoblastomas summarized in Table 23.2 are based on analysis of 128 cases. These submucosal lesions may have several particularities: infiltration (2.4% of cases), prolapse of the tumor into the duodenum (0.8%), or pyloric stenosis (1.6%) (Conte et al. 1973). Intratumoral calcifications are rare (Ozoktay et al. 1979).

Barium examinations detect 89.5% of lesions, but can determine the degree of extension for only 75.8% of these cases. Tumor ulceration is not visible in 7.8% of cases; a dumbbell image is not recognized and an intramural or intraluminal tumor is diagnosed in 7% of cases; an extragastric lesion is not recognized and an intramural tumor is diagnosed in 9.4% of cases (Figure 23.1). Barium studies cannot differentiate leiomyoblastomas from other connective tissue tumors, and in particular from leiomyoma, leiomyosarcoma, schwannoma, or granular cell myoblastoma (Faegenburg et al. 1975; Lecomte et al. 1981).

Review of the literature revealed only 14 cases for which *angiographic findings* were available. Pizzimbono et al. (1973) performed hepatic

Table 23.2. Radiographic features of gastric leiomyoblastoma (128 literature cases)

Intramural	41.4%
Intraluminal	22.7%
Subserosal	25.7%
Dumbbell	10.2%
Ulceration[a]	31.3%
[a] False negative for ulceration	25%

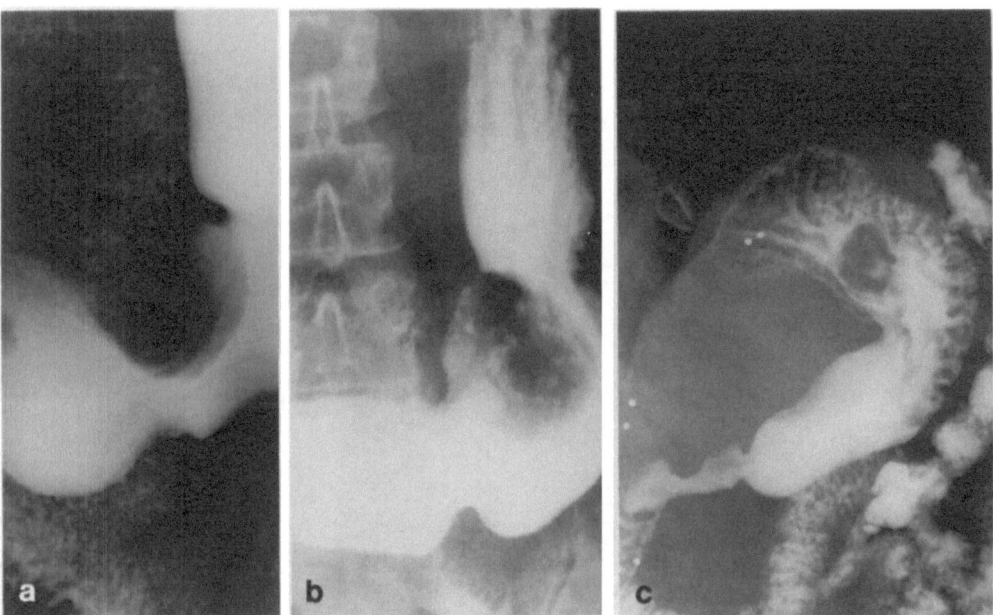

Fig. 23.1a-c. Barium study of leiomyoblastomas. **a** Intramural lesion. **b** Intramural lesion with small ulcerations. **c** Ulcerated intramural lesion

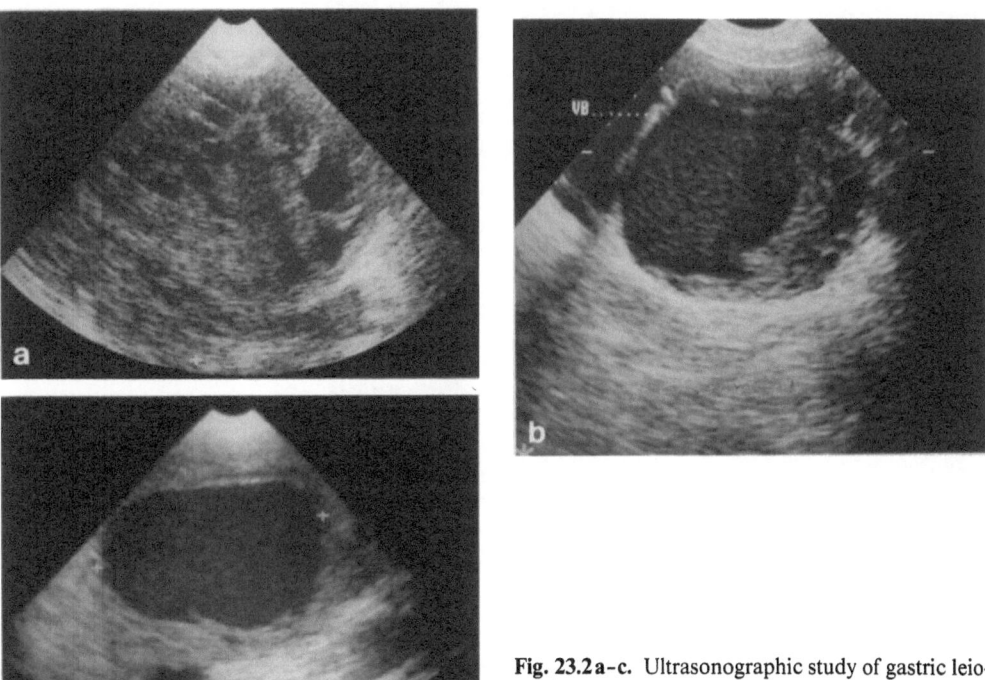

Fig. 23.2a-c. Ultrasonographic study of gastric leiomyoblastomas. **a** Solid lesion with small areas of necrosis. **b** Lesion with a large fluid component. *VB*, bile duct. **c** Necrotic lesion

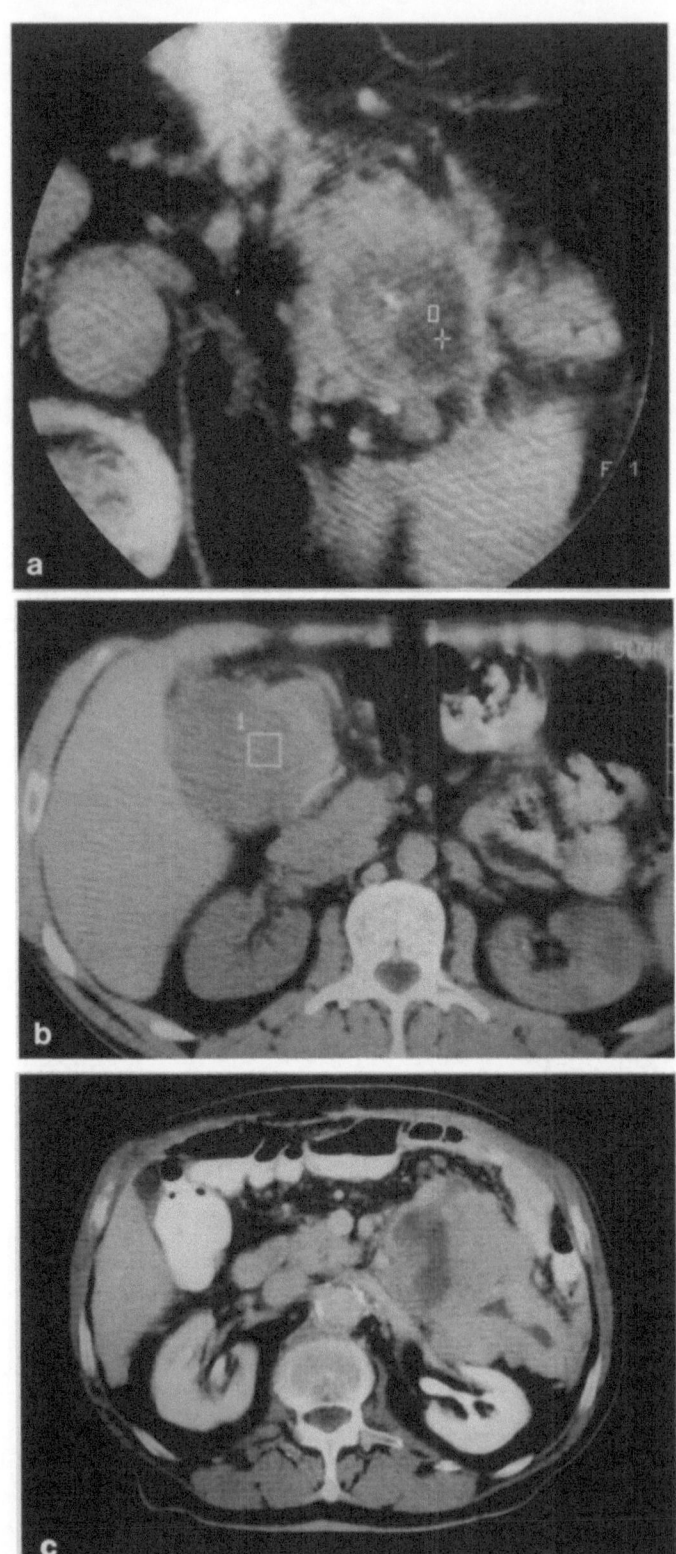

angiography in a patient who had already undergone treatment in order to arrive at a diagnosis of liver metastases, which were hypervascularized. Of the 14 cases reviewed, arteriography was negative in two cases (Conte et al. 1973; Salazar and Totten 1970). Eight of the 12 positive cases were hypervascular tumors (seven benign, one malignant); the other four positive cases were all hypovascular (2 benign, 2 malignant). Angiography does not appear indicated for pretherapy staging of this type of muscular gastric lesion because benign and malignant leiomyoblastoma can present a number of angiographic patterns.

Results with *ultrasonography* are variable, but examination of the stomach is usually satisfactory (Figure 23.2). Few reports have been published in the literature (Langley 1976; Sandler et al. 1978; Choi et al. 1988; Worlicek et al. 1986; Pignon et al. 1984; Striffing et al. 1984; Slasky et al. 1982). The lesions have a very variable echostructure: solid, mixed, or extensively necrotic. Malignant tumors may be associated with sonographically visible celiac adenopathies (Worlicek et al. 1986). *CT* demonstrates the polymorphism of these lesions (Figure 23.3): solid, homogeneous tumor; central necrosis, massive cyst formation with a multilocular appearance (Choi et al. 1988; Pignon et al. 1984; Pillari et al. 1983; Postma and Gerlag 1986; Slasky et al. 1982; Stanley et al. 1986; Striffling et al. 1984). Subserosal lesions that are missed or poorly analyzed by endoscopy may suggest extragastric tumoral or cystic etiologies (especially pancreatic lesions) (Choi et al. 1988; Pignon et al. 1984). The submucosal nature of gastric leiomyoblastoma explains why biopsies are often disappointing: the resected tissue is often uninvolved mucosa or non-diagnostic tissue from an ulcer crater (Graham et al. 1987; Mann et al. 1975).

◄ **Fig. 23.3a–c.** CT study of gastric leiomyoblastomas: examination is disappointing for lesions of the lower edge of the stomach because of the transverse plane of the scans. **a** Partially necrotic tumoral lesion. **b** (Courtesy of Dr. Padovani, Nice, France) Extensively necrotic lesion (fluid density in the *square*) **c** Partially necrotic degenerated lesion with small peripheral adenopathies

23.2 Extragastric Sites

Extragastric gastrointestinal sites of leiomyoblastoma are exceedingly rare (Lavin et al. 1972; Mouroux 1986; Ranchod and Kempson 1977; Wilson 1975). Their imaging patterns are similar to lesions in the stomach: tumor hypervascularity, solid and occasionally necrotic masses on ultrasound and CT scans.

23.3 References

Bose B, Landy J (1970) Gastric leiomyoblastoma. Gut 11: 875–880

Carney JA (1979) The triad of gastric epithelioid leiomyosarcoma, functioning extra-adrenal paraganglionoma and pulmonary chondroma. Cancer 43: 374–382

Choi BI, Ok ID, Im JG, Man Ch, Eun SY, Yong IK (1988) Exogastric cystic gastric leiomyoblastoma with unusual CT appearance. Gastrointest Radiol 13: 109–111

Conte M, Conte-Marti J, Benistry H (1973) Les tumeurs myoïdes de l'estomac (léiomyoblastomes). A propos de cinq observations. Sem Hop 49: 537–544

De Castro FJ, Olsen WR, Littler ER (1972) Gastric leiomyoblastoma in an adolescent. Am J Surg 123: 614–616

Faegenburg D, Farman J, Dallemand S, Schelter LS, Rosen Y, Chiat H (1975) Leiomyoblastoma of stomach. Radiology 117: 297–300

Graham SM, Ballantyne GH, Modlin IM (1987) Gastric epithelioid leiomyomatous tumors. Surg Gynecol Obstet 164: 391–397

Gupta RK, Chandler JP (1965) Leiomyoblastoma of stomach; case report. Ann Surg 161: 562

Hadju SI, Erlandson RA, Plagia MA (1982) Light and electron microscopic studies of a gastric leiomyoblastoma. Arch Pathol 93: 36–41

Kay S, Still WJ (1969) A comparative electron microscopic study of a leiomyosarcoma and bizarre leiomyoma of the stomach. Am J Clin Pathol 52: 403–413

Kelsey JR (1966) Leiomyoblastoma of the stomach presenting as acute intraperitoneal hemorrhage. Gastroenterology 51: 539–541

Knake JE, Gross MD (1979) Extraadrenal paraganglioma, pulmonary chondroma, and gastric leiomyoblastoma: triad in young females. AJR 132: 448

Langley JR (1976) Gastric and extragastric leiomyoblastoma: report of six new cases with a review of the literature. Am Surg 42: 369

Lavin P, Hajdu SI, Foote FW (1972) Gastric and extragastric leiomyoblastomas: clinicopathologic study of 44 cases. Cancer 29: 305–311

Lecomte P, Bruneton JN, Sicart M (1981) Leiomyo-blastoma of the stomach. Fortschr Geb Roent-genstr 135: 57-60

Leger H, Dubarry JJ, Darmaillacq R, Kermarec J, Planes A (1962) Tumeur myoïde intramurale de l'estomac. Bordeaux Chir 4: 186

Leger L, Hamel D, Lemaigre G, Delaitre B (1972) Tumeurs myoïdes de l'estomac (à propos de 3 cas). J Chir 103: 205

Lenne Y, Delumeau G (1973) Etude anatomo-cli-nique de 26 tumeurs myoïdes de l'estomac. Arch Med Quest 5: 207

Loiseau JP, Le Fur M, Conte-Marti M, Conte M (1968) A propos de 13 tumeurs bénignes de l'es-tomac. Sem Hop 44: 1561

Maaouni A, Benmansour A, Hamiani O, El Alaoui M, Outarahout O, Souadka A, Mellouki M, Am-mar F, Haffa D (1980) Les tumeurs gastrointesti-nales d'origine musculaire. A propos de 11 obser-vations. Chirurgie 106: 630-635

Maillet P, Cuche J, Croizat B (1969) Tumeur myoïde de l'estomac. Lyon Chir 65: 135

Mann NS, Sachdev AJ, Agrawal AB, Krecker EC (1975) Leiomyoblastoma of the stomach. South Med J 68: 1350-1352

Martin JF, Bazin P, Feroldi J, Cabanne F (1960) Tumeurs myoïdes intramurales de l'estomac. Con-sidérations microscopiques à propos de 6 cas. Ann Anat Pathol 5: 484-497

Mignon M, Le Quintrec Y, Potet F, Alaoui A, Belghiti A, Lambling A (1968) Tumeurs myoïdes de l'estomac. Presse Med 76: 1628

Mouroux J, Frapier JM, Durand ML, Deixonne B, Baumel H (1986) Une étiologie rare de rectorra-gie: léiomyoblastome du Meckel. Intérêt de l'arté-riographie coeliomésentérique. J Chir (Paris) 123: 239-241

Muller M, Rugsegger CH, Pettavel J, Gardiol D (1972) Evolution et pronostic des léiomyoblastomes gas-triques (tumeurs myoïdes). Revue de la littérature à propos de 5 cas. Arch Fr Mal Appar Dig 61: 181

Nahas V (1969) Tumeur myoïde de l'estomac. Lyon Chir 65: 123

Naidech HJ, Axelrod RS, Seliger C (1971) Granular cell tumor (myoblastoma) of the stomach. AJR 113: 245

Nardi C, Benhamou G, Marche C, Avenier F (1973) La tumeur myoïde de l'estomac. A propos de deux nouvelles observations. Chirurgie 99: 898

O'Brien SE, Shier KJ (1974) Leiomyoblastoma of the stomach. Can J Surg 17: 105

Osterras GR, Chandor SB (1971) Malignant leio-myoblastoma: report of ninth case. Hawaii Med J 30: 89

Ozoktay S, Alexander L, Yoon S, Deshpande V (1979) Unusual leiomyoblastoma of the stomach. Gastrointest Radiol 4: 227-230

Pignon JP, Travers B, Zerbib M, Louvel A, Coutu-rier O, Guerre J, Legall R (1984) Volumineuse tu-meur myoïde exogastrique. Apports de l'écho-tomographie et de la tomodensitométrie. J Radiol 65: 463-466

Pillari G, Weinreb J, Vernace G, Kumari S, Marc JA, Phillips G, Cruz V, Pochaczevsky R (1983) CT of gastric masses: image patterns and a note on potential pitfalls. Gastrointest Radiol 8: 11-17

Pizzimbono C, Higa AE, Wise L (1973) Leiomyo-blastoma of the lesser sac: case report and review of the literature. Am Surg 39: 692-699

Postma CT, Gerlag PGG (1986) Leiomyoblastoma of the stomach. Neth J Med 29: 126-128

Rachman R, Meranze DR, Zibelman CS, Leto F (1968) Malignant leiomyoblastoma. Am J Clin Pa-thol 49: 556

Ranchod M, Kempson RL (1977) Smooth muscle tumors of the gastrointestinal tract and retroperi-toneum. Cancer 39: 255-262

Regensberg C, Veillefond A, Paillas J, Frileux C (1972) Les tumeurs myoïdes de l'estomac. His-togénèse et indications thérapeutiques. Chirurgie 98: 172

Salazar H, Totten RS (1970) Leiomyoblastoma of the stomach. An ultrastructural study. Cancer 25: 176-185

Salmela H, Kohler R (1969) Roentgenological char-acteristics of mesenchymal tumours of the sto-mach. A retrospective study of 59 patients. Ann Clin Res 1: 57

Sandler MA, Ratanaprakarn S, Madrazo BL (1978) Ultrasonic findings in intramural exogastric le-sions. Radiology 128: 189-192

Saubier E (1969) A propos de deux observations de tumeurs myoïdes de l'estomac dont une dégéné-rée ayant nécessité une hépatectomie droite élar-gie; résultat éloigné. Lyon Chir 65: 128

Sautot J, Tommassi M, Vauzelle JL (1965) Tumeur myoïde intramurale de l'estomac. Lyon Chir 61: 567

Sava P, Billerey C, Camelot G, Opperman R, Gissel-drecht H (1979) Les tumeurs myoïdes gastriques. Etude de 4 cas et revue de la littérature. Gastro-enterol Clin Biol 3: 29-36

Schmitt EL, Heidelberger KP (1976) Gastric leio-myoblastoma in a child. J Can Assoc Radiol 27: 115-117

Schofield PF, Fox H (1965) Leiomyoblastoma of stomach. Br J Surg 52: 928

Schwartz DT, Gatz HP (1965) Multiple granular cell myoblastomas of stomach. Am J Clin Pathol 44: 453

Sehgal B, Nayak NC, Hingotani V, Bapna BC (1966) Bizarre leiomyoblastoma of the stomach. Indian J Pathol Bacteriol 9: 90

Sinnreich M, Friedman R, Dacso MR (1966) Bizarre gastric leiomyoblastoma simulating a pedunculat-ed uterine fibromyoma. Obstet Gynecol 27: 690

Slasky BS, Denese L, Skilnick ML (1982) Exogastric leiomyoblastoma: diagnosis by CT and ultrason-ography. South Med J 75: 1275-1277

Smithwick W, Biesecken JL, Leand PM (1969) Leio-myoblastoma: behavior and prognosis. Cancer 24: 996-1003

Soustelle J, Bertocchi R, Sauvage Y (1969) Tumeur myoïde de l'estomac. Lyon Chir 65: 127

Stanley JH, Ravenel D, Parker TH, Vujic I (1986) Exogastric leiomyoblastoma; a rare gastric neo-plasm mimicking left hepatic mass on computed tomography. CT 10: 187-190

Stout AP (1962) smooth muscle tumors of the sto-mach. Cancer 15: 400-409

Striffling V, Sala JJ, Briet S, Duchat A, Piard F (1984) Les tumeurs myoïdes de l'estomac. Apport diagnostique de l'échographie et de la tomodensi-tométrie. A propos d'un cas. Ann Gastroenterol Hepatol (Paris) 20: 17-20

Tallqvist G, Salmela H, Linstrom BL (1967) Leio-myoblastoma of the stomach. A clinicopathologic study of 10 cases. Acta Pathol Microbiol Scand 71: 194-202

Tanghe W, Brackman J, Desmet V, Noyez D (1970) The leiomyoblastoma of the stomach. Tijdschr Gastroenterol 13: 244

Viard H, Cabanne F, Klepping C (1975) Les tu-meurs myoïdes intramurales de l'estomac. Quatre nouvelles observations. Lyon Chir 71: 44-49

Wilson JM (1975) Benign small bowel tumors. Ann Surg 181: 247-250

Wolf JS (1968) Massive leiomyoblastoma of sto-mach. Arch Surg 96: 284-288

Woodington GF, Carter KL (1966) Leiomyoblasto-ma of the stomach. Wis Med J 65: 173

Worlicek H, Lederer P, Lux G (1986) Ultrasonogra-phic evaluation of the wall of the fluid-filled sto-mach. Case report of a leiomyoblastoma. Hepato-gastroenterology 33: 184-186

Yannopoulos K, Stout AP (1962) Smooth muscle tu-mors in children. Cancer 15: 958-971

Hemangiopericytoma is a rare vascular tumor that usually affects the soft tissues of the extremities; intra-abdominal sites represent only 10% of all published cases. In addition to its rarity, hemagiopericytoma is unusual in hav-᷉ an uncertain evolutionary potential: it may be malignant from the outset; a "benign" lesion associated with local or distant, benign or malignant recurrence; or a truly benign tumor. Except for those hemangiopericytomas that are malignant from the start, follow-up of these lesions can be difficult.

24.1 General Features

Hemangiopericytoma develops from the pericyte of Zimmerman, a cell that surrounds the blood capillaries (Stout 1949). This pericyte corresponds to the smooth muscle cells around arteries and veins.

Gross examination reveals a firm, well-delimited solid tumor with a pseudocapsule. Histologically, hemangiopericytomas are made up of three components: (a) a vascular component corresponding to numerous mature capillaries of unequal diameter that are always separated from the peripheral tumor cells; (b) tumor cells which originate from the pericytes; (c) sparse intercellular substance which divides the tumoral mass into small groups of cells (Stout 1949).

Criteria for malignancy include a large tumor with necrosis, presence of an increased number of cells, and more than four mitoses per field (Enzinger and Smith 1956). The differential histologic diagnoses include sarcomatous connective tissue tumors and such rare vascu-

lar tumors as capillary hemangioma and hemangioendothelioma.

Multiple lesions are infrequent (Rau 1977), but associations have been described with other pathologies, and in particular fibrosarcoma (Hiersche et al. 1979).

Involvement of the soft tissues of the extremities predominates, accounting for one-half of all published cases. Subdiaphragmatic sites, including the pelvis and the retroperitoneum, account for 21.2% of all cases for Dal-Col (1977). In fact, purely intraperitoneal sites represent only 10% of cases in adults and in children (Neumann 1983). The most frequent gastrointestinal site is the stomach (Berner and Streicher 1977; Bonhof et al. 1983; Piard et al. 1972; Reigner et al. 1966; Tabghe et al. 1969). Esophageal (Burke and Ranchod 1981; Fernandez Lloret et al. 1983), intestinal (Binder et al. 1973; Olsen and Wellwood 1970; Torner Garcia et al. 1983; Veyssiere et al. 1968; Wagner et al. 1985), colonic (Genter et al. 1982), and rectal sites of involvement (Kay and Warthen 1960) are very rare.

As mentioned earlier, hemangiopericytoma may follow one of four different courses: malignant from the outset, lesion with an indeterminate evolutionary potential, benign lesion with a local or distant benign or malignant recurrence, or benign form without recurrence. Regardless of the anatomic site, over 50% of all hemangiopericytomas are malignant from the beginning (Genter et al. 1982; McMaster et al. 1975). Indeterminate lesions (borderline malignancy) represent 25% of all cases. One-quarter of all hemangiopericytomas are therefore benign at diagnosis: two-thirds of them never recur. The remaining third recur either locally or at a distance, as either benign or malignant relapses (Neumann 1983).

The incidence of benign and malignant forms, as well as the frequency of recurrence, appear

---

* Written in collaboration with A. Rogopoulos.

related to the site of the lesion. Intra-abdominal sites, except those in the stomach and the pelvis, have a higher than average rate of malignancy (70%) (Backwinkel and Diddams 1970).

Clinical symptoms are a function of the site: dysphagia in patients with esophageal involvement, hemorrhage with certain gastric lesions, intussusception or perforation with intestinal involvement. A more specific finding is the hypoglycemic syndrome without pancreatic involvement described in certain patients with hemangiopericytoma; this condition disappears after surgery or hepatic arterial embolization of the secondary lesion in the liver (Bell and Buist 1981).

Wide surgical resection, the only curative therapy at present, is not always possible (Backwincel and Diddams 1970; Mira et al. 1977).

24.2 Imaging (Figs. 24.1–24.4)

The oldest reports of gastrointestinal hemangiopericytoma describe *barium studies*. Pe-

dunculated lesions have been observed in the esophagus (Burke and Ranchod 1981; Fernandez-Lloret et al. 1983) while Piard et al. (1972) reported prolapse of a sessile gastric lesion into the duodenum which caused intussusception.

The scarcity of *sonographic descriptions* is related to the rarity of intra-abdominal hemangiopericytomas (Bonhof et al. 1983; Grant et al. 1982). Predominantly fluid density lesions appear to be most common. They combine a solid, irregular rim of variable thickness with a central, fluid-like center which makes up over 80% of the tumor. Intratumoral septae are possible (Grant et al. 1982; Parker et al. 1985; Roesler et al. 1985). Solid lesions appear more or less homogeneous. These generally well-limited tumors merely displace adjacent organs, without invasion, thereby often permitting complete surgical resection regardless of the maligant or benign etiology.

Several distinctive *computed tomographic* patterns have been identified, including inconstant calcifications (Alpern et al. 1986) and

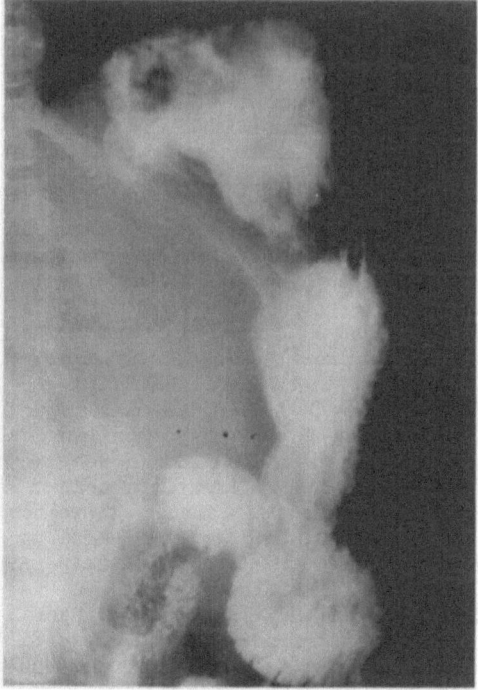

Fig. 24.1. Hemangiopericytoma of the upper third of the stomach (multinodular tumoral lesion)

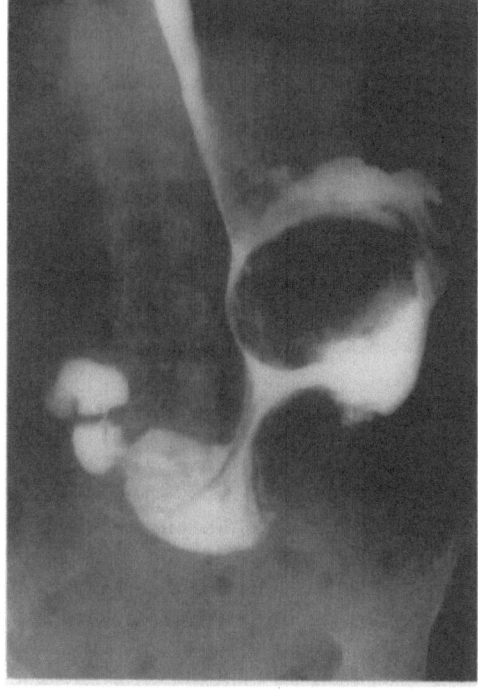

Fig. 24.2. Bifocal hemangiopericytoma in the upper and middle thirds of the stomach

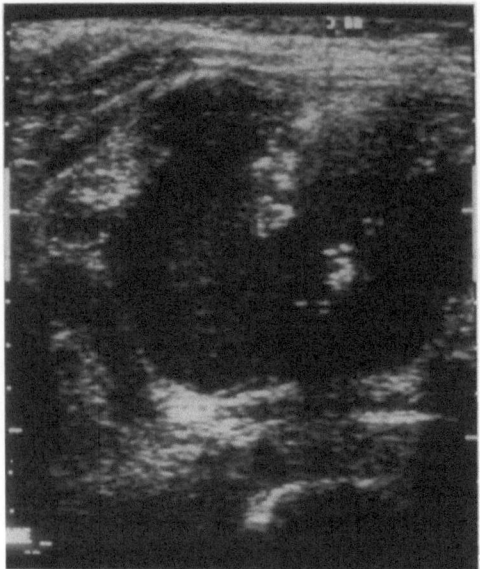

Fig. 24.3. Intestinal hemangiopericytoma: ultrasonography demonstrated extensively necrotic lesions

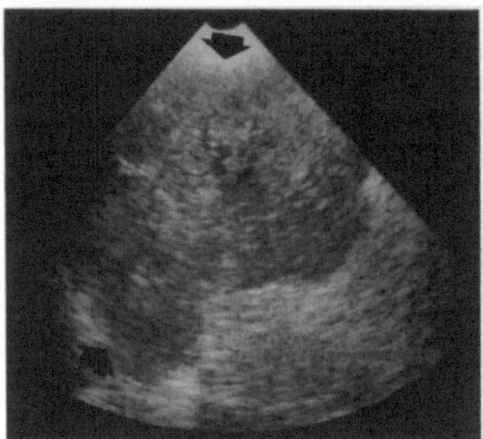

Fig. 24.4. Recurrence of a gastric hemangiopericytoma: solid lesion (23 cm between the *two arrows*)

bone lysis in continuity with an intra-abdominal lesion (Grant et al. 1982). As on sonograms, low-density lesions are most prevalent (Parker et al. 1985; Roesler et al. 1985; Trulock et al. 1982). Solid lesions are less common. Abdominal CT scans can define the relations of these often large lesions with adjacent organs. Hemangiopericytoma is not usually di-

agnosed from ultrasound or CT scans because of the rarity of this etiology. The most common diagnoses are cystic lymphangioma of the mesentery or a connective tissue tumor.

Angiography frequently demonstrates hypervascularity, but there are no specific features (Berner and Streicher 1977; Grant et al. 1982).

24.3 Conclusion

Intra-abdominal hemangiopericytoma generally has a very poor prognosis, regardless of whether it is malignant from the outset or an early recurrence. Imaging techniques allow satisfactory disease staging but cannot predict the evolutionary potential of these tumors. Similarly, neither imaging studies nor laboratory tests can predict the course of the so-called indeterminate and benign hemangiopericytomas. Twice-yearly sonographic and CT follow-up examinations thus appear justified for these patients, at least for the first 5 years after diagnosis.

24.4 References

Alpern LB, Thorsen MR, Kellman GM, Pojumas K, Lawson TL (1986) CT appearance of hemangiopericytoma. J Comput Assist Tomogr 10: 264–267

Angervall L, Kindblom LG, Nielsen JM, Stener B, Svenden P (1978) Hemangiopericytoma. A clinicopathologic, angiographic and microangiographic study. Cancer 42: 2412–2427

Atkinson JB, Mahour GH, Isaacs H, Ortega JA (1984) Hemangiopericytoma in infants and children. A report of six patients. Am J Surg 148: 372–374

Aubert J, Dore B, Touchard G, Salzard C (1981) Une tumeur rare: l'hémangiopéricytome pelvien paravésical. J Urol (Paris) 87: 219–226

Backwinkel KD, Diddams JA (1970) Hemangiopericytoma: report of a case and comprehensive review of the literature. Cancer 25: 896–901

Bell GM, Buist TAS (1981) Arterial embolization in the management of liver tumour with recurrent hypoglycemia. Postgrad Med J 57: 534–536

Berner H, Streicher HJ (1977) Das Hamangiopericytom des Magens. Chirurgie 48: 400–402

Binder SC, Wolfe HJ, Deterling RA (1973) Intra-abdominal hemangiopericytoma. Report of four cases and review of the literature. Arch Surg 107: 536–543

Bonhof JA, Kremer H, Schuman G, Damm G, Zollner N (1983) Sonographische Befunde bei einem

Hämangiopericytom des Magens. Fallbericht. Ultraschall 4: 49–51

Burke JS, Ranchod M (1981) Hemangiopericytoma of the esophagus. Hum Pathol 12: 96–100

Conroy B, Gunn A (1981) Malignant haemangiopericytoma presenting as an insulinoma. J R Coll Surg Edinb 26: 178–180

Dal-Col JL (1977) L'hémangiopéricytome. A propos de 6 observations (place de la radiothérapie et de la chimiothérapie). Medical thesis, no 457, University of Lyons

Enzinger FM, Smith BH (1956) Hemangiopericytoma: an analysis of 106 cases. Hum Pathol 7: 61–82

Fernandez Lloret S, Garcia Gil JM, Alonso J, Lopez Cantarero M, Marfil Lizana JM (1983) Hemangiopericytoma de localization esofagica. Rev Esp Enferm Appar Dig 63: 451–455

Genter B, Mir R, Strauss R, Flint G, Levin L, Lowy R, Wise L (1982) Hemangiopericytoma of the colon: report of a case and review of literature. Dis Colon Rectum 25: 149–156

Grant EG, Gronvall S, Sarosi TE, Borts FT, Holm HH, Schellinger D (1982) Sonographic findings in four cases of hemangiopericytoma. Radiology 142: 447–451

Grosser S, Dreyer M, Kuhnau J, Kloppel G, Polonius MJ, Klose G (1985) Erfolgreiche Therapie rezidivierender Hypoglykämien durch operative Entfernung eines malignen Hämangioperizytoms. Dtsch Med Wochenschr 110: 1212–1215

Hammoudi SM, Corkery JJ (1985) Congenital hemangiopericytoma of duodenum. J Pediatr Surg 20: 559–560

Hiersche HD, Dobberstein HH, Godtel R (1979) Unerwartete Situationen bei der Laparotomie II. Eine Klinisch-morphologische Stellungnahme zum malignen Hämangioperizytom. Geburtshilfe Frauenheilkd 39: 294–296

Kauffman SL, Stout AP (1960) Hemangiopericytoma in children. Cancer 13: 695–710

Kay S, Warthen HJ (1953) Hemangiopericytoma of the rectum. Cancer 6: 167–169

Maillet P, Lamesch A, Dawagne MP (1985) L'hémangiome congénital. A propos de 2 cas personnels. Revue de la littérature. Chir Pediatr 26: 22–25

Marre P, Sibertin-Blanc M, Nassif N, Topolanski F (1979) Hypoglycémie organique spontanée par hémangiopéricytome pelvien. Nouv Presse Med 8: 2621–2622

Mc Master MJ, Soule EH, Ivins JC (1975) Hemangiopericytoma. A clinicopathologic study and long-term followup of 60 patients. Cancer 36: 2232–2244

Mira JG, Chu FCH, Fortner JG (1977) The role of radiotherapy in the management of malignant hemangiopericytoma. Report of eleven new cases and review of the literature. Cancer 39: 1254–1259

Neumann H (1983) Morphologie und Klinik des Hämangioperizytoms. Eine Analyse von 84 Fällen mit einem eigenen Beitrag. Pathologe 4: 64–70

Olsen EGJ, Wellwood JM (1970) Haemangiopericytoma of the small intestine. A report of three cases. Br J Surg 57: 66–69

Parker LA, Vincent LM, Mauro MA (1985) Hemangiopericytoma metastatic to liver: sonographic appearance. J Clin Ultrasound 13: 347–349

Piard A, Mabille JP, Ferry C, Putelat R, Michiels R, Peres J, Chatelain P (1972) Hémangiopéricytome gastrique invaginé dans le duodénum. Med Chir Dig 1: 203–206

Rau JBV (1977) Multiple malignant intraabdominal hemangiopericytomas. Rare sites. Am J Gastroenterol 67: 148–151

Reigner J, Lemaire JP, Fekete F (1966) Deux cas d'hémangiopéricytome gastroduodénal. Mem Acad Chir 14–15: 363–368

Roesler A, Schreyer T, Keller E, Storkel S (1985) Hemangiopericytom der Leber. Roentgenblatter 38: 58–59

Stout AP (1949) Hemangiopericytoma. A study of twenty-five new cases. Cancer 2: 1027–1035

Tabghe W, Desmet V, Vermeulen J, Noyez D, Tytgat G (1969) Haemangiopericytoma of the stomach. Trop Gastroint 12: 159–167

Torner Gracia J, Fernandez Alonso A, Agundez Basterra M (1983) Hemangiopericytoma de intestino delgado. Presentacion de un caso y revision de la literatura. Rev Esp Enferm Apar Dig 64: 523–528

Trulock TS, Gould RA, Glenn JF (1982) Massive pelvic hemangiopericytoma. J Urol (Balt) 127: 1197–1199

Veyssiere C, Smadja A, Vives P, Baillet J (1968) Les hémangiopéricytomes du grêle. A propos d'une observation. Arch Fr Mal Appar Dig 57: 801–808

Wagner M, Dibos H, Bertling J (1985) Intestinale Manifestation eines Hämangiopericytomes. Chirurgie 56: 663–665

Wong PP, Yagoda A (1978) Chemotherapy of malignant hemangiopericytoma. Cancer 41: 1256–1260

Yaghmai I (1978) Angiographic manifestation of soft-tissue and osseous hemangiopericytomas. Radiology 126: 653–659

Subject Index